CLINICAL ATLAS OF AIRWAY DISEASES:

Bronchoscopy, Radiology, and Pathology

David R. Duhamel, M.D.
Director of Pulmonary Special Procedures Unit
Director of Lung Cancer Center
Virginia Hospital Center
Arlington, Virginia

James H. Harrell, M.D.
Professor of Medicine
Chief, Pulmonary Special Care Unit
Director, Pulmonary Diagnostic and Nd:YAG Laser Unit
University of California, San Diego, Medical Center
San Diego, California

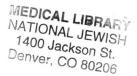
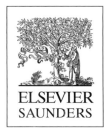

ELSEVIER
SAUNDERS

ELSEVIER | SAUNDERS

The Curtis Center
170 S Independence Mall W 300E
Philadelphia, Pennsylvania 19106

CLINICAL ATLAS OF AIRWAY DISEASES: BRONCHOSCOPY,
RADIOLOGY, AND PATHOLOGY   ISBN 0-7216-0007-7
Copyright ©2005, Elsevier Inc.

NOTICE

Respiratory Medicine is an ever-changing field. Standard safety precautions must be followed,
but as new research and clinical experience broaden our knowledge, changes in treatment and
drug therapy may become necessary or appropriate. Readers are advised to check the most
current product information provided by the manufacturer of each drug to be administered to
verify the recommended dose, the method and duration of administration, and
contraindications. It is the responsibility of the treating physician, relying on experience and
knowledge of the patient, to determine dosages and the best treatment for each individual
patient. Neither the Publisher nor the editor assumes any liability for any injury and/or
damage to persons or property arising from this publication.

The Publisher

Library of Congress Cataloging-in-Publication Data

Duhamel, David R.
    Clinical atlas of airway diseases: bronchoscopy, radiology, and pathology/David R.
    Duhamel, James H. Harrell—1st ed.
        p. ; cm.
    Includes bibliographical references and index.
    ISBN 0-7216-0007-7
    1. Respiratory organs—Diseases—Atlases. 2. Respiratory organs—Cancer—Atlases. I.
    Harrell, James H. II. Title.
    [DNLM: 1. Respiratory Tract Diseases—diagnosis—Atlases. 2. Diagnostic Techniques,
Respiratory System—Atlases. 3. Respiratory Tract Diseases—therapy—Atlases. WF 17
D869c 2005]
RC732.D848 2005
616.2'0022'2—dc22   2003069361

Acquisitions Editor: Dolores Meloni and Todd Hummel
Developmental Editor: Marla Sussman
Publishing Services Manager: Frank Polizzano
Project Manager: Lee Ann Draud
Design Coordinator: Gene Harris

Printed in China
Last digit is the print number: 9 8 7 6 5 4 3 2 1

This book is dedicated to our wives, Karen and Terrie, for their constant support and understanding throughout our careers. We are also indebted to those friends and mentors who have given so much of themselves to make us the physicians we are, especially Dr. Kenneth Moser, Dr. Eugene Braunwald, Dr. Charles Read, and Dr. Steven Zimmet. Finally, this book would not be possible without the endless compassion and devotion of the nurses, respiratory therapists, secretaries, and patients of our Pulmonary Special Procedure Units.

CONTRIBUTORS

Gehan Devendra, M.D.
Assistant Clinical Professor of Medicine, University of California, Davis, School of Medicine; Davis; Pulmonary and Critical Care Medicine, The Permanente Medical Group, Sacramento, California

Small Cell Carcinoma; Kaposi's Sarcoma; Extrinsic Compression of the Trachea from the Thyroid; Coccidioidomycosis of the Airway; Behçet's Disease of the Airway; Pseudomembranous Disease of the Airway; Candidal Tracheobronchitis; Manifestations of Fibrosing Mediastinitis on the Airway; Endobronchial Aspergillosis

David R. Duhamel, M.D.
Director of Pulmonary Special Procedures Unit and Director of Lung Cancer Center, Virginia Hospital Center, Arlington, Virginia

Diagnostic and Therapeutic Bronchoscopy; Squamous Cell Carcinoma; Carcinoma in Situ; Adenoid Cystic Carcinoma; Bronchial Carcinoids; Mucoepidermoids; Benign Fibrous Tumors and Tumor-like Lesions; Carcinomas with Pleomorphic, Sarcomatoid, and Sarcomatous Elements; Metastatic Thyroid Cancer; Metastatic Esophageal Cancer; Metastatic Ovarian Cancer; Metastatic Renal Cell Cancer; Metastatic Melanoma; Metastatic Breast Cancer; Metastatic Colorectal Cancer; Sarcomas; Endobronchial Lymphoma; Lipoma; Papillomatosis; Tumors of Nerve Sheath Origin; Plasma Cell Granuloma; Granular Cell Tumor; Smooth Muscle Tumors Related to the Human Immunodeficiency Virus; Pleomorphic Adenoma; Chondroma; Tracheal Stenosis; Idiopathic Subglottic Stenosis; Granulation Tissue; Radiation Stenosis; Tuberculous Stenosis; Bronchopleural Fistulas; Tracheoesophageal Fistulas; Foreign Body Aspiration; Inhalation Injury; Wegener's Granulomatosis; Tracheobronchial Amyloidosis; Tracheopathia Osteoplastica; Relapsing Polychondritis; Rhinoscleroma; Herpes Tracheobronchitis; Radiation Necrosis of the Airway; Tracheobronchomalacia; Bronchial Webs and Adhesions

David P. Kapelanski, M.D.
Clinical Professor of Surgery, Division of Cardiothoracic Surgery, University of California, San Diego, Medical Center, San Diego, California

Surgical Management of Airway Disease

David L. Levin, M.D.
Assistant Professor, Department of Radiology, University of California, San Diego, School of Medicine; La Jolla; Radiologist, Department of Radiology, University of California, San Diego, Medical Center, San Diego, California

Radiographic Methods for Imaging of the Large Airways

Jeffrey S. Prince, M.D.
Adjunct Assistant Professor, Department of Radiology, University of Utah School of Medicine; Department of Medical Imaging, Primary Children's Medical Center, Salt Lake City, Utah

Large Cell Carcinoma; Hamartoma; Papillomatosis; Tumors of Nerve Sheath Origin; Leiomyoma; Tracheal Stenosis; Idiopathic Subglottic Stenosis; Post-transplant Stricture; Sarcoidosis; Inflammatory Bowel Disease of the Airway; Saber Sheath Trachea

Eunhee S. Yi, M.D.
Associate Professor, Department of Pathology, University of California, San Diego, Medical Center, San Diego, California

PREFACE

State of the art management of diseases of the airway relies on a fusion of knowledge and skills from multiple specialties in the field of medicine. Whether it is the radiologist identifying a lesion on a radiographic study, the bronchoscopist evaluating the lesion and performing a biopsy, the pathologist making the definitive diagnosis, or the interventional bronchoscopist, thoracic surgeon, and oncologist performing therapy, each contributes a vital component to the complex care of patients with airway diseases. No reference text on airway disease would be complete without addressing the subject from each of these viewpoints. Just as we approach each case clinically, with advice and input from our radiologists, pathologists, and surgeons, so we have created this book, *Clinical Atlas of Airway Diseases.*

The trachea and central bronchi are subject to many unique and diverse disorders. These range from neoplastic to traumatic, infectious, inflammatory, infiltrating, and autoimmune. Many of these processes are extremely unusual and difficult to diagnose and treat. With the development of the flexible bronchoscope by Shigeto Ikeda in the early 1970s, physicians were presented with an ideal instrument for examining and diagnosing the airways. As the popularity of the flexible bronchoscope has grown over the last three decades, so too have the tools and technologies available to the bronchoscopist. Physicians are now able to diagnose a premalignant lesion with autofluorescence, evaluate paratracheal lymph nodes with endobronchial ultrasound, vaporize an obstructing tumor with a YAG laser, remove a foreign body with cryotherapy, or treat a carcinoma with brachytherapy.

The tools and technologies available to the radiologist and pathologist have continued to progress as well. The radiologist is now able to perform three-dimensional reconstructions of the tracheobronchial tree or virtual bronchoscopies to see beyond an obstructing lesion when a flexible bronchoscope cannot be passed. The interventional radiologist can selectively embolize the blood supply to a metastatic airway tumor, allowing for a safer endoscopic resection. The pathologist now has available a whole library of diagnostic tests, assays, stains, and probes to make diagnoses more accurately and definitively.

As one might expect, the influx of tools, techniques, and technologies available to diagnose and treat the various diseases of the airway has sparked a strong interest among physicians from many disciplines. Pulmonologists, otolaryngologists, thoracic surgeons, anesthesiologists, and interventional radiologists utilize these procedures and techniques. In the last two decades, interventional bronchoscopy has been clearly established as a vital and potentially lifesaving treatment option. Previously, nothing could be done for patients with many of these disease processes who faced a miserable death by asphyxiation. Now, with minimal invasiveness, patients can have effective palliation or even cure of their diseases.

It is unfortunate, however, that as the number of physicians skilled in the diagnosis and management of the various disorders of the airway has grown significantly, our knowledge and understanding of many of the diseases and the effectiveness of intervention has stagnated. It is not unusual when reviewing the literature on one of these processes to find only isolated case reports, small series, or anecdotal experiences. *Clinical Atlas of Airway Diseases* is an attempt to remedy this void in our medical literature. We have drawn on more than 30 years of clinical experience treating diseases of the trachea and bronchi to create this book. This atlas offers a unique and valuable resource to clinicians who treat diseases of the airway.

The book is designed to be a reference for practitioners who are involved in the care of patients afflicted by one of these disorders, regardless of their particular area of expertise. Starting with an overview of interventional bronchoscopic techniques, it proceeds to radiographic evaluation and surgical management, followed by a chapter-by-chapter analysis of more than 70 disease processes that affect the airways. It is a unique case-based collection of bronchoscopic, radiographic, and pathologic images accompanied by a thorough review of the literature on each subject. Included in each summary is information on the incidence, etiology, and prognosis, as well as detailed descriptions of the pertinent bronchoscopic, radiographic, and pathologic manifestations. Each chapter concludes with a discussion of prognosis as well as current management approaches for the individual disease entities.

The CD-ROM that accompanies the book was inspired by our more than four decades of experience teaching medical students, residents, and fellows. The field of interventional bronchoscopy is frequently criticized for its lack of training opportunities for physicians. Many of the procedures are so highly specialized that they are performed in only a handful of tertiary institutions. This prevents many trainees from obtaining an adequate procedural experience. The CD is designed as an educational supplement for physicians interested in learning the basic diagnostic procedures as well as advanced interventional treatment techniques. Included in the CD are 16 digital video segments showing various diagnostic and interventional procedures. These procedures include thoracentesis, flexible bronchoscopy with transbronchial biopsy, rigid bronchoscopy with YAG laser ablation, and percutaneous tracheostomy. The videos are accompanied by a detailed narration of all aspects of the procedure as well as digital images of the various instruments and devices used to perform the procedure.

The creation of this atlas marks the culmination of one author's career in treating airway diseases and the initiation of the other's. Although no textbook is a substitute for the clinical experience gained in a 40-year career, we have attempted to incorporate as much of it as possible in our book. It is our sincere hope that this atlas will prove vitally beneficial to all physicians providing care and treatment to patients afflicted with these disorders.

DAVID R. DUHAMEL
JAMES H. HARRELL

CONTENTS

CHAPTER 1

Diagnostic and Therapeutic Bronchoscopy

David R. Duhamel

As a new century in medical technology begins, the diagnostic and therapeutic armamentarium available to the bronchoscopist is expanding rapidly. What began in the 1970s with Strong and Jako[1] using the carbon dioxide (CO_2) laser to treat laryngeal disorders has grown into a vast array of technologies including Nd:YAG laser photoresection, endobronchial stents, argon plasma coagulator, cryotherapy, electrocautery, lung imaging fluorescent endoscopy (LIFE), and photodynamic therapy. Over the past 20 years, the use of lasers for treating endobronchial disease has been tested and accepted as an important therapeutic option. As the epidemic of bronchogenic lung cancer continues,[2] the skills and techniques of the interventional bronchoscopist are increasingly in demand. Although their role in the oncology patient is predominantly a palliative one, in carefully selected patients these bronchoscopic techniques can improve the quality of life, lower the level of care, allow withdrawal from mechanical ventilation, and on occasion prolong survival.[3]

Laser Therapy

Laser (light amplification by stimulated emission of radiation) has been used in the field of medicine since the early 1960s.[4] The Nd:YAG laser is commonly accepted as the "workhorse" for the laser bronchoscopist (Fig. 1-1). Owing to many of its inherent characteristics, the Nd:YAG laser is felt to be a superior choice over other medical lasers when treating endobronchial lesions. Because of the wavelength of the Nd:YAG laser, its energy is poorly absorbed by quartz material, allowing it to be transmitted through a flexible fiber (Fig. 1-2). This pliable laser fiber can be passed through either a flexible or rigid bronchoscope, allowing the laser energy to be delivered with pinpoint accuracy to fairly distal lesions. The variable laser energy characteristics of the Nd:YAG laser also make it ideal for hemostasis and tissue coagulation at low power and vaporization of tissue at high power. The classic approach to laser photoresection of an obstructing endobronchial lesion is to first "paint" the entire surface of the lesion with a series of short low-energy laser pulses. We have found that 0.5-second pulses at 45 watts of energy are best at minimizing complications while successfully obtaining hemostasis. Next, the tip of the rigid bronchoscope can be used to shear off large pieces of the lesion, which are than removed with forceps. Some endoscopists prefer to use the laser to vaporize the entire lesion; this technique, however, leads to a higher rate of complication including airway fire, perforation, or fistula formation.

Laser photoresection can be performed with either a rigid or flexible bronchoscope. The choice of instrument depends on the expertise of the operator and anatomic factors related to the lesion and its location. The author's preference, however, is the rigid bronchoscope because of several distinct advantages (Fig. 1-3). These advantages include a shortened procedure time, greater optical clarity, greater suction capacity, maintenance of an airway with the ability to oxygenate and ventilate, ability to resect tissue with the beveled tip of the bronchoscope, better instruments for débridement, inability to ignite with a laser, and ability to tamponade a bleeding lesion.[3] The flexible bronchoscope does have a few advantages when used to apply laser therapy. Its use does not require general anesthesia or an operating room, and it can reach distal lesions, especially in the upper lobes. In addition, the flexible bronchoscope is increasingly becoming the vehicle of choice for delivering many of these newer endoscopic therapies, such as cryotherapy and photodynamic therapy.

Electrocautery

Electrocautery is a new technology for the interventional bronchoscopist but one that has been used with great success in the fields of gastroenterology and urology. It relies on high-frequency electrical current to cut, coagulate, and vaporize the obstructing tissue in the tracheobronchial tree.[4] The electrical current is delivered through various probes or snare or loop devices that have been passed through the working channel of a flexible bronchoscope into the airway. A separate high-frequency current generator supplies the electricity to these various tools and devices. When compared with the costs of the Nd:YAG laser, the lower equipment and maintenance costs of electrocautery make it very attractive to the interventionalist with a limited budget. The device can be used in various modes depending on the desired effect on the tissue. The current generator can be set to "coagulate" at high amperage and low voltage, "cut" at low amperage and high voltage, or "blend" at a setting midway between cut and coagulate.[4] There are two techniques for performing electrocautery. One technique utilizes a cutting snare, which is essentially a wire loop used to encircle a portion of the lesion and cut off large pieces. This tool works particularly well for pedunculated lesions because the stalk can be easily ensnared and cut. The other technique uses a blunt probe to deliver the electrical energy. The probe is positioned adjacent to the lesion and causes "electrodestruction" of the tumor tissue at the point of contact.

One disadvantage of electrocautery is that it requires direct contact with the lesion to work. Also, if there is any blood or secretions in the procedural field, the electrocautery is much less effective. A recent advance in the field of electrocautery has allowed it to be used in a noncontact mode. This technique, called *argon plasma coagulation*, uses a stream of ionized argon gas as a conductor to transmit electrical current from the source to the lesion. Argon plasma coagulation does not require direct contact to be effective and can be used in the setting of mild to moderate hemorrhage. The argon gas jet distributes electrical energy evenly to the tissues and dissipates any pooled blood or secretions.[5] However, the electrical effect with argon plasma coagulation tends to be superficial, therefore limiting its use in large or vascular tumors.

Cryotherapy

Whereas the YAG laser, electrocautery, and argon plasma coagulators rely on heat to induce cell death and tissue destruction, cryotherapy relies on cold temperatures. The cryotherapy device induces tissue necrosis though hypothermic cellular crystallization and microthrombosis.[6] Cryotherapy utilizes a relatively inexpensive and simple piece of equipment. The essential components include a tank of compressed nitrous oxide and a blunt probe device. The probe is passed through the working channel of a flexible bronchoscope, and when it is activated the flow of gas supercools the probe tip and an ice ball forms. This probe tip can be plunged into an endobronchial lesion and supercooled to induce tissue destruction. Cryotherapy has also proved to be extremely useful in the removal of foreign bodies. The probe tip can be placed in soft gelatinous or partially dissolving foreign bodies such as aspirated food, blood clots, or vegetable matter. These items typically crumble if grasped with the usual foreign body forceps. When the tip is supercooled, a semisolid congealed mass is created on the tip of the probe, which can be removed easily along with the bronchoscope. The probe tip can also be frozen to the rough angular surfaces of difficult-to-remove objects such as teeth and thumbtacks. Although the role for cryotherapy is somewhat limited, in certain situations it seems to prove invaluable.

Brachytherapy

Brachytherapy is a form of radiation therapy that relies on the temporary placement of a potent radioactive source adjacent to a malignant lesion. This technique is particularly well suited for the treatment of endobronchial, submucosal, or peribronchial malignant lesions. It is a simple procedure and can be performed in an outpatient setting. A flexible bronchoscope is inserted into the airway and a closed-end hollow plastic catheter is passed through the working channel (Fig. 1-4). The bronchoscope is removed after positioning the catheter adjacent to the lesion. Next, the catheter is attached to an afterloader device, which is responsible for safely storing the radioactive source and advancing or retracting it through the catheter (Fig. 1-5). A computer program tells the afterloader where to position the source and how long to keep it there. The end result is a very intense but localized dose of radiation to the lesion.[7] A recent advance in the field includes the use of high-dose-rate (HDR) brachytherapy, which delivers up to 500 cGy per hour of radiation. This shortens the duration of the procedure to minutes and allows it to be performed in an outpatient setting. Typically, the patient returns two or three times for repeat fractionated doses. Brachytherapy offers a few pertinent advantages over routine external beam radiation: delivery of a very high dose of radiation directly to the tumor, thus avoiding radiation damage to healthy tissue; rapid drop in radiation outside the treatment region; precise dose localization; and adaptability to the tumor's shape.[4] However, it is important to remember that the major goal of brachytherapy is the palliation of symptoms and not the cure of malignant disease. In general, HDR brachytherapy is 85% successful in relieving the symptoms of airway obstruction.[8]

A stent is a hollow, cylindric prosthesis that maintains the luminal patency of a cylindric object by opposing extrinsic compressive forces and providing intrinsic support. Stents are used throughout medicine, and the field of pulmonary disease is no exception. The primary indication for stent placement is in the setting of extrinsic compression of the trachea or mainstem bronchi from either benign or malignant disease. Stents are also placed in the setting of endoluminal stenosis or obstruction. A stenotic lesion from either inflammation or infection is first "opened up" with either balloon dilation using angioplasty balloons or mechanical dilation using a rigid bronchoscope. Once the lesion has been dilated, a stent can be placed to maintain luminal patency. In the setting of endobronchial obstruction from a tumor, the airway is first opened up using YAG laser therapy or electrocautery to remove the obstruction. Next, a stent can be placed to prevent the regrowth of tumor and subsequent airway obstruction. The final indication for stenting is in the setting of tracheobronchomalacia, when the airway is dilated and floppy from weakening or loss of cartilaginous support.

There are two main categories of airway stents: Silastic and metal (Fig. 1-6). Both types of stent come in multiple different shapes, sizes, and configurations. Each category of stent has certain positive and negative attributes that must be weighed when determining which stent to use for treating a certain airway lesion. The ideal tracheobronchial stent should possess the following characteristics: ability to maintain airway patency and conform to airway tortuosity, ease of insertion and removal, low cost, minimal granulation tissue formation, no interference with mucociliary clearance, and no tendency to migrate.[4] No current stent is capable of doing all this, but the author relies predominantly on the Silastic stents for their minimal granulation response and ease of removal and repositioning. A major limiting factor to the widespread use of Silastic stents, however, is the need for general anesthesia and rigid bronchoscopy for insertion. Metallic stents are gaining popularity because they can be inserted with a flexible bronchoscope under topical anesthesia and conscious sedation. Whichever stent is used, the decision should be based on the anatomic structure and pathologic characteristics of the lesion as well as the comfort level of the bronchoscopist.

Photodynamic Therapy

The concept of photosensitization has been around since the early 1900s, but only recently has the clinical potential of photodynamic therapy been explored in the lung. Photodynamic therapy involves the injection of a photosensitizing agent that preferentially concentrates in neoplastic tissue and is quickly cleared from normal healthy tissue. The neoplastic tissue is then exposed to laser light of a specified wavelength, which triggers the intracellular activation of the photosensitizing agent and subsequent release of toxic oxygen free radicals. It is these free radicals that are responsible for the eventual tissue necrosis and cell death.[9] The indication for photodynamic therapy is endobronchial obstruction from neoplastic tissue, both benign and malignant. Because the effect on the tumor tends to be somewhat superficial, photodynamic therapy works particularly well after initial tumor debulking with either a YAG laser therapy or electrocautery. Photodynamic therapy is also ideally suited for treatment of the superficial but diffusely pervasive lesions of carcinoma in situ. It has also been found to be extremely useful in the treatment of endobronchial papillomatosis.

The technique of photodynamic therapy requires an initial outpatient injection of the photosensitizing agent porfimer sodium, a hematoporphyrin derivative. For the next 4 weeks it is imperative that the patient remain completely shielded from any exposure to sunlight. Sunlight is capable of activating the photosensitizing agent and causing severe sunburn. Forty to 50 hours after the initial injection, the patient undergoes a flexible bronchoscopy, and the endobronchial lesion is exposed to 630-nm wavelength laser light. The most common laser used to generate this specific wavelength laser light is the argon pump–dye laser. The laser light triggers the photochemical reaction, which causes tumor necrosis through cellular destruction from superoxide and hydroxyl radicals as well as vascular obstruction from thromboxane-A_2 release.[10] A follow-up bronchoscopy is typically necessary 2 to 4 days later to débride the necrotic tumor tissue. The entire procedure can be performed multiple times in a patient's lifetime.

LIFE Bronchoscopy

No discussion of diagnostic and therapeutic bronchoscopy would be complete without at least a brief mention of LIFE. LIFE bronchoscopy relies on the fact that there is a difference in the autofluorescence spectrum of normal endobronchial mucosa and carcinoma in situ. Normal tissue has a high intensity of autofluorescence at 500 nm, whereas carcinoma in situ demonstrates low-level autofluorescence at this level.[9] This simple observation is the basis for the LIFE bronchoscopy system. The device uses helium-cadmium laser light and fluorescence imaging cameras in combination with a flexible bronchoscope to screen for cancerous and precancerous lesions of the airway. Of course no screening device is 100% specific, so all suspicious lesions must be biopsied to pathologically confirm the diagnosis. The clinical value of this device has yet to be determined, but the theoretic potential is enormous.

Because the lung cancer epidemic shows no signs of abating, little doubt exists that the need for interventional bronchoscopists will persist for many years to come. As the technologies in this field continue to advance, so too will the benefits we can offer our patients. It is unclear what the role of these new technologies might prove to be; therefore, prospective controlled studies must be done to clarify these questions. Currently, these are mostly palliative procedures and our focus has been on alleviating symptoms and improving quality of life. The future may lie in combining these various technologies to maximize therapeutic, palliative, and possibly even curative effect. As the experience of the medical community with interventional bronchoscopy continues to grow, and as more health care professionals are made aware of its therapeutic capability, fewer patients with cancer will need to suffer and die with complications of airway obstruction.[3]

REFERENCES

1. Strong MS, Jako GJ: Laser surgery in the larynx: Early clinical experience with continuous CO₂ laser. Ann Otol 81:791-798, 1972.
2. American Cancer Society: Cancer 34:1-43, 1984.
3. Duhamel DR, Harrell JH: Laser bronchoscopy. Surg Clin North Am 11:769-789, 2001.
4. Lee P, Kupeli E, Mehta AC: Therapeutic bronchoscopy in lung cancer. Clin Chest Med 23:241-256, 2002.
5. Storek D, Grund KE, Gronbach G, et al: Endoscopic argon gas coagulation—Initial clinical experiences. Z Gastroenterol 31:675-679, 1993.
6. Seijo LM, Sterman DH: Interventional pulmonology. N Engl J Med 344:740-748, 2001.
7. Villanueva AG, Lo TC, Beamis JF: Endobronchial brachytherapy. Clin Chest Med 16:445-454, 1995.
8. Lo TC, Girshovich L, Healey GA, et al: Low dose rate versus high dose rate intraluminal brachytherapy for malignant endobronchial tumors. Radiother Oncol 35:193-197, 1995.
9. Edell ES, Cortese DA: Photodynamic therapy. Its use in the management of bronchogenic carcinoma. Clin Chest Med 16:455-463, 1995.
10. Dougherty TJ, Marcus SL: Photodynamic therapy. Eur J Cancer 28:1734-1742, 1992.

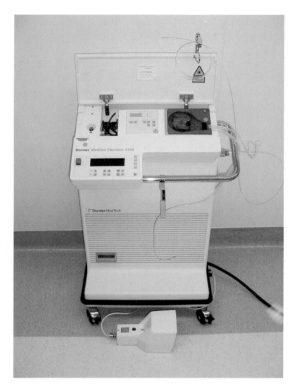

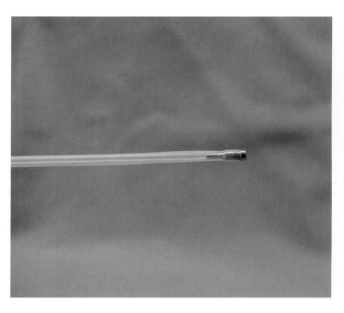

Figure 1-2. A close-up of the laser fiber tip. The laser fiber is made of flexible plastic and can be easily passed through a flexible or rigid bronchoscope.

Figure 1-1. A typical Nd:YAG laser unit (Dornier, Wessling, Germany). Note the foot pedal on the ground in front of the unit, which is used to control each laser pulse.

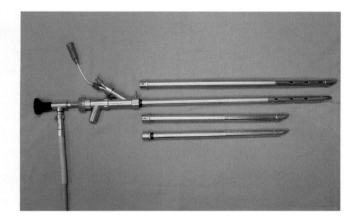

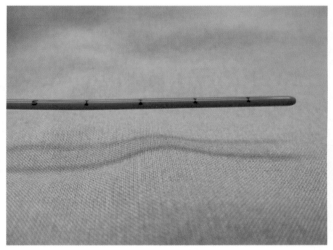

Figure 1-3. The Dumon-Harrell rigid bronchoscope (Bryan Corp., Woburn, Mass.). There are multiple interchangeable barrels of various size and diameter. A telescope attached to a light source is passed through one of the barrels. Note the side ports for suction catheters, laser fibers, and to oxygenate and ventilate the patient.

Figure 1-4. A close-up of the distal tip of the brachytherapy catheter (Cook Catheter, Bloomington, Ind.). The catheter is easily passed through a flexible bronchoscope, and the external markings are used to position it adjacent to the lesion.

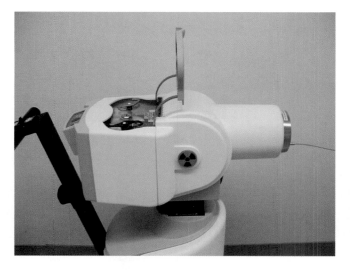

Figure 1-5. The afterloader device (Nucletron, Columbia, Md.) that houses the radioactive source and inserts or retracts it during treatment procedures. Note the proximal end of the brachytherapy catheter, which is inserted into the afterloader device.

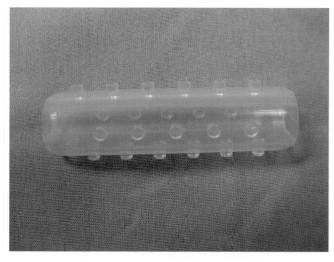

Figure 1-6. A side view of the Dumon-style Silastic stent. The multiple knobs seen protruding along the outer surface of the stent are helpful for anchoring it in the airway.

CHAPTER 2

Radiographic Methods for Imaging of the Large Airways

David L. Levin

Diseases of the large airways are often difficult to visualize radiographically. The initial study for the evaluation of suspected airway disease is typically chest radiography. A conventional radiograph is limited, however, in its ability to evaluate the trachea and proximal bronchi. This limitation may reflect suboptimal technique because poor penetration of the mediastinum limits visualization of the large airways. More frequently, the limitation reflects a failure on the physician's part to evaluate the airways carefully. Studies have reported detection rates of tracheal neoplasms to be as low as 23% using conventional radiography.[1] When evaluating the posteroanterior (PA) and lateral chest radiographs, the trachea and central bronchi should be evaluated for abnormalities of contour or regions of focal or diffuse narrowing (Fig. 2-1). A thorough evaluation is especially important if symptoms referable to large airway disease are present.

Computed tomography (CT) is superior to chest radiography in the identification of large airway disease. Again, the airways need to be carefully evaluated for focal lesions or regions of narrowing. Kwong and colleagues[2] found that CT had a sensitivity to detection of tracheal disease of greater than 90% compared with a sensitivity of only 66% for conventional radiography in the same patient population. However, once an abnormality was detected, both techniques were equal in classifying disease as either focal or diffuse (>90%) and as likely to be benign or malignant (~80%).

Diseases of the large airways can be evaluated using non-contrast technique CT with a slice thickness of 5 to 7 mm. Advanced imaging techniques, such as three-dimensional reconstruction and virtual bronchoscopy, may be helpful in the evaluation of specific lesions (Fig. 2-2). These usually require the use of different protocols, with a slice thickness of 1 to 3 mm. CT also can be used to demonstrate dynamic changes in the airways, such as collapse during expiration (Fig. 2-3).

Bronchoscopy remains the definitive method for the evaluation of the airways. However, radiographic evaluation remains an important supplement to the bronchoscopic examination. A thorough radiographic evaluation will help to characterize imaging findings as diffuse or focal and may provide specific imaging criteria to narrow the differential diagnosis in patients with diseases of the airways. These details can give important prebronchoscopic information to aid in the planning of the procedure and any therapeutic intervention that may be considered.

REFERENCES

1. Stark, P: Radiology of the Trachea. New York, Thieme Medical Publishers, 1991.
2. Kwong JS, Muller NL, Miller RR: Diseases of the trachea and main-stem bronchi: Correlation of CT and pathological findings. Radiographics 12:645, 1992.

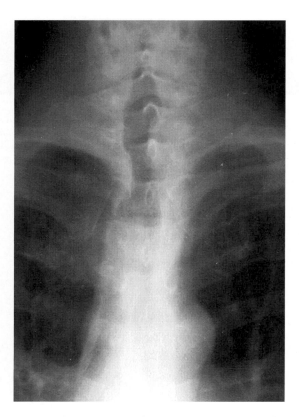

Figure 2-1. Short segmental narrowing of the trachea at the level of the thoracic inlet secondary to post-intubation stenosis.

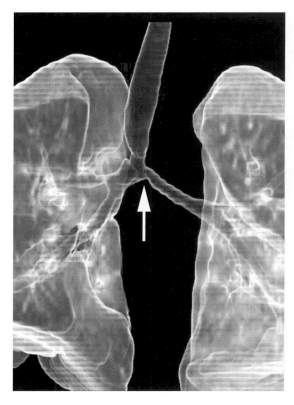

Figure 2-2. Volume rendered CT imaging demonstrates a complex narrowing (*arrow*) of the distal trachea and proximal left mainstem bronchus secondary to Wegener's granulomatosis.

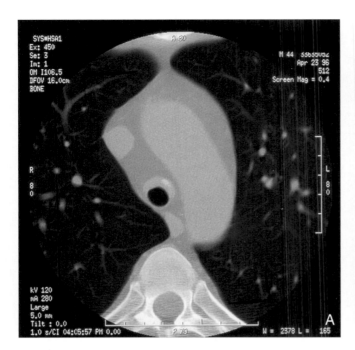 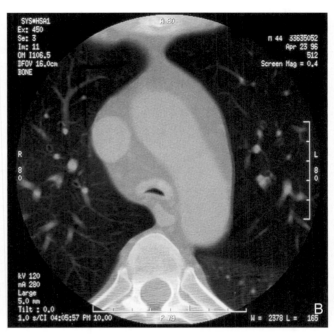

Figure 2-3. A and **B**, Change in tracheal caliber from end-inspiration (**A**) to midexpiration (**B**) in patient with relapsing polychondritis.

CHAPTER 3

Surgical Management of Airway Disease

David P. Kapelanski

Even though many of the diseases described elsewhere in this atlas are not managed operatively, many of the disorders herein depicted are best treated by resection with reconstruction of the central airway. The rationale and considerations for airway reconstruction are as diverse as the disorders depicted in this book. In the setting of traumatic airway disruption, surgical management is the only option because no suitable endoscopic treatment exists. When benign obstruction of the central airway is identified, surgery in selected patients affords a more durable and satisfactory option than dilation and stenting. For malignant disease, reconstructive surgery offers the best opportunity for definitive treatment. For neoplasms originating in the proximal bronchi, parenchyma-sparing procedures offer an outcome essentially identical to more extensive resections of equivalently staged lesions, provide a better immediate functional outcome, and, in a population at heightened risk for additional malignancy, may preserve a future operative option.

This chapter describes the general institutional approach we have developed to select, prepare, and care for operative candidates. It should be emphasized from the outset that

optimal results cannot be achieved without close collaboration and communication among the pulmonary specialist, radiologist, and surgeon.

Operative Preparation

The sequence and number of diagnostic and preliminary therapeutic interventions are largely contingent on the presentation of the patient, but the goals of operative preparation are uniform. Foremost, an adequate airway must be ensured. The nature and extent of intraluminal disease must next be determined, and the status of the distal airway and pulmonary parenchyma characterized. Any extraluminal disease extension must be identified, and involvement of adjoining structures characterized.

If the patient has a stable airway, the initial diagnostic endeavors are generally radiographic, and the varied findings are richly illustrated elsewhere in this atlas. It is worth emphasizing that the conventional radiograph is often normal even with very high-grade obstruction, and computed tomography and magnetic resonance imaging are the primary diagnostic imaging tools. Recent improvements in both tomographic modalities have enhanced the fidelity of both conventional sections and three-dimensional reconstructions, allowing for very precise definition of the primary process as well as the collateral effect of any obstruction on more distal components of the airway and lungs, including atelectasis, pneumonia, and bronchiectasis. With neoplastic disease, regions suspicious for contiguous extension can be readily identified, and the potential for mediastinal and parenchymal metastatic disease assessed with considerable accuracy. Associated disorders, such as emphysema, which might influence the determination to undertake conservative resection, are similarly demonstrated.

Notwithstanding the utility of radiographic techniques, the most essential diagnostic method is endoscopic visualization of the pathologic lesion by the surgeon, even if bronchoscopy had been performed previously. In cases of traumatic airway disruption or high-grade stenosis, endoscopically guided intubation of the distal airway using a preloaded armored tube secures the airway and provides an interval within which to stabilize the patient and obtain other essential diagnostic studies. As illustrated elsewhere in this atlas, many of the lesions amenable to airway reconstruction are easily diagnosed by visual inspection, and biopsy, if not already submitted, should be obtained as necessary to differentiate between benign and malignant lesions. The adjoining mucosa proximal and, if possible, distal to the lesion should be scrutinized carefully, and a biopsy should be performed on any area that is suspicious for extension. The extent, if any, of distal bronchiectasis should be characterized, and cultures of distal purulent secretions should be obtained.

In patients with bronchogenic carcinoma, PET scanning is an as yet unproven diagnostic adjunct. Without question, those patients identified as having stage IV disease would be saved an unnecessary resection. However, the resolution of current generation scanners may not allow spatial discrimination between hilar nodal metastasis and a proximal bronchial primary, nor differentiation between locoregional metastasis and postobstructive nodal inflammation. That said, we advocate this modality, because any positive scan would provoke additional staging modalities including mediastinoscopy, mediastinotomy, or thoracoscopy, and would exclude patients with stage IIIB disease from resection altogether. Those patients with stage IIIA disease would be offered neoadjuvant therapy in accord with current cooperative protocols, and because the risk of anastomotic complications is judged to be greater in patients so treated, conventional resection would be undertaken in those deemed to have adequate pulmonary reserve. Conversely, those patients with marginal function and regionally advanced disease would be offered conventional chemoradiation. Similarly, PET-negative patients found at surgery to have significant perihilar nodal disease and adequate pulmonary reserve would undergo conventional resection, because the amount of peribronchial dissection may jeopardize bronchial vascularity and compromise anastomotic healing, leading either to postoperative stricture or frank dehiscence.

In addition to the aforementioned, patients undergoing planned airway reconstruction undergo routine screening mechanics, supplemented by exercise testing and radionuclide ventilation perfusion scanning in those with marginal reserve. Cardiac screening is routine in older patients and those with known cardiac disease to limit comorbid risk. In elective cases, patients with limited function are routinely encouraged to undergo preoperative cardiopulmonary rehabilitation. Because of the known adverse effects on healing, steroids are tapered before surgery, and patients with prior radiation, type 1 diabetes, or steroid dependence are excluded from surgery.

One important consideration is the desirability of endoscopic resection, dilation, and temporary stenting in advance of any contemplated airway reconstruction for postinfectious airway stenosis or neoplastic obstruction. As a general policy, despite the delay this may impose on a definitive procedure, we have generally advocated this approach for numerous reasons. First, it allows immediate control of the airway to be regained, and for many central tumors may in fact represent the sole available operative therapy. Second, it facilitates a rapid transition to spontaneous ventilation in those patients transferred on ventilators. In concert with appropriately tailored antimicrobial therapy, postobstructive infection can be brought under control, and atelectasis alleviated, allowing a more realistic appraisal of anatomically functioning parenchyma. We believe that the risk of postresection anastomotic dehiscence, already low, is further reduced by the elimination of distal infection before surgery. Direct observation of the airway distal to the lesion allows a more accurate assessment of the extent of airway resection that will be requisite and, in addition, facilitates a preliminary determination of the need for parenchymal resection, either to achieve complete control of neoplastic disease or to preclude future infection originating in lobes or segments destroyed by long-standing obstruction. Finally, for proximal airway lesions, preliminary management of the airway at the time of reconstruction is greatly simplified.

When stenting is performed, we employ studded Silastic stents and remove them a few days in advance of surgery to allow local inflammation to subside, allowing a more accurate intraoperative assessment of the airway mucosa and cartilaginous integrity. In general, the interval between endoscopic intervention and definitive reconstruction has averaged about 1 month, but in benign inflammatory stricture, particularly tuberculous stenosis with broncholithiasis, we have paused several months for antimicrobial therapy to control the infectious process and for the airway inflammation to stabilize.

Operative Considerations

The general techniques employed in airway reconstruction have been known for several decades although they are generally available at only a few centers. However, with practical experience in lung transplantation available in many training programs, the capability to undertake such procedures with confidence is much more widely disseminated. An excellent and comprehensive resource, with several chapters dedicated to various specific aspects of this broad field, should be within the personal library of any practitioner of these methods.[1]

At whatever level of the airway the reconstruction is undertaken, the surgical goal is identical and can be summarized briefly: to construct a barostatic, tension-free anastomosis between macroscopically (and, in neoplastic disease, microscopically) normal and well-vascularized airway components. With distal reconstruction, a secondary goal is to preserve functional lung parenchyma whenever possible; accordingly, in younger patients we believe that the preservation of lobes with even moderate bronchiectasis is a preferred alternative to resection. To this end, dissection about the airway is limited to just that which will allow disease-free airway margins, verified by intraoperative frozen section in reconstructions for malignant disease, preserving the maximal length and caliber of the airway.

None of the release maneuvers that extend the length of trachea that can be safely resected, no matter how well executed, compensates for an anastomosis within which vascularity has been compromised. Similarly, pedicled vascular grafts, an essential adjunct to surgery conducted in a presumed or known infected field, as occurs when undertaking repair of traumatic airway disruption, tracheo-innominate fistula, or postintubation tracheoesophageal fistula, can substitute for meticulous resection or débridement and accurate apposition of the airway margins.

Keeping the preceding essentials always in mind, the sole remaining consideration during airway reconstructive procedures is airway management.

Airway management for reconstruction is contingent on location and nature of the lesion. For lesions distal to the carina, direct contralateral bronchial intubation using an armored tube is a satisfactory alternative to intubation with a dual lumen tube, and may be accomplished more readily in patients with smaller airways or when cervical immobility limits oropharyngeal exposure. If necessary, when resection abuts the carina, the armored tube can be advanced further into the contralateral bronchus under direct vision to preclude accidental disruption of the balloon during the repair. A further alternative is the use of balloon occlusion catheters, endoscopically guided into the ipsilateral mainstem bronchus, although their utility is generally confined to use for lesions several centimeters distal to the carina.

Airway management for reconstruction of the proximal trachea, accomplished through cervical incision, is similarly straightforward. An armored tube is advanced under endoscopic guidance beyond the lesion, if possible, and dissection up to the point of airway entry accomplished. The site of tracheal entry is then selected. If it proved impossible to pass the lesion with the armored tube, entry distal to the lesion is essential, and the distal trachea is intubated through the operative field with a sterile armored tube, which is immediately secured with suture to prevent inadvertent dislodgment. If the tracheal tube has been passed beyond the pathologic lesion, the airway can be entered either proximal or distal; if the indwelling tube hinders dissection, the distal trachea is intubated as above. If the dissection can be accomplished without restriction, the armored tube is withdrawn into the proximal trachea, and the resected specimen removed. The distal trachea can then be intubated, as above, or the orotracheal tube advanced under direct vision into the distal trachea. For very proximal tracheal lesions, an umbilical tie is secured to the side hole of the armored tube before withdrawal to facilitate easy retrieval. If repair of the membranous trachea is at all hindered by a translaryngeal armored tube bridging the gap between the resected tracheal margins, there should be no hesitation in conversion to intubation of the distal trachea through the operative field, as described above. If intubation through the operative fields has been necessary, we generally withdraw this tube and advance the orotracheal tube into the distal airway as the resected margins are opposed with stay sutures, believing this limits tension on the repair as the membranous sutures are tied.

For reconstruction of the distal trachea, an armored orotracheal tube is advanced under endoscopic guidance into the left mainstem bronchus, allowing absorption atelectasis of the right lung to commence before right thoracotomy. After the principal dissection has been completed, the distal trachea is opened, and the left main bronchus intubated across the operative field. During the repair, this tube can be withdrawn briefly, as necessary, to facilitate precise suturing. After all sutures have been placed, the tube placed across the operative field is withdrawn, and the orotracheal tube again advanced into the left mainstem bronchus.

Carinal reconstructions provide the most challenging problems in intraoperative airway management. For reconstruction via right thoracotomy, the approach described immediately above is simplest. Airway control in reconstructions through a left thoracotomy can be handled in a roughly analogous fashion, with an armored orotracheal tube advanced into the right mainstem bronchus, although this generally occludes the right upper lobe orifice and may cause significant impairment of ventilation. For this reason, as well as the limited exposure of the carina from the left even when the aortic arch is mobilized, this approach is rarely favored. The greatest flexibility is available when a clamshell incision is employed, because mainstem bronchus can be readily intubated either from within the operative field or by advancement of the orotracheal tube.

Postoperative Considerations

Immediately following the procedure, endoscopic assessment of the airway is performed to verify the integrity of the reconstruction, to assess mucosal vascularity, and to aspirate secretions and blood from the distal airway. Any possible technical flaws should be remedied at this juncture because a subsequent anastomotic failure may be neither correctable nor survivable. In almost all elective procedures, the patient can be extubated immediately. When emergency surgery is undertaken, this may not be feasible, and in such circumstances, in those undergoing tracheal repair, the balloon of the endotracheal tube should be endoscopically positioned distal to the reconstruction, if possible.

We perform routine endoscopic inspection of the reconstruction on the morning following surgery, both to assess the vascularity and integrity of the anastomosis and to evacuate blood and secretions that often elude clinical and radiographic examination. This examination is a daily routine until such time as secretions are no longer problematic.

With few exceptions, the postoperative care of these patients is no different from that of others undergoing conventional intrathoracic procedures, provided the patient has been selected and prepared properly for surgery and the reconstruction meticulously performed. Drainage catheters, either in the neck or pleura, are removed according to conventional criteria. If employed, the cervical fixation suture is removed 1 week following surgery. Delayed complications of the reconstruction—primarily granulation tissue and stricture—are uncommon. Accordingly, fiberoptic inspection is performed at 6 to 8 weeks following surgery, and any necessary therapy is initiated.

REFERENCE

1. Pearson FG, Cooper JD, Deslauriers J, et al (eds): Thoracic Surgery, 2nd ed. New York, Churchill Livingstone, 2002.

CHAPTER 4

Squamous Cell Carcinoma

David R. Duhamel

The percentage of pulmonary neoplasms that are of the squamous cell subtype has been decreasing over recent years. Adenocarcinoma is now believed to be the most common subtype, followed by squamous cell at 30%. However, squamous cell carcinoma originates most frequently in the segmental or lobar bronchi[1] and is the subtype that most often leads to endobronchial obstruction. As a result of this endobronchial growth, airway obstruction is a common presenting feature of squamous cell carcinoma, with distal atelectasis, lobar collapse, bronchiectasis, and obstructive pneumonitis being frequently present as well. Almost all patients are current or former smokers.

Squamous cell carcinoma is also the most common cause of tracheal neoplasm and accounts for 50% of all cancers arising in the trachea.[2] It should be pointed out, however, that tracheal cancers are very rare, with one tracheal tumor being identified for every 180 lung cancers.[2] Tracheal tumors often manifest with dyspnea, which is paradoxic in nature and tends to be worse at night when the patient is recumbent. Localized wheezing may be heard over the trachea, which can be inspiratory or expiratory depending on the tumor location.

The early bronchoscopic appearance of squamous cell carcinoma is that of carcinoma in situ or minimally invasive carcinoma. These lesions may appear as raised whitish plaques, subtle mucosal granularity, or erythematous thickening of a bronchial spur. They may extend for a considerable distance within the mucosa without significant growth into the airway lumen.[3] These lesions are often overlooked by less experienced bronchoscopists. Not all carcinoma in situ lesions go on to become invasive carcinomas; however, many grow into the bronchial lumen as an obstructing mass. The bronchoscopic appearance is highly variable, but most lesions will be described as a polypoid or papillary infiltrative growth with superficial ulcerations or erosions.[4] On occasion a cancer will be discovered with significant endobronchial obstruction but little or no invasion of the bronchial wall. The tumor seems to grow along the path of least resistance within the bronchial lumen until it has completely occluded the airway with a cast of tumor tissue, secretions, blood, and necrotic debris. However, it is much more common to have extensive submucosal and peribronchial invasion at the time of presentation. These tumors are capable of extensive local invasion, with destruction of tracheal cartilage and involvement of adjacent lymph nodes, lung, pericardium, vena cava, nerves, and occasionally esophagus.[2]

The radiographic findings in squamous cell carcinoma are diverse. Because endobronchial obstruction is a frequent occurrence, the radiographic manifestations of segmental atelectasis, lobar collapse, and obstructive pneumonitis are common. The squamous cell tumor mass is typically centrally located because the site of origin is usually within the bronchus. As the tumor enlarges and outgrows its blood supply, it can become necrotic and cavitate—a classic radiographic appearance most often associated with squamous cell carcinomas. Squamous cell tumors of the trachea are much less common, and unfortunately their radiologic manifestations are subtle and often overlooked. The malignant tracheal tumors tend to manifest with focal or circumferential tracheal narrowing or as a sessile or polypoid mass, 2 to 4 cm in length.[5] The lower third of the trachea is the most frequent site of occurrence at 44%.[2] Associated findings include a paratracheal mass due to extratracheal extension, lymphadenopathy, metastatic parenchymal nodules, and rarely a tracheoesophageal fistula. In general, radiography is not very sensitive for detecting tracheal tumors, because only 23% to 45% of tracheal lesions are detected with the standard posteroanterior and lateral chest radiographs.[5] A 30-degree anterior oblique film is sometimes useful when evaluating the trachea because it may separate the tracheal air shadow from the vertebral column.

Histologically, carcinoma in situ appears as a thickened epithelium of squamous cells in which nuclear atypia is present from the most basal to the most apical cells.[6] A true squamous cell carcinoma is classified based on the presence of two microscopic findings; intercellular bridging and keratinization. One or both of these findings should be present to make a definite diagnosis. The tumor cells may be well differentiated with clear evidence of intercellular bridging and keratinization or be poorly differentiated without the pathognomonic findings of squamous cell carcinoma and difficult to distinguish from small cell or adenocarcinoma.[7] Within the subtype of squamous cell carcinoma, there exist a few histologic variants. These are identified by their unique histologic pattern and include papillary, clear cell, basaloid, and small cell.[6] The last pattern is very easily confused with small cell carcinoma and can cause a serious diagnostic dilemma.

The prognosis for endobronchial squamous cell carcinoma is best if the lesion can be surgically resected. Isolated tracheal neoplasms without significant tissue invasion are very amendable to surgical resection with a better overall prognosis. The majority of patients, however, who present with endobronchial obstruction already have extensive disease and are not candidates for surgery. In these patients, the focus should be on palliation of symptoms. External beam radiation has not been found to be very effective at relieving endobronchial obstruction, whereas Nd:YAG laser ablation and mechanical débridement with the rigid bronchoscope are known to be safe and effective. The relief of the luminal obstruction significantly improves the patient's symptoms of obstruction including cough, dyspnea, hemoptysis, and obstructive pneumonitis. Once the obstruction has been cleared, other endobronchial therapies such as bronchial stenting, brachytherapy, and photodynamic therapy may be valuable in maintaining lumenal patency. As these endoscopic treatments and techniques continue to improve, the goal of complete patient palliation or even cure seems an ever increasing possibility.

REFERENCES

1. Lisa JR, Trinidad S, Rosenblatt MB: Site of origin, histogenesis, and cytostructure of bronchogenic carcinoma. Am J Clin Pathol 44:375-380, 1965.
2. Houston HW, Payne WS, Harrison EG Jr, et al: Primary cancers of the trachea. Arch Surg 99:132-138, 1969.
3. Nagamoto N, Saito Y, Suda H, et al: Relationship between length of longitudinal extension and maximal depth of transmural invasion and roentgenographically occult squamous cell carcinoma of the bronchus (nonpolypoid type). Am J Surg Pathol 13:11-19, 1989.
4. Hajdu SI, Huvos A, Goodner JT, et al: Carcinoma of the trachea. Clinicopathologic study of 41 cases. Cancer 25:1448-1456, 1970.
5. McCarthy MJ, Rosado-de-Christenson ML: Tumors of the trachea. J Thorac Imaging 10:180-198, 1995.
6. Carter D: Squamous cell carcinoma of the lung. An update. Semin Diagn Pathol 2:226-239, 1985.
7. Edwards C, Carlile A: Poorly differentiated squamous carcinoma of the bronchus: A light and electron microscopic study. J Clin Pathol 39:284-291, 1985.

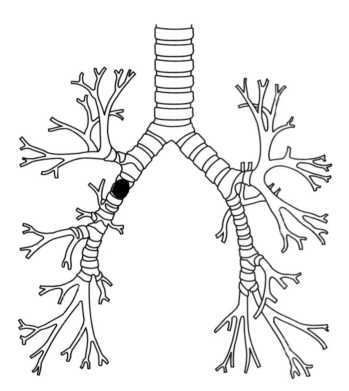

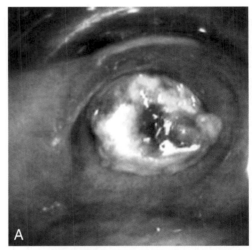

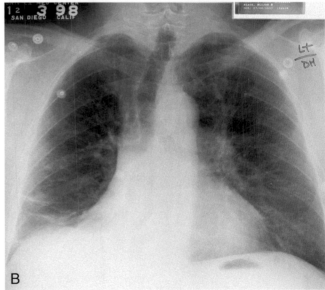

Figure 4-1. **A**, A necrotic mass of endobronchial squamous cell carcinoma completely occluding the right mainstem bronchus. Note the central area of hemorrhage. **B**, A frontal radiograph demonstrating volume loss and collapse of the right middle and lower lobes. The right bronchial air column appears truncated just below the opening to the right upper lobe.

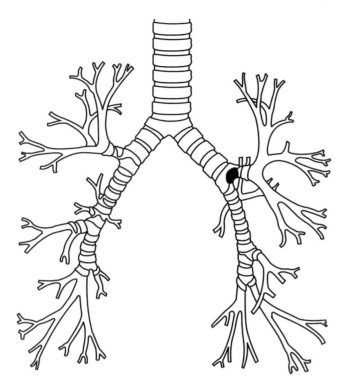

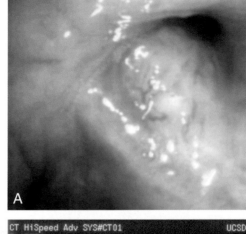

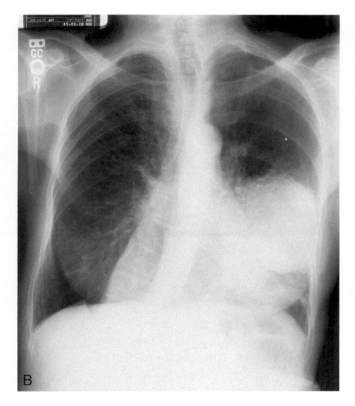

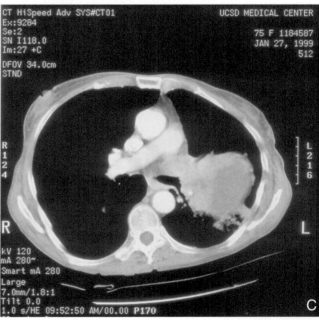

Figure 4-2. A, Extensive submucosal and lymphangitic infiltration from squamous cell carcinoma with partial obstruction of the left upper lobe orifice. Note the thickened and splayed bifurcation between the upper and lower lobes. **B,** A frontal radiograph demonstrating a large parenchymal lung mass nearly replacing the left lower lobe. **C,** A computed tomography scan demonstrating a large necrotic-appearing mass with invasion of the left lower lobe bronchus. The bronchial lumen is narrowed and has an irregular appearance.

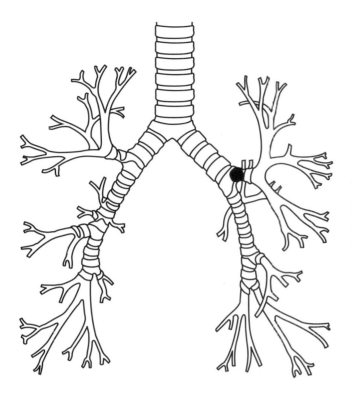

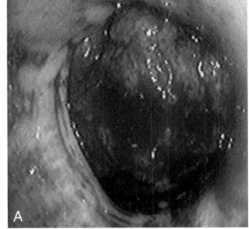

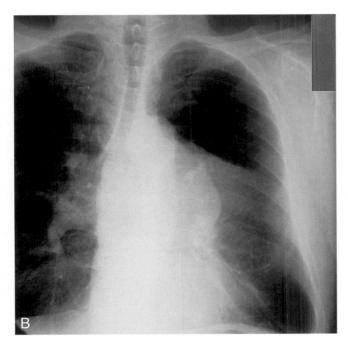

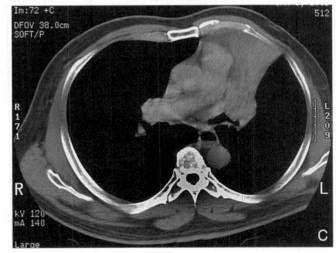

Figure 4-3. **A,** A hemorrhagic squamous cell tumor obstructing the left upper lobe orifice. The bronchial mucosa does not appear to be infiltrated by tumor, suggesting that the tumor may have grown up from the lung parenchyma rather than arising in the bronchus. **B,** A frontal radiograph demonstrating complete left upper lobe collapse along with left hilar fullness. **C,** A computed tomography scan demonstrating consolidation and collapse of the left upper lobe, with an irregular soft tissue mass occluding the left upper lobe bronchus.

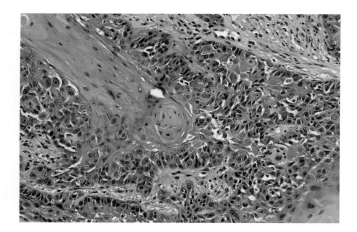

Figure 4-4. Malignant squamous cells invading the tissue stroma and showing evidence of squamous differentiation, including intercellular bridges and keratin pearl formation (H&E, ×200, original magnification).

CHAPTER 5

Carcinoma in Situ

David R. Duhamel

Carcinoma in situ is defined as the presence of atypical cells in all layers of the epithelium without evidence of invasion of the basement membrane.[1] Occult bronchial carcinoma in situ is found at necropsy in 6% of smokers[2] and in more than a third of specimens resected for another broncho-genic carcinoma.[3] Surprisingly, it remains a rarely diagnosed clinical entity. The vast majority of patients are asympto-matic, and the presence of carcinoma in situ is discovered only when a screening sputum cytology result is positive or the abnormality is noted on bronchoscopy performed for other indications. Significant risk factors include the expo-sure to tobacco and asbestos for more than 10 years. This is demonstrated by the findings of Auerbach and co-workers, who found bronchial dysplasia in 40% of heavy smokers.[4]

The diagnosis of carcinoma in situ can be difficult to make by conventional bronchoscopy because the lesions are only a few cell layers thick (0.2 to 1 mm) and a few millimeters in surface diameter.[5] In a study by Woolner and colleagues, carcinoma in situ was visible by conventional bronchoscopy in less than 30% of patients.[6] The mucosal changes observed with conventional white-light bron-choscopy can be subtle and easily overlooked by the less experienced bronchoscopist. These subtle changes include increased redness, thickening of the spur, or mucosal granularity. Occasionally, more obvious findings are seen, including exophytic, polypoid, or papillary growth.

A recent bronchoscopic development that aids in the diagnosis of these more obscure lesions is called lung imaging fluorescent endoscopy (Xillix Technologies Corp., Vancouver, B.C.), or LIFE. Fluorescence endoscopy is based on the observation that premalignant and malignant lesions of the bronchial epithelium fluoresce less than normal epithelium when excited by violet (405 nm) or blue (442 nm) light.[7] This allows an area of abnormal mucosa to be iden-tified and biopsied. The potential benefits of this technology appear impressive. Lam and colleagues, using fluorescence bronchoscopy in a group of 53 patients with known or suspected lung cancer, found synchronous carcinoma in situ in 15%.[5] It is important to temper these impressive results, however, with the understanding that the technique is not very specific. Approximately one third of all biopsies taken from areas labeled as "abnormal" during fluorescence do not show any histologic abnormality.[8]

A second bronchoscopic technology, which may prove extremely useful in the workup and staging of these pre-malignant lesions, is endobronchial ultrasound. By defini-tion, carcinoma in situ lacks basement membrane invasion, and when this finding is present the lesion is considered an invasive carcinoma. A routine bronchoscopy gives little information about the depth of tissue invasion; however, in a recent article endobronchial ultrasound delivered through a flexible bronchoscope was found to determine the depth of tumor invasion with a 95.8% accuracy.[9] Currently, both photodynamic therapy and brachytherapy have been shown to be curative of carcinoma in situ, whereas invasive carcinoma still must be treated with surgical resection. Therefore, the ability to accurately determine in vivo which lesions are potentially curable with nonsurgical therapy represents a major benefit.

The role of radiology in the diagnosis and workup of this disease is very limited. The vast majority of these lesions are considered radiographically occult. The role of CT scan is limited as well. On occasion, a polypoid or exophytic lesion may be observed, but in general these lesions are too small to be properly characterized by CT scan. CT may also be obtained to look for adenopathy or distant metastases.

It has been proposed that squamous cell carcinoma of the bronchus arises after a series of progressive histologic changes in the epithelium. These histologic changes are, in order of increasing severity, basal cell hyperplasia; squamous metaplasia; mild, moderate, and severe dysplasia; and carcinoma in situ.[7] Carcinoma in situ is still considered a preneoplastic change and the last step before invasive carcinoma. This is not to imply that all carcinoma in situ lesions go on to become invasive carcinomas; in fact, some premalignant lesions actually regress when the irritant exposure discontinues. A prospective study to determine the percentage of carcinoma in situ lesions that progress to invasive carcinoma is difficult to design for obvious ethical reasons. In an observational study of nine patients undergoing treatment for carcinoma in situ, five (56%) were found to have lesions that progressed to invasive carcinoma.[10] The microscopic findings include extreme cytologic aberration, mitoses throughout all layers of the epithelium, and the absence of maturation.[8] Various cytogenetic (p53, bcl-2, k-*ras*) and chromosomal alterations (28-32, 34) have also been found to play an important role in carcinogenesis and the development of carcinoma in situ.[8]

The ability to treat and potentially cure carcinoma in situ with endoscopic therapies has been realized recently with the development of photodynamic therapy. The therapy is based on the concept that hematoporphyrin derivatives can be injected into the vein and disseminated throughout the entire body. It is cleared rapidly by normal cells but remains longer in tumor tissue. Because it is a dye, it preferentially absorbs light of a certain wavelength. The absorption of light activates a photochemical reaction and releases free radicals, causing cell death. Because the tumor cells concentrate the dye, they are the only ones affected by the reaction.[11] Radiation has also been used successfully to treat these lesions, both external beam and endoscopic brachytherapy. Surgical resection, including sleeve resection, segmentectomy, lobectomy, and even pneumonectomy, also has been used to treat carcinoma in situ.[12] The rationale for this more aggressive therapy includes the existence of metachronous and synchronous lesions, the high rate of progression to invasive carcinoma, and the inability to definitively confirm the lack of invasion without a surgical specimen. However, as these new endoscopic therapies are further studied and refined, it is hoped that we can create a vital array of tools to screen, diagnose, and treat this, the earliest of cancerous lesions.

REFERENCES

1. Infield M, Gerblich A, Subramanyan S, et al: Focus of bronchial carcinoma in situ eradicated by endobronchial biopsy. Chest 94:1107-1109, 1988.
2. Auerbach O, Stout AP, Hammond EC, et al: Changes in bronchial epithelium in relation to cigarette smoking and in relation to lung cancer. N Engl J Med 165:253-267, 1961.
3. Black H, Ackerman LV: The importance of epidermoid carcinoma in situ in the histogenesis of carcinoma of the lung. Ann Surg 136:44-55, 1952.
4. Auerbach O, Hammond EC, Garfinkel L: Changes in bronchial epithelium in relation to smoking. N Engl J Med 300:381-386, 1979.
5. Lam S, MacAulay C, Hung J, et al: Detection of dysplasia and carcinoma in situ with a lung imaging fluorescence endoscope device. J Thorac Cardiovasc Surg 105:1035-1040, 1993.
6. Woolner LB, Fontana RS, Cortese DA, et al: Roentgenographically occult lung cancer: Pathologic findings and frequency of multicentricity during a 10 year period. Mayo Clin Proc 59:453-466, 1984.
7. Bota S, Auliac JB, Paris C, et al: Follow-up of bronchial precancerous lesions and carcinoma in situ using fluorescence endoscopy. Am J Respir Crit Care Med 164:1688-1693, 2001.
8. Kerr KM: Pulmonary preinvasive neoplasia. J Clin Pathol 54:257-271, 2001.
9. Kurimoto N, Murayama M, Yoshioka S, et al: Assessment of usefulness of endobronchial ultrasonography in determination of the depth of tumor invasion. Chest 115:1500-1506, 1999.
10. Venmans BJW, van Boxem TJM, Smit EF, et al: Outcome of bronchial carcinoma in situ. Chest 117:1572-1576, 2000.
11. McCaughan JS, Williams TE, Bethel B: Photodynamic therapy of endobronchial tumors. Lasers Surg Med 6:336-345, 1986.
12. Nagamoto N, Saito Y, Sato M, et al: Clinicopathological analysis of 19 cases of isolated carcinoma in situ of the bronchus. Am J Surg Path 17:1234-1243, 1993.

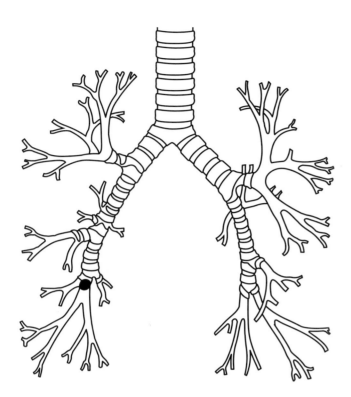

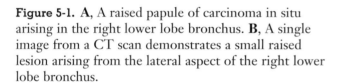

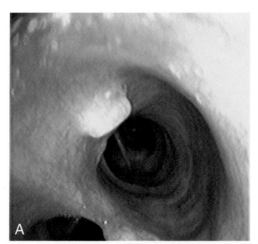

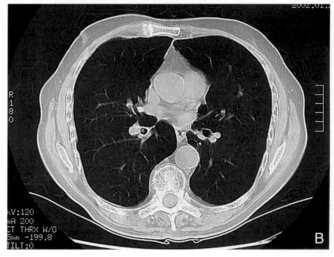

Figure 5-1. A, A raised papule of carcinoma in situ arising in the right lower lobe bronchus. **B,** A single image from a CT scan demonstrates a small raised lesion arising from the lateral aspect of the right lower lobe bronchus.

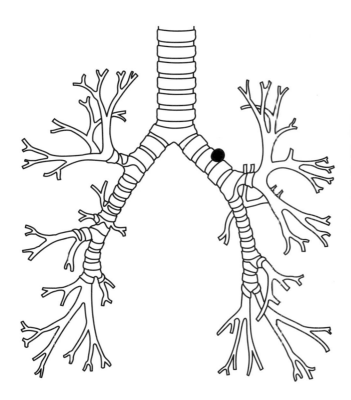

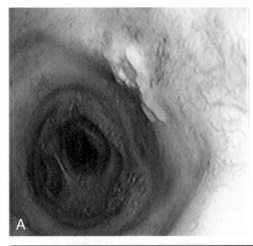

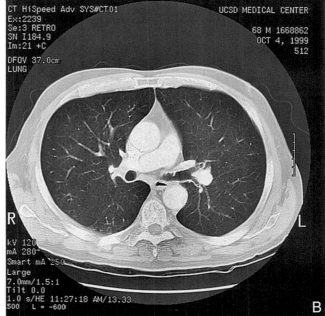

Figure 5-2. A, An ulcerative carcinoma in situ lesion on the lateral wall of the left mainstem bronchus, with a prominent vascular pattern seen in the surrounding mucosa. **B,** No discrete lesion is seen on this CT scan, but slight irregularity is present within the distal left main bronchus.

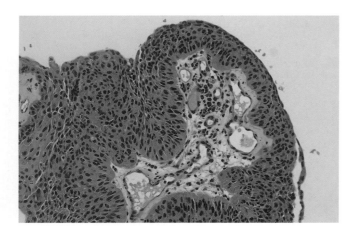

Figure 5-3. Dysplastic squamous cells replace the full thickness of bronchial mucosa. However, the basement membrane is intact with no evidence of stromal invasion (H&E, ×200, original magnification).

CHAPTER 6

Adenoid Cystic Carcinoma

David R. Duhamel

Adenoid cystic carcinoma, or cylindroma, is an uncommon histologic variant of adenocarcinoma, which usually arises from the salivary, lacrimal, or other exocrine glands.[1] Occasionally, this uncommon tumor is seen in the lung, where it classically develops in the larger bronchi and trachea. Originally classified as a bronchial adenoma, this tumor is now described more accurately as a *neoplasm of the tracheobronchial glands*. The adenoid cystic carcinoma is the most common tumor in this family, but other types include mucoepidermoids, acinic cell tumors, and oncocytomas. Tracheobronchial gland tumors account for 0.5% of all lung neoplasms, of which 75% to 80% are adenoid cystic carcinomas.[2] The tumors tend to invade surrounding tissues, recur locally, and have a prolonged clinical course. Although adenoid cystic carcinoma is very rare, it remains one of the most common primary tracheal tumors. In a series of 198 primary tracheal tumors by Grillo and Mathison, it represented 40% of the lesions.[3] The etiology is unknown, and there are no clear risk factors, although it was reported in an 18-year-old who had received thoracic radiation therapy.[4] Most tumors are discovered in patients aged 40 to 45 years, with no sex predominance.

Bronchoscopically, the lesion is fairly unique. It characteristically arises along the lateral and posterolateral wall of the trachea, where the rigid cartilaginous structures join the posterior membrane. The mucous glands are highly concentrated in this area. The lesion grows into the lumen and has a smooth, lobulated, polypoid or fusiform shape. The lesions are apt to be disturbingly large by the time the diagnosis is made. The surface is covered with a prominent vascular pattern, and there is frequently submucosal extension a considerable distance from the primary lesion. The lesion occasionally grows circumferentially within the tracheal lumen, giving rise to the historical term *cylindroma*.

The radiographic findings include an endobronchial or endotracheal smooth hemispheric mass that occludes the airway lumen to varying degrees. The report of a normal chest radiograph result is a recurring theme in most of the large case series; therefore, clinicians should have a high index of suspicion and pursue other means of diagnosis. CT scanning is very useful for making the diagnosis as well as for evaluating mediastinal lymphadenopathy but is relatively insensitive for assessing the extent of submucosal or perineural lymphatic involvement.

Histologically, the tumor consists of uniform cells with scant cytoplasm arranged in well-defined nests. The cystic spaces separating the cells contain a mucinous substance that stains strongly with alcian blue. Mitotic activity and tissue necrosis are unusual. The tumor can be divided into the histologic subtypes of solid, tubular, and cribriform. Tumors of the solid subtype exhibit more extensive and invasive extraluminal growth and a greater tendency for distant metastasis. The tubular and cribriform patterns are associated with a higher frequency of local recurrence due to their tendency to infiltrate the adjacent submucosa and perineural lymphatics.[5] Occasionally, these tumors metastasize to distant sites such as the liver, kidneys, and bone marrow, and their metastases exhibit the same histologic features as the primary tumor. Spread of adenoid cystic carcinomas is mainly by direct infiltration, and incomplete removal results in local recurrence.

Although adenoid cystic carcinoma is a malignant neoplasm capable of metastasizing, the clinical course tends to be indolent and prolonged. Survival rates are estimated at between 65% and 79% for 5 years and 53% and 57% at 10 years. Surgical resection of the tumor is the treatment of choice, but the number of patients who are able to undergo complete resection is typically low. According to the Mayo experience, only 3 of 13 patients were able to undergo complete resection because of extension into surrounding tissues.[6] Therefore, radiation therapy plays an important role as adjuvant therapy to treat residual tumor or as primary therapy to treat inoperable lesions. Additional localized radiation can also be given with brachytherapy. There have been multiple case reports of successful endobronchial resection with the Nd:YAG laser followed by irradiation in inoperable patients as well.[7] Metastases are uncommon and usually appear late in the course of disease, with death resulting from thoracic complications. Local recurrence is unfortunately common and can develop as late as 30 years after initial discovery of the tumor.[8] Therefore, prolonged close bronchoscopic follow-up is a necessity.

REFERENCES

1. Cleveland RH, Nice CM Jr, Ziskind J: Primary adenoid cystic carcinoma (cylindroma) of the trachea. Radiology 122:597-600, 1977.

2. Spencer H: Bronchial mucous gland tumors. Virchows Arch (Pathol Anat Histol) 383:101-109, 1979.

3. Grillo HC, Mathison DJ: Primary tracheal tumors: Treatment and results. Ann Thorac Surg 49:69-77, 1990.

4. Hajdu SI, Huvos AG, Goodner JT, et al: Carcinoma of the trachea. Clinicopathologic study of 41 cases. Cancer 25:1448-1456, 1970.

5. Nomori H, Kaseda S, Kobayashi K, et al: Adenoid cystic carcinoma of the trachea and main-stem bronchi. J Thorac Cardiovasc Surg 96:271-277, 1988.

6. Conlan AA, Payne WS, Woolner LB, Sanderson DR: Adenoid cystic carcinoma (cylindroma) and mucoepidermoid carcinoma of the bronchus. J Thorac Cardiovasc Surg 76:369-377, 1978.

7. Aggarwal A, Tewari S, Mehta AC: Successful management of adenoid cystic carcinoma of the trachea by laser and irradiation. Chest 116:269, 1999.

8. Houston HE, Payne WS, Harrison EG, et al: Primary cancers of the trachea. Arch Surg 99:132-148, 1969.

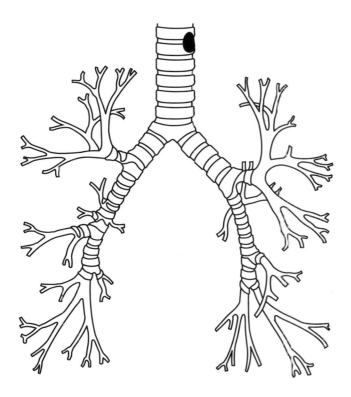

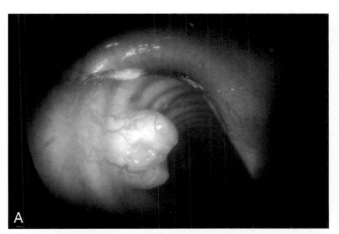

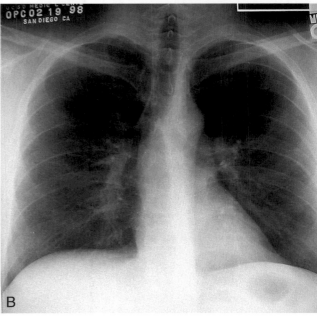

Figure 6-1. A, A raised nodule of adenoid cystic carcinoma arising from the proximal left lateral tracheal wall and extending into the lumen. **B,** The chest radiograph demonstrates slight narrowing of the tracheal air column in the midtracheal region.

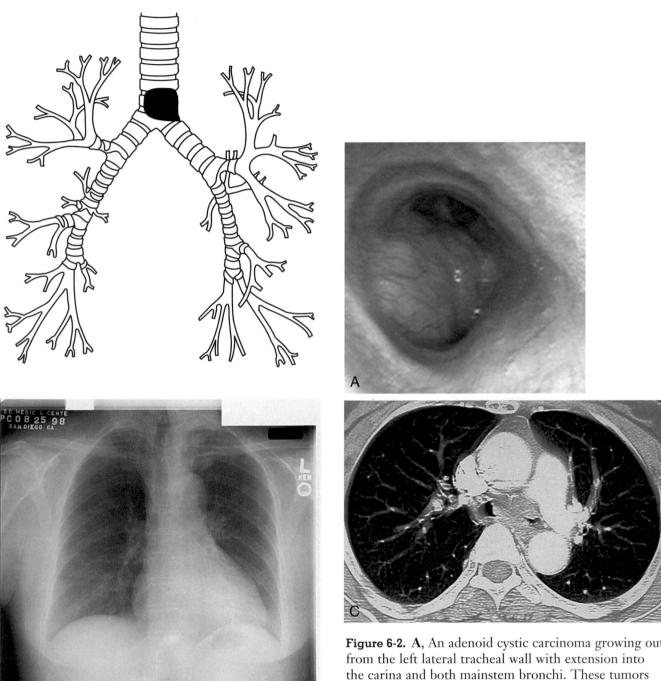

Figure 6-2. A, An adenoid cystic carcinoma growing out from the left lateral tracheal wall with extension into the carina and both mainstem bronchi. These tumors arise most commonly from the lateral tracheal walls, where the salivary glands are most densely concentrated. **B,** The chest radiograph demonstrates increased density in the subcarinal region, with narrowing of the proximal main bronchi. **C,** The CT image demonstrates a large mass in the subcarinal region, narrowing the left main and right main bronchi.

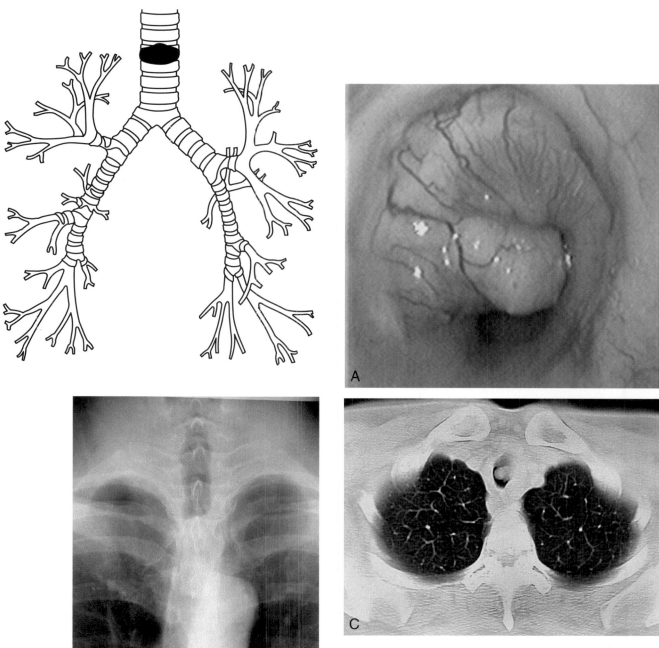

Figure 6-3. A, An adenoid cystic carcinoma arising from the left lateral wall of the trachea. The classic vascular pattern on the tumor surface is easily seen. **B,** A close-up of the trachea demonstrates abrupt termination of the air column. **C,** The CT scan demonstrates a large mass arising from the left lateral aspect of the trachea.

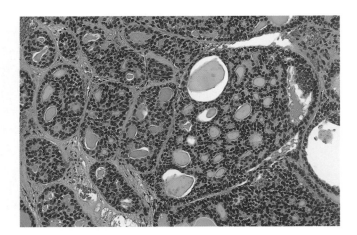

Figure 6-4. Adenoid cystic carcinoma, showing monotonous tumor cells with the characteristic cribriform pattern (H&E, ×200).

CHAPTER 7

Bronchial Carcinoids

David R. Duhamel

Bronchial carcinoids were first described in the 1800s, but it was not until 1907 that Seigfried Oberndorfer coined the term *Karzinoide* to describe a tumor "resembling carcinoma."[1] They were originally grouped along with adenoid cystics and mucoepidermoids as bronchial adenomas because of their good prognosis. More recently, it has become apparent that there exists a subgroup of carcinoids called *atypical carcinoids* that exhibit a much greater malignant potential when compared with that of a typical carcinoid. The atypical carcinoid exhibits a higher mitotic index per high-powered field, an increased rate of nodal metastasis, a higher recurrence rate, and a worse overall 5-year prognosis. It is now felt that carcinoids are of neuroectodermal origin and arise from the Kulchitsky cells of respiratory epithelium. Small cell carcinoma of the lung has similar neuroectodermal origins, and this has given rise to a concept of a spectrum of neuroendocrine tumors of the lung.[2] On one end of the spectrum is the benign typical carcinoid, and on the other end is the malignant small cell carcinoma. Somewhere in between are the more malignant atypical carcinoids.

Bronchial carcinoids can occur in a wide age range, but most clinical series show a median age in the mid 40s. There are about 2000 new cases of bronchial carcinoids diagnosed each year, which represents 2% of all primary lung tumors.[3] Of these 2000 new lesions, 50% to 70% are located centrally within the trachea and mainstem bronchi and are reachable with the flexible bronchoscope.[4,5] The others are located peripherally within the lung parenchyma. The patients with central lesions are much more likely to be symptomatic on presentation. These symptoms classically include cough (42%), hemoptysis (20%), stridor or wheeze (15%-25%), or postobstructive pneumonia (20%).[4] Symptoms of carcinoid syndrome are very rare and are seen only with atypical carcinoids that have metastasized to the liver. A significant majority of patients are completely asymptomatic on presentation, and their tumors are discovered after a routine chest radiograph. There is no known relationship to smoking or other inciting factors.[6]

Fiberoptic bronchoscopy plays a major role in diagnosis of carcinoids. A raised, pinkish, vascular, lobulated lesion is classically seen endobronchially. On occasion, a lesion is pedunculated, but the majority of lesions have a sessile base, which is firmly attached to the bronchial wall. There had been concerns in the past about endobronchial biopsy for fear of uncontrollable hemorrhage. These concerns have been put to rest by multiple case series that documented a very low bleeding risk from endobronchial biopsy.[7,8,9] Bronchial brushings, sputum specimens, and lavage fluid rarely provide adequate tissue to make a diagnosis.[6] A large piece of tissue is frequently needed to make a definitive diagnosis because there is often difficulty distinguishing between carcinoid and small cell carcinoma.

Most patients have an abnormal chest radiograph result either because of visualization of the tumor itself or as a consequence of airway obstruction. A rounded, smooth-surfaced, highly vascular, and well-demarcated endobronchial lesion is typically seen on CT scan. Although common in the larger bronchi, carcinoids are infrequent in the trachea.[10] Less than 10% of the lesions are calcified. Extraluminal extension, mediastinal invasion, and lymph node metastases are infrequently seen.

The treatment is typically surgical, with particular focus on lung sparing or bronchoplastic surgery. Many patients with suitable lesions do extremely well with a bronchial sleeve resection surgery. This entails removal of a small section of diseased airway with reanastomosis of the two ends without loss of lung parenchyma. Endoscopic Nd:YAG laser resection through a rigid bronchoscope also has a role. This is best utilized for certain patients who are not surgical candidates or who refuse surgery as well as for patients with postobstructive pneumonia. In the setting of postobstructive pneumonia, the lesion is removed endoscopically, and the infection is treated with antibiotics. This greatly improves the chances of successful surgical resection. In one study Sutedja and colleagues[11] demonstrated a curative role for endoscopic therapy in carcinoids. They treated 11 patients with laser therapy for intraluminal typical carcinoids. Six of the 11 patients then went on to surgical resection, including lobectomy or sleeve resection. Amazingly, all six surgical specimens were found to be disease free. Radiation therapy has a palliative role in disseminated disease, but its value as a curative therapy is limited.[12]

The clinical course of bronchial carcinoids is highly variable. The median 5- and 10-year disease-free survival for a carcinoid is 100% and 87%, respectively.[5] The best outcomes are associated with tumors smaller than 2 cm, complete resection, and typical pathology. Patients with atypical pathology, systemic symptoms, nodal involvement, and male gender have the worst outcome. The 5- and 10-year disease-free survival for atypical carcinoid is 69% and 52%, respectively.[5]

REFERENCES

1. Oberndorfer S: Karzinoide. Ergebnisse der allgemeinen Pathologie und pathologischen. Anatomie des Menschen und der Tiere 13:527-535, 1909.
2. DeCaro LF, Paladugu R, Benfield JR, et al: Typical and atypical carcinoids within the APUD tumor spectrum. J Thorac Cardiovasc Surg 86:528-536, 1983.
3. Kulke MH, Mayer RJ: Carcinoid tumors. N Engl J Med 340:858-868, 1999.
4. Soga J, Yakuwa Y: Bronchopulmonary carcinoids: An analysis of 1875 reported cases with special reference to a comparison between typical carcinoids and atypical varieties. Ann Thorac Cardiovasc Surg 5:211-219, 1999.
5. McCaughan BC, Martini N, Bains MS: Bronchial carcinoids. J Thorac Cardiovasc Surg 89:8-17, 1985.
6. Luce JA: Lymphoma, lymphoproliferative diseases, and other primary malignant tumors. *In* Murray JF, Nadel JA (eds): Textbook of Respiratory Medicine, Vol 2, 3rd ed. Philadelphia, WB Saunders, 2000, pp 1460-1462.
7. Okike N, Bernatz PE, Woolner LB: Carcinoid tumors of the lung. Ann Thorac Surg 22:271-277, 1976.
8. Todd TR, Cooper JD, Weissberg D, et al: Bronchial carcinoid tumors. J Thorac Cardiovasc Surg 79:532-536, 1980.
9. Lawson RM, Ramanathan L, Hurley G, et al: Bronchial adenoma. Review of an 18 year experience at the Brompton Hospital. Thorax 31:245-252, 1976.
10. Felson B: Neoplasms of the trachea and mainstem bronchi. Semin Roentgenol 18:23-37, 1983.
11. Sutedja TG, Schreurs AJ, Vanderschueren RG, et al: Bronchoscopic treatment of intraluminal typical carcinoids. Chest 107:556-558, 1995.
12. Schupak KD, Wallner KE: The role of radiation therapy in the treatment of locally unresectable or metastatic carcinoid tumors. Int J Radiat Oncol Biol Phys 20:489-495, 1991.

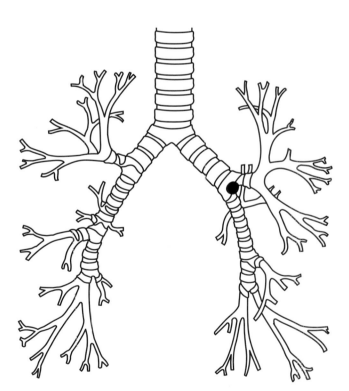

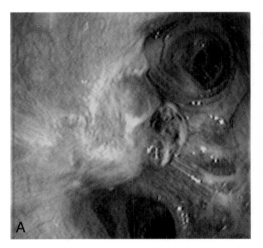

Figure 7-1. A, A raised reddish brown growth of carcinoid tumor in the distal left mainstem bronchus. The lesion appears to be infiltrating the bronchial wall and on biopsy was determined to be an atypical carcinoid.

Continued

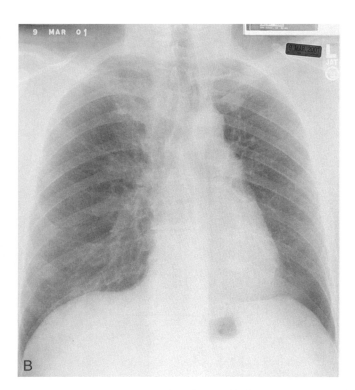

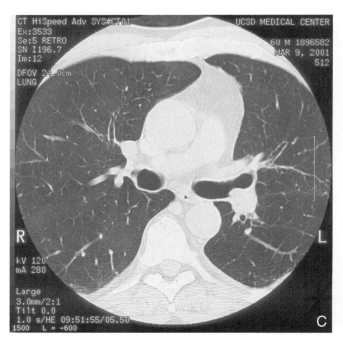

Figure 7-1, *cont'd.* **B,** Frontal radiograph demonstrates no definite abnormality. **C,** Single CT image demonstrates a raised lesion arising from the distal left main bronchus.

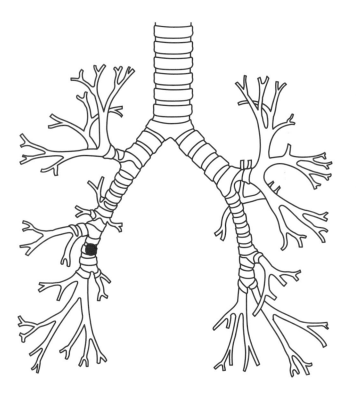

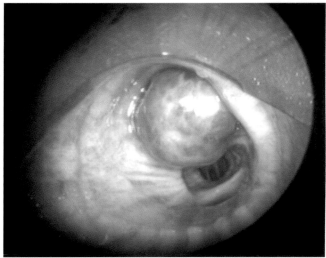

Figure 7-2. A typical reddish, smooth, pedunculated carcinoid tumor arising from a stalk in the right lower lobe superior segment.

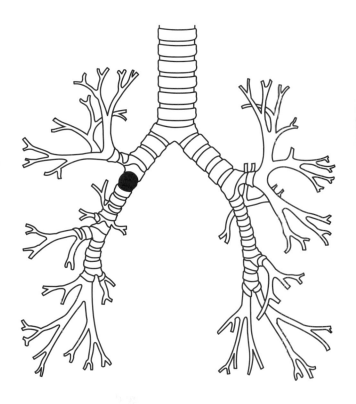

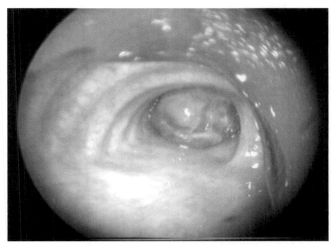

Figure 7-3. A typical reddish smooth ball of carcinoid tumor completely obstructs the right mainstem bronchus.

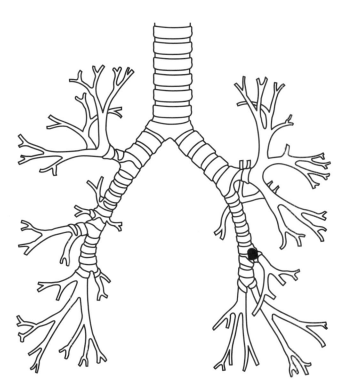

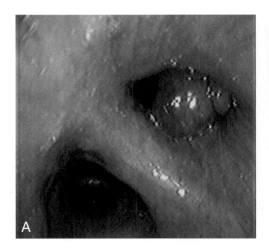

Figure 7-4. A, A small reddish carcinoid tumor obstructs the superior segment bronchus of the left lower lobe. Note the surrounding mucosal inflammation, which raises concern for tumor infiltration but actually is related to a postobstructive pneumonia. *Continued*

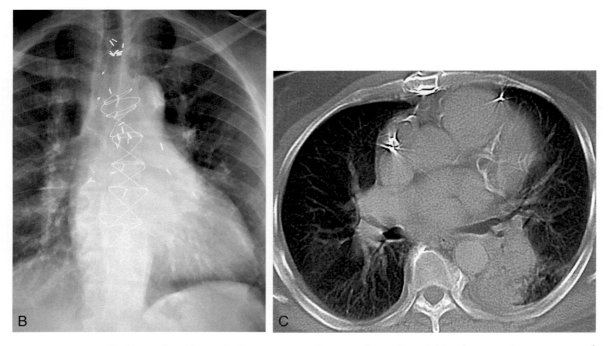

Figure 7-4, *cont'd.* **B,** Frontal radiograph demonstrates increased opacity within the superior segment of the left lower lobe. **C,** CT image demonstrates irregularity and narrowing of the superior segmental bronchus on the left with distal airspace opacity.

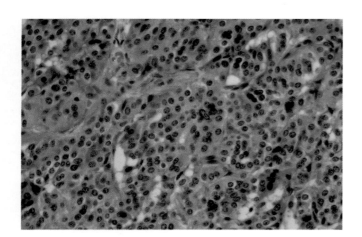

Figure 7-5. Typical bronchial carcinoid without increased mitoses or necrosis (H&E, ×20, original magnification).

CHAPTER 8

Mucoepidermoids

David R. Duhamel

Mucoepidermoid tumors of the tracheobronchial tree are rare entitles that arise from the excretory ducts of the submucosal bronchial glands.[1] They were first described in 1952 by Smetana and colleagues and account for about 1% to 5% of all neoplasms of the tracheobronchial glands (previously called bronchial adenomas).[2] In a large series of 4250 primary pulmonary carcinomas, only 7 (0.16%) cases of mucoepidermoids were reported.[1] There is a slight female preponderance and an age range from 4.5 to 78 years. There are no known risk factors, including tobacco. Mucoepidermoid tumors tend to be slow-growing and may be present for many years before a diagnosis is made. Pathologically, they are divided into low-grade or high-grade lesions. The behavior of the tumor and its prognosis directly correlate with the histologic grade of the lesion. However, low-grade tumors have shown aggressive behavior with lymph node metastasis and tissue invasion.[3] The majority of tumors remain localized to the bronchus of origin, with extrabronchial spread seen in only 25% of cases.[4]

The low-grade tumor classically manifests as an exophytic, endobronchial, polypoid lesion with a thin, smooth mucosal covering. These tumors are well circumscribed and occlude the bronchial lumen to varying degrees. The majority of lesions are located in the main or lobar bronchi. Only rarely do they involve the trachea and then usually in a supracarinal location.[5] It is unusual to see hilar lymph node involvement or metastatic disease with a low-grade tumor. The high-grade tumors manifest as larger lesions with significant tissue infiltration being seen in 46% of cases.[6] The tumor is known to metastasize by lymphangitic and hematogenous spread to lymph nodes, lung, brain, bone marrow, adrenals, and skin.

The radiographic appearance reported with mucoepidermoid carcinoma ranges from normal to the presence of solitary masses. Focal nodular areas of pneumonic consolidation, partial or complete atelectasis, and peripheral subpleural tumors are also occasionally seen. In a series of 58 cases reviewed in the Armed Forces Institute of Pathology, 41 had roentgenographic evidence of a solitary nodule or mass, 17 had evidence of postobstructive pneumonia, 16 had focal pneumonic consolidation, 10 had partial or complete atelectasis, and only 1 was considered normal.[7] There are no specific radiographic features to determine whether a tumor will be low grade or high grade.

Histologically, they are composed of a mixture of well-differentiated mucus-containing cells arranged in a glandular structure adjacent to sheets of "epidermoid" cells with keratinization and intercellular bridges. It is this intimate association of mucus secreting and epidermoid cells that gives rise to the designation mucoepidermoid. Nuclear pleomorphism is mild, and necrosis and mitotic figures are rare in the low-grade tumor. The high-grade lesion, on the other hand, shows areas of cytologic atypia, frequent mitoses, and focal areas of necrosis. Of note, some authors argue that the entity of high-grade mucoepidermoid tumors does not exist and this represents misdiagnosed adenosquamous carcinoma.[7]

Surgical resection of the low-grade tumor has an excellent long-term prognosis.[8] A conservative lung-sparing approach, such as sleeve resection, is recommended. After complete surgical resection, the incidence of local recurrence or late metastasis has been extremely small. Postoperative chemotherapy or radiation therapy is rarely indicated. The tumors are not very radiosensitive. High-grade tumors carry a worse prognosis and should be treated similar to non–small cell cancer with radical surgical resection when appropriate. Radiation and chemotherapy may be beneficial in nonsurgical candidates or those with metastatic disease. Endobronchial therapy with the Nd:YAG laser has proved to be extremely useful in nonsurgical candidates and in those who refuse an operation.

REFERENCES

1. Leonardi HK, Legg MA, Legg Y, Neptune WB: Tracheobronchial mucoepidermoid carcinoma. J Thorac Cardiovasc Surg 76:431-438, 1978.
2. Smetana HF, Iverson L, Swan LL: Bronchogenic carcinoma: An analysis of 100 autopsy cases. Mil Surgeon 111:335-351, 1952.
3. Axelsson C, Burcharth F, Johansen F: Mucoepidermoid lung cancers. J Thorac Cardiovasc Surg 65:902-908, 1973.
4. Wolf KM, Mehta D, Claypool WD: Mucoepidermoid carcinoma of the lung with intracranial metastases. Chest 94:435-438, 1988.
5. Turnbull AD, Huvos AG, Goodner JT, et al: Mucoepidermoid tumors of the bronchial glands. Cancer 28:539-544, 1971.
6. Patel RG, Norman JR: Unilateral hyperlucency with left lower lobe mass in a patient with bronchial asthma. Chest 107:569-570, 1995.
7. Yousem SA, Hochholzer L: Mucoepidermoid tumors of the lung. Cancer 60:1346-1352, 1987.
8. Breyer RH, Dainauskas JR, Jenik RJ, Faber LP: Mucoepidermoid carcinoma of the trachea and bronchus: The case for conservative resection. Am Thorac Surg 29:197-204, 1980.

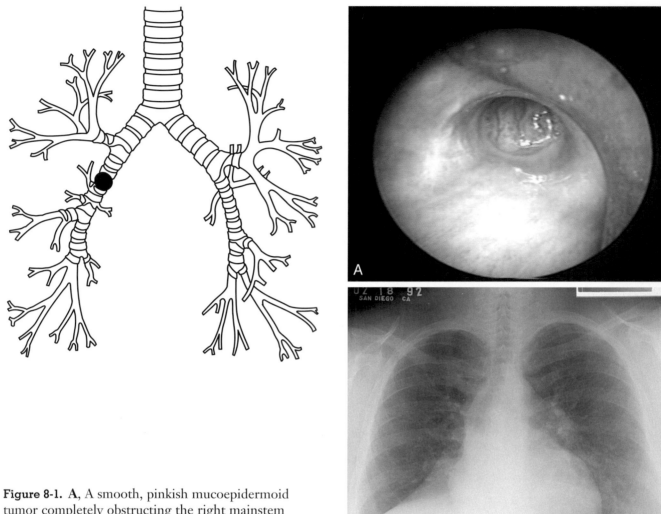

Figure 8-1. **A,** A smooth, pinkish mucoepidermoid
tumor completely obstructing the right mainstem
bronchus. Note the characteristic vascular pattern on
the tumor surface. **B,** Frontal radiograph demonstrates
obliteration of the airway just distal to the takeoff of the
right upper lobe bronchus with partial collapse of the
right lower and middle lobes.

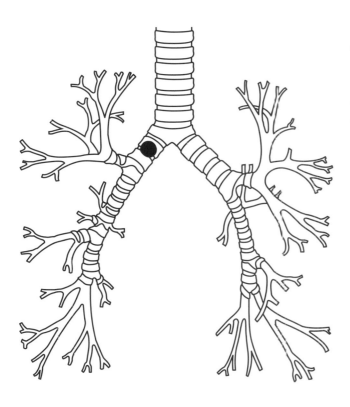

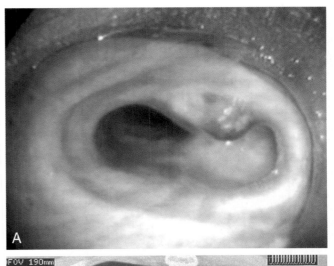

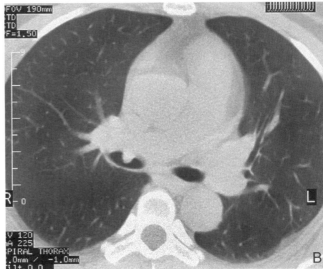

Figure 8-2. A, A raised pinkish growth of mucoepidermoid tumor tissue arising from the anterior surface of the proximal right mainstem bronchus. **B,** CT image demonstrates a 7-mm raised mass arising from the anterior surface of the right mainstem bronchus.

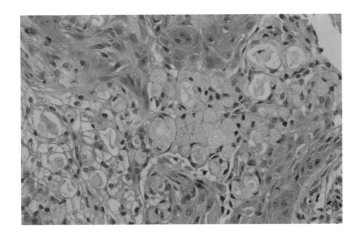

Figure 8-3. The tumor shows a combination of well-differentiated mucinous glands and squamoid cells (H&E, ×200).

CHAPTER 9

Benign Fibrous Tumors and Tumor-like Lesions

David R. Duhamel

A fibroma is a rare benign tumor believed to arise from pulmonary mesenchymal tissue. The first known report of an airway fibroma was described in 1767 by Lieutaud. The typical manifestation is a slow-growing polypoid endobronchial or endotracheal lesion. Less commonly, it appears as an asymptomatic parenchymal lung mass.[1] These tumors are extremely rare, with only 21 endobronchial fibromas having been reported in the world literature as of 1982.[2] The age distribution ranges from 10 months to 84 years, with an average of 55 years. All cases have been reported in whites, and there was a 2:1 male predominance.[3]

The tumors are evenly distributed throughout the trachea and proximal bronchi and are easily accessible to bronchoscopic biopsy. They are typically singular with a pinkish-gray color and have been described as being nodular or polypoid, pedunculated or sessile, soft or firm. They are typically covered with epithelium and exhibit various degrees of vascularization.

Radiographically, pulmonary fibromas arising within the parenchyma appear as solitary nodules within the lower lobes. Endobronchial and endotracheal fibromas are difficult to see on plain radiographs but can be visualized easily on CT scan. Their appearance is similar to that of most other benign airway lesions, and fibromas frequently manifest with atelectasis or postobstructive pneumonitis. Calcifications are a common finding.

The histologic origin of these lesions remains unclear at this point. Because of their similar histologic appearance, Yousem and Flynn[4] propose an association with the localized fibrous mesothelioma of the visceral pleura. Parenchymal fibromas frequently contain connections to the pleural surface, which supports this theory but does not account for the origin of an endobronchial fibroma. Another explanation assumes the pluripotent nature of mesenchymal tissue.[5] A fibroma most likely represents tumor growth of a single mesenchymal cell line. Microscopically, fibromas are composed of intermingling collagen fibers and spindle-shaped fibroblasts capable of fatty, mucoid, or malignant degeneration. Mitotic figures are rare and nuclear atypia is uncommon. The possibility of a fibrosarcoma should be raised if these findings are anything but minimal.

The tendency of fibromas to be insensitive to radiation, cause bronchial obstruction, recur if not completely excised, and undergo malignant degeneration requires the complete removal of the tumor for adequate treatment. Rigid bronchoscopic therapy with the Nd:YAG laser has been performed with success on endobronchial lesions. Surgical resection with a bronchoplastic procedure, however, is the more commonly used treatment.

Fibrous tumors of the airway are not always derived solely from fibrous tissue but frequently contain mixtures of various mesenchymal tissue components. They are named according to the components that are most predominant, with fibrolipomas being one of the most common. Like fibromas, they are considered benign and typically are discovered during the fifth and sixth decades of life. About 50 reports of fibrolipomas of the airway exist, with the vast majority being located in the bronchi. They are typically singular isolated lesions; however, case reports exist of multiple synchronous lesions occurring in the airway called *tracheobronchiolipomatosis*.[6]

During bronchoscopy, the lesion appears as a yellowish, smooth, and pedunculated mass. Fibrolipomas are often mobile and can create a ball-valve effect within the lung, leading to hyperinflation and emphysema. They typically vary in size between 1 and 3 cm. The diagnosis can be entertained on CT scan, because the lesion appears heterogeneous with a large proportion of tissue at fat density. A histologic diagnosis is made by fiberoptic biopsy about 50% of the time. This low yield is most likely due to the hard fibrous outer capsule or the overlying layer of squamous metaplasia.[7] The microscopic appearance is that of mature adipose cells divided into lobules by fibrous trabeculae and covered with respiratory epithelium.

Fibromyxomas are included in the family of benign fibrous tumors of mesenchymal origin. Like fibromas, they are composed of spindle-shaped fibroblasts, but they also contain a large component of intercellular myxoid material. To date, there exist a single case report of an endotracheal fibromyxoma[8] and two references to endobronchial fibromyxomas[9,10] within the world literature. The lesion presented here is the fourth reported endobronchial fibromyxoma. Parenchymal fibromyxomas have also been described. As with fibromas, lipomas, and chondromas, these lesions are thought to derive from pluripotent mesenchymal cells. Mesenchymal cell tumors were typically grouped under the nonspecific diagnosis of hamartoma in the past, but recently pathologists have attempted to specify these lesions according to their histologic components.[5]

Bronchoscopically, the tracheal fibromyxoma is described as a smooth, white, glistening, pedunculated lesion arising lateral to the posterior membrane. The lesion is located in the distal third of the trachea, which is the typical location for more than half of all benign tracheal tumors. Radiographically, there are no unique or identifiable characteristics. A high index of suspicion is needed to diagnose this tumor on plain radiograph alone. Microscopically, the tumor is composed of monotonously similar spindle cells set in a myxomatous matrix interspersed with collagen fibrils. Typically, there are no mitoses or pleomorphism seen. Of importance, the myxomatous matrix stains for hyaluronic acid with alcian blue.[6]

The tracheal tumor described in the case report was treated successfully by surgical resection of the affected tracheal segment. The Nd:YAG laser was used successfully to endoscopically resect this most recent fibromyxoma. Although very few examples exist, the fibromyxoma appears to behave in a benign manner without recurrence and carries an excellent prognosis.

REFERENCES

1. Engelman RM: Pulmonary fibroma: A rare benign tumor. Am Rev Respir Dis 96:1242-1245, 1967.

2. Halttunen P, Meurala H, Standertskjold-Nordenstam CG: Surgical treatment of benign endobronchial tumours. Thorax 37:688-692, 1982.

3. Sauk JJ, Pliego M, Anderson WR: Primary pulmonary fibroma. Minn Med 55:220-223, 1972.

4. Yousem SA, Flynn SD: Intrapulmonary localized fibrous tumor: Intraparenchymal so-called localized fibrous mesothelioma. Am J Clin Pathol 89:365-369, 1988.

5. Tomashefski JF: Benign endobronchial mesenchymal tumors: Their relationship to parenchymal pulmonary hamartomas. Am J Surg Pathol 6:531-540, 1982.

6. Taviot B, Coppere B, Pacheco Y, et al: Lipomatose tracheo-bronchique: A propos d'un cas. Rev Pneumol Clin 43:42-45, 1987.

7. Baharloo F, Corhay JL, Hoterman G, et al: A case of tracheal fibrolipoma. Acta Clinical Belgica 49:23-25, 1994.

8. Pollak ER, Naunheim KS, Little AG: Fibromyxoma of the trachea. Arch Pathol Lab Med 109:926-929, 1985.

9. Wang NS, Morin J: Recurrent endobronchial soft tissue tumors. Chest 85:787-791, 1984.

10. MacLachlan RF: Tracheal fibroma in a child. J Laryngol 82:565-570, 1968.

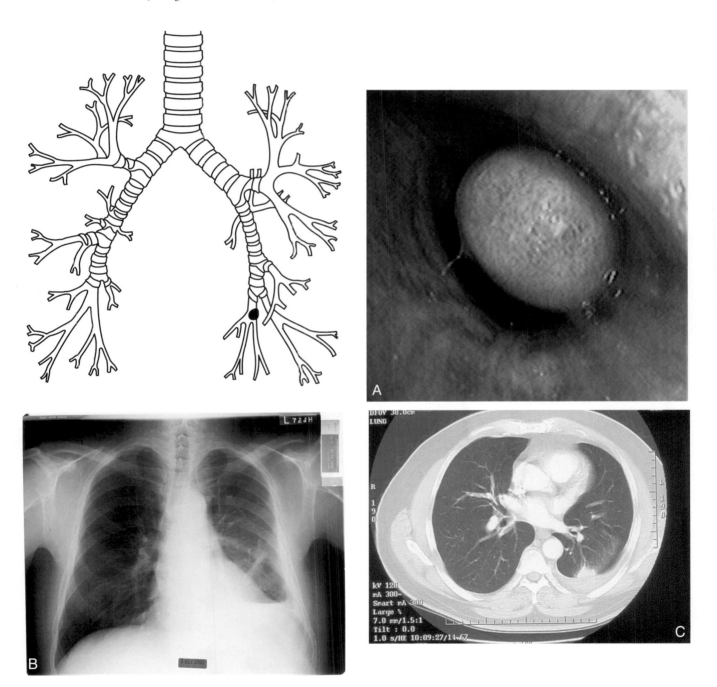

Figure 9-1. A, A smooth white fibrous tissue growth, arising from a long stalk in the posterior basilar subsegment of the left lower lobe that was found to be a fibrolipoma on endoscopic resection. **B,** Frontal radiograph demonstrates a left pleural effusion and left lower lobe volume loss. **C,** Computed tomography also demonstrates a small lesion within the left lower lobe bronchus.

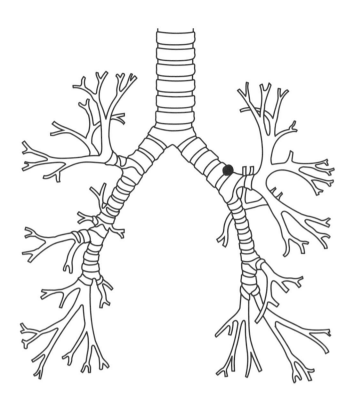

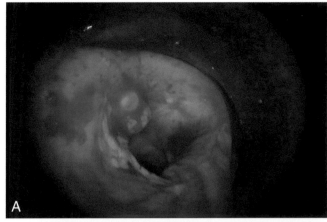

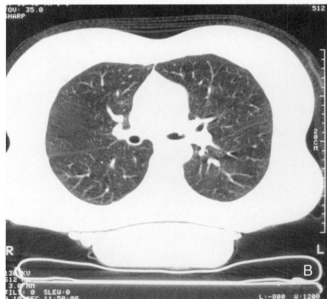

Figure 9-2. A, A small hemorrhagic growth of tissue in the left mainstem bronchus is consistent with a fibroma on biopsy. **B,** A CT image demonstrates a small nodule along the anterior surface of the left main bronchus.

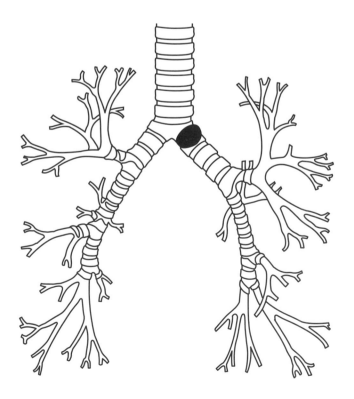

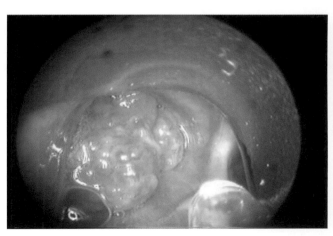

Figure 9-3. A large, lobulated, pinkish fibrous tumor completely obstructs the left mainstem bronchus. This lesion was pathologically identified as a fibroma.

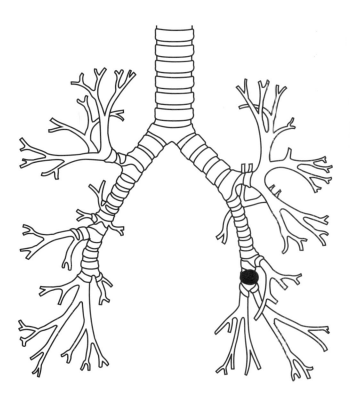

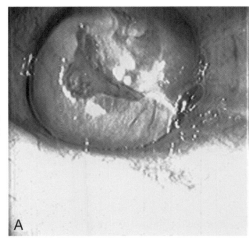

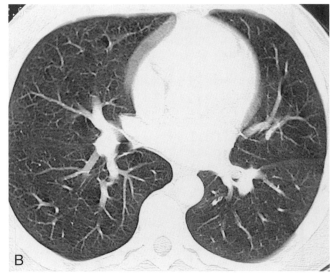

Figure 9-4. A, A smooth rounded tumor growth in the left lower lobe contains both fibrous and myxomatous tissue and is classified as a fibromyxoma. Note the area of ulceration in the overlying fibrous capsule. **B,** A CT image demonstrates a small nodule within the left lower lobe with slight left lower lobe atelectasis.

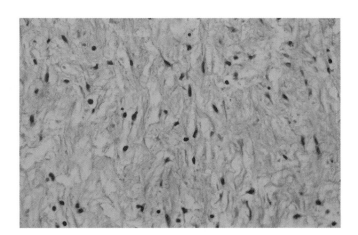

Figure 9-5. Fibromyxoma: bland-appearing fibrous spindle cells in a slightly myxoid background (H&E, ×200, original magnification).

CHAPTER 10

Carcinomas with Pleomorphic, Sarcomatoid, and Sarcomatous Elements

David R. Duhamel

The category of carcinomas with pleomorphic, sarcomatoid, and sarcomatous elements carries a rather broad definition and includes many different types of tumors. In actuality, all of these tumors are rare and represent a very small percentage of lung malignancies. The World Health Organization defines this category as a group of poorly differentiated non–small cell carcinomas that contain a component of sarcoma or sarcoma-like elements.[1] Included in this group are tumors described under a variety of terms including pleomorphic carcinoma, spindle cell carcinoma, sarcomatoid carcinoma (monophasic and biphasic), giant cell carcinoma, and carcinosarcoma. The variability in the terminology used to describe these lesions, the lack of uniform diagnostic criteria, and the subtle pathologic characteristics used to delineate these tumors have led to much confusion in the literature. However, as early as 1938, Saphir and Vass[2] proposed an explanation for the development of this type of tumor, which still stands today. They felt that these tumors represented a primary epithelial malignancy that had undergone divergent differentiation or metaplasia as it developed. The confusion arises from the fact that a spectrum of divergent differentiation occurs. Not all components of the tumor have differentiated to the same degree or by the same route. However, it is clear that all varieties of tumors in this category are characterized pathologically by a combination of epithelial and mesenchymal elements. In an attempt to minimize potential confusion, we have elected to discuss examples of pleomorphic carcinoma, spindle cell carcinoma, and carcinosarcoma together in one chapter.

The term *pleomorphic carcinoma* has been used to describe tumors that contain malignant spindle cells, giant cells, or both in association with squamous cell carcinoma, adenocarcinoma, or large cell carcinoma.[3] A giant cell is described as having abundant cytoplasm containing multiple nuclei or a single large pleomorphic nucleus, whereas the malignant spindle cell has a fusiform appearance with an eosinophilic cytoplasm. These two cell types are considered the most basic components of mesenchymal tissue. The spindle and giant cell components should constitute at least 10% of the tumor and will frequently stain positive for epithelial markers such as keratin, carcinoembryonic antigen, and epithelial membrane antigen. Pleomorphic carcinomas are felt to account for 0.3% of all lung malignancies.[4] In a series of 78 pleomorphic carcinomas,[3] Fishback and co-workers found the mean age at diagnosis was 62 years, the ratio of men to women was 2.7:1, and the majority of patients who presented with symptoms were smokers. The tumors tended to be large peripheral masses ranging from 2.2 to 18 cm,

with 24% exhibiting invasion of the chest wall. Only 2 of the 78 were considered truly endobronchial, with an additional 3 having an endobronchial component. The endobronchial appearances are highly variable, ranging from white to gray to a yellow-tan and have a smooth, bosselated, or even lobular appearance. The tumor frequently contains areas of necrosis or infarction. In Fishback's series of pleomorphic carcinomas, the epithelial cellular component was found to be adenocarcinoma 46% of the time, followed by large cell at 24%, and squamous cell at 8%. In a study of the molecular characteristics of these tumors,[5] the identical *p53* gene mutation was found in both the epithelial and spindle cell components of the tumor, thus giving strong support to the monoclonal histogenesis theory proposed by Saphir in 1938. The overall survival of patients with pleomorphic carcinoma is poor, with a median survival of 10 months and a 10% 5-year survival.

On occasion, a tumor is discovered that consists solely of spindle cells. These spindle-shaped tumor cells stain positive for epithelial immunohistochemical markers but histologically epithelial tumor cells are absent; therefore, the tumor is called a spindle cell carcinoma. Because it represents a pathologic continuum with pleomorphic carcinoma and shares the same aggressive behavior, it is grouped with this class of tumors.[1] If any component of squamous cell carcinoma, large cell carcinoma, or adenocarcinoma is present along with the spindle cells, it is better classified as a pleomorphic carcinoma. A pure collection of spindle-shaped cells can be easily confused with a sarcoma, but the immunoreactivity to epithelial markers helps to differentiate. The pure form of spindle cell carcinoma is extremely rare. Histologically, spindle cell carcinomas exhibit cellular pleomorphism and abnormal mitoses in a background of non-neoplastic connective tissue elements. No large series of pure spindle cell carcinomas exists, but in general it is safe to assume that they exhibit the same biologic activity and carry the same prognosis as pleomorphic carcinomas.

A carcinosarcoma is defined as a tumor containing a mixture of malignant epithelial and mesenchymal components. It is distinguished from a pleomorphic carcinoma by the presence of specific differentiation of the mesenchymal tissue into bone, cartilage, or muscle. If a spectrum of mesenchymal tissue differentiation exists, than carcinosarcomas are on the well-differentiated end, whereas pleomorphic carcinomas are on the poorly differentiated end. Carcinosarcomas are also known to be extremely rare, representing 0.2% of all lung malignancies.[6] In a study of 66 cases, Koss and colleagues found a 7.25:1 male-to-female ratio with a median age of 65 years and a high incidence of smoking.[7] The distribution of tumor location is much different from that seen in pleomorphic carcinoma. An endobronchial component was found in 34% to 46% of cases in the literature, with 12% to 17% being purely endobronchial. The endobronchial lesions were polypoid and frequently pedunculated, gray-white to tan-red, and had areas of hemorrhage and necrosis. Owing to the high rate of endobronchial involvement, two thirds of patients present with symptoms of obstruction. The most frequent epithelial component found in association with the sarcomatous tissue was squamous cell carcinoma followed by adenocarcinoma.

It is curious that squamous cell carcinoma is most frequently seen with carcinosarcomas, whereas adenocarcinoma is seen most frequently in pleomorphic carcinomas. One explanation is the tendency of carcinosarcomas to arise in the major airways, whereas pleomorphic carcinomas tend to arise in the peripheral lung. The most frequent sarcomatous elements included rhabdomyosarcoma, chondrosarcoma, osteosarcoma, or some combination. Metastases are common and can be carcinomatous, sarcomatous, or both. Survival of patients with carcinosarcoma of the lung is poor, with a 5-year survival rate of 21.3%. The ideal therapy is surgical resection, but most patients are not candidates for this at the time of presentation. Adjunctive irradiation and chemotherapy have been used to treat many cases, but in general these therapies have little beneficial effect.[8]

REFERENCES

1. Travis WD, Colby TV, Corrin B, et al: WHO Histological Typing of Lung and Pleural Tumors, 3rd ed. Berlin, Springer, 1999.

2. Saphir O, Vass A: Carcinosarcoma. Am J Cancer 33:331-359, 1938.

3. Fishback NF, Travis WD, Moran CA, et al: Pleomorphic (spindle/giant cell) carcinoma of the lung: A clinicopathologic correlation of 78 cases. Cancer 73:2936-2945, 1994.

4. Travis W, Travis L, Devesa S: Lung cancer. Cancer 75: 191-202, 1995.

5. Holst VA, Finkelstein S, Colby TV, et al: p53 and K-ras mutational genotyping in pulmonary carcinosarcoma, spindle cell carcinoma, and pulmonary blastoma: Implications for histogenesis. Am J Surg Path 21:801-811, 1997.

6. Davis MP, Eagan RT, Weiland LH, et al: Carcinosarcoma of the lung: Mayo Clinic experience and response to chemotherapy. Mayo Clin Proc 59:598-603, 1984.

7. Koss MN, Hochholzer L, Frommelt RA: Carcinosarcomas of the lung: A clinicopathologic study of 66 patients. Am J Surg Path 23:1514-1526, 1999.

8. Wick MR, Ritter JH, Humphrey PA: Sarcomatoid carcinomas of the lung: A clinicopathologic review. Am J Clin Pathol 108:40-53, 1997.

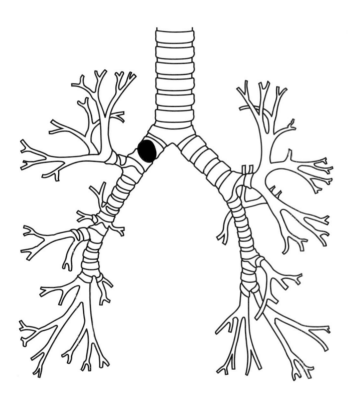

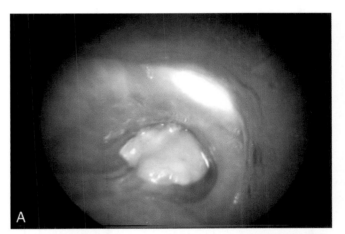

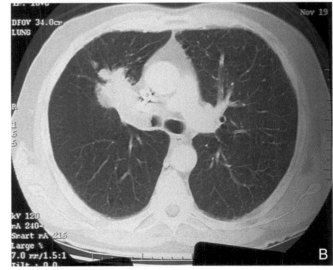

Figure 10-1. A, A soft white fleshy tumor obstructing the right mainstem bronchus. On endoscopic resection, this lesion was found to be a spindle cell carcinoma. **B,** A CT scan demonstrates a large right hilar mass with tumor extension within the right main bronchus.

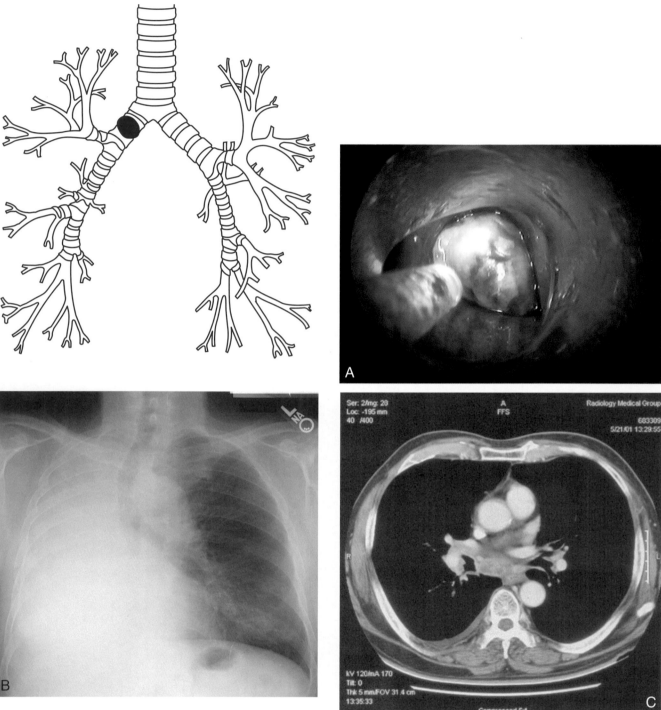

Figure 10-2. A, A white, firm, fibrous pleomorphic carcinoma that completely obstructs the right mainstem bronchus is shown. The suction catheter from the rigid bronchoscope is seen in the foreground. **B,** The frontal radiograph demonstrates complete opacification of the right hemithorax. The airway terminates abruptly within the right main bronchus. **C,** A CT image following intervention demonstrates re-expansion of the right lung with subcarinal lymph node and right pleural effusion present.

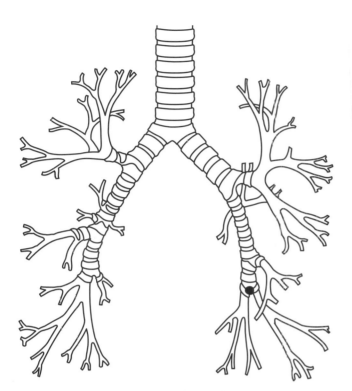

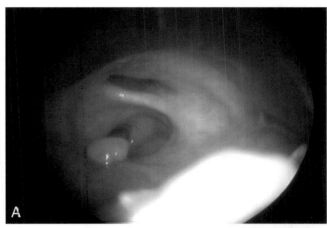

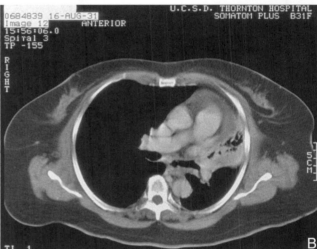

Figure 10-3. A, A smooth pink nodule of carcinosarcoma tumor tissue arises in the left lower lobe. Not well visualized is the extensive infiltration of the distal left mainstem bronchus by the carcinosarcoma. **B,** The CT image demonstrates a small mass at the left upper lobe orifice, with consolidation and bronchiectasis present within the left upper lobe.

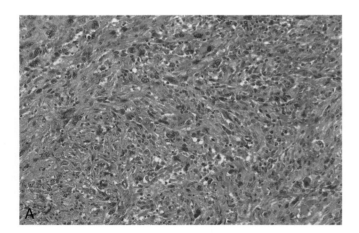

Figure 10-4. A, Spindle cell carcinoma: A poorly differentiated carcinoma containing predominantly spindle cells (H&E, ×200, original magnification).

Continued

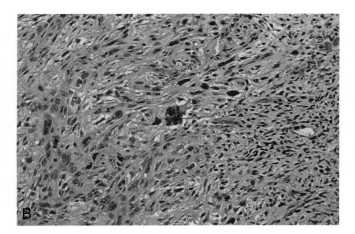

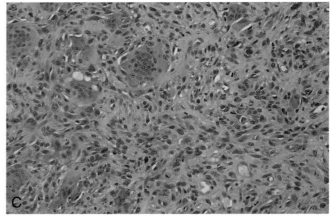

Figure 10-4, *cont'd.* **B,** Carcinosarcoma: The tumor has a mixture of malignant spindle cells and giant cells (H&E, ×200, original magnification). **C,** Pleomorphic carcinoma: The tumor has a mixture of malignant spindle cells and giant cells (H&E, ×200, original magnification).

CHAPTER 11

Adenocarcinoma

Jeffrey S. Prince

Adenocarcinoma is the most common histologic class of bronchogenic carcinoma. It accounts for 30% to 35% of all cases. It typically arises in a peripheral parenchymal location, which is explained by its origin from alveolar epithelium. Subsequently, involvement of the trachea and bronchi is an unusual finding. Centrally originating adenocarcinomas have been described, but their histogenesis is less well defined. It is thought that they may arise from bronchiolar surface epithelium, which exhibits glandular differentiation in the form of goblet cells.[1] Others have hypothesized that these more proximal adenocarcinomas may arise from the bronchial mucus glands.[2] Adenocarcinomas are known to originate in the trachea as well. Of the primary malignant tumors of the trachea, multiple series have shown that adenocarcinoma is the third most common histology behind squamous cell carcinoma and adenoid cystic carcinoma.[3,4,5]

The clinical presentation of patients with adenocarcinoma of the airway is similar to that seen in other forms of neoplasia. Hemoptysis is a common first symptom. Other presenting symptoms include dyspnea, wheezing, stridor, or dysphagia. As with other endobronchial masses, obliteration of approximately 70% of the airway lumen is required before respiratory symptoms manifest.[6]

Viewed bronchoscopically, a centrally occurring adenocarcinoma is indistinguishable from a squamous cell carcinoma. The tumor is seen as an intraluminal mass with an irregular or ulcerated surface. The lesions can be a singular raised nodular growth or multiple infiltrating and ulcerating extensions arising from the submucosa. Lymphangitic spread into the bronchial mucosa is not uncommon.

Typically, it is characterized by mucosal erythema and thickening as well as a prominent meshlike vascular pattern. Laser resection can be used for palliative treatment, but in general it is not curative. Radiation treatment can be used both preoperatively and postoperatively. Surgical resection of the trachea, if possible, continues to be the most favored treatment.[7]

On radiographs, these lesions have an appearance similar to that of other airway masses. On plain radiographs, adenocarcinoma may be identified as mass or filling defect in the trachea. Secondary signs include atelectasis or hyperinflation due to obstruction and air trapping. On CT scan, these masses are of soft tissue density with either a smooth or an irregular surface. Often the mass has a "tip of the iceberg" appearance with only a small portion of the mass seen within the lumen and extensive extraluminal extent. Calcifications are not normally present. The tumor may extend over long segments of the trachea. Differentiation of adenocarcinoma from other malignant or even benign neoplasms based on radiographic characteristics is not reliable. The only significant differentiating characteristic is size. Masses greater than 4 cm are more likely to be malignant, whereas those less than 2 cm are more likely benign.[8]

Adenocarcinoma is divided into four histologic subgroups: acinar, solid, papillary, and bronchoalveolar. More than 50% of adenocarcinomas of the lung are the acinar subtype, but it is unclear whether any one subtype has a predilection for developing in the airway. The microscopic appearance varies with subtype and degree of differentiation. In general, the tumors consist of columnar and cuboidal cells arranged in a glandular formation with numerous microvilli on the external membrane surface. The presence of apical tight junctions and numerous cytoplasmic secretory granules is also characteristic. Many adenocarcinomas characteristically express certain cellular markers, including carcinogenic embryonic antigen, keratin, and vimentin, but typically do not express the neuroendocrine markers chromogranin and synaptophysin.

REFERENCES

1. Dermer GB: Autoradiography of cellular glycoproteins reveals histogenesis of bronchogenic adenocarcinomas. Cancer 47:2000-2004, 1981.
2. Kimula Y: A histochemical and ultrastructural study of adenocarcinoma of the lung. Am J Surg Pathol 2:253-262, 1978.
3. Li W, Ellerbroek NA, Libshitz HI: Primary malignant tumors of the trachea: A radiologic and clinical study. Cancer 66:894-899, 1990.
4. Weber AL, Grillo HC: Tracheal tumors: A radiological, clinical, and pathological evaluation of 84 cases. Radiol Clin North Am 16:227-246, 1978.
5. Makarewicz R, Mross M: Radiation therapy alone in the treatment of tumours of the trachea. Lung Cancer 20:169-174, 1998.
6. Felson B: Neoplasms of the trachea and main stem bronchi. Semin Roentgenol 18:23-37, 1983.
7. Schneider P, Schirren J, Muley T, Vogt-Moykopf I: Primary tracheal tumors: Experience with 14 resected patients. Eur J Cardiothorac Surg 20:12-18, 2001.
8. Stark P: Radiology of the Trachea. New York, Thieme Medical Publishers, Inc, 1991.

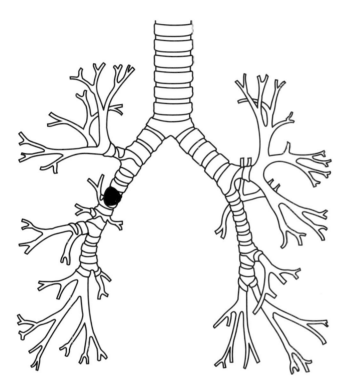

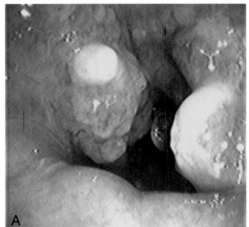

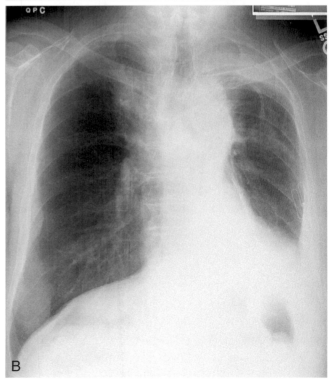

Figure 11-1. A, Multiple fungating nodules of adenocarcinoma filling the lumen of the right mainstem bronchus. **B,** A frontal radiograph showing volume loss and shift to the left, with mediastinal fullness and bilateral hilar lymphadenopathy. Note the fully aerated lung on the right despite extensive airway involvement of the right mainstem bronchus. *Continued*

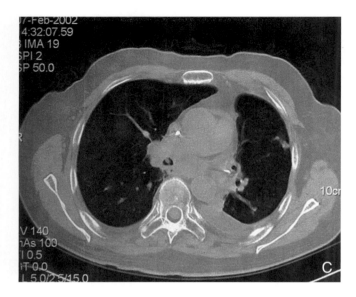

Figure 11-1, *cont'd.* **C,** A small nodule is present within the right mainstem bronchus on CT scan.

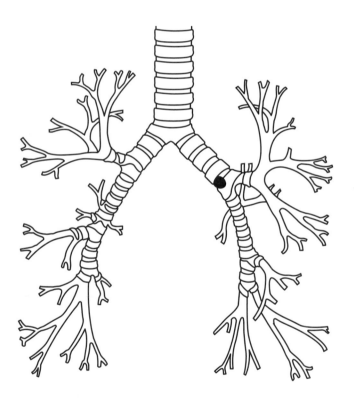

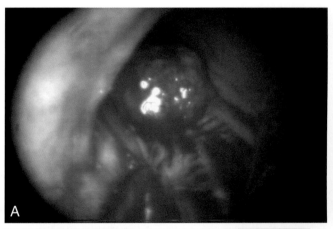

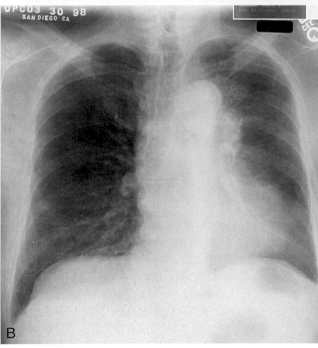

Figure 11-2. A, A hemorrhagic growth of adenocarcinoma arising from the left mainstem bronchus. **B,** A frontal radiograph demonstrates loss of an air column within the left main bronchus.

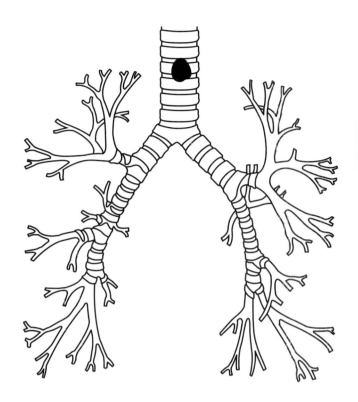

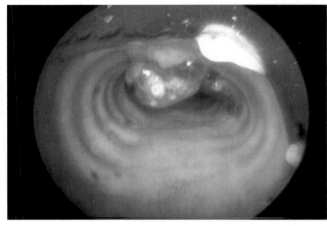

Figure 11-3. A raised, friable outgrowth of adenocarcinoma arising from the anterior wall of the midtrachea.

Figure 11-4. Well- to moderately differentiated adenocarcinoma characterized by well-formed glands and highly malignant-appearing cells (H&E, ×200, original magnification).

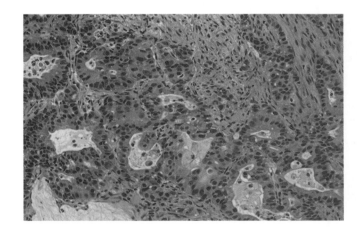

CHAPTER 12

Small Cell Carcinoma

Gehan Devendra

Small cell lung cancer (SCLC) was described initially in 1926 by W. C. Barnard and accounts for approximately 14% of lung carcinomas. SCLC has a strong association with tobacco, as does non–small cell lung cancer, but overall SCLC has a more aggressive course. It tends to occur near major airways and blood vessels, thereby having a more centralized location with frequent endobronchial involvement. SCLC tends to manifest with distant metastasis and has a median survival time without treatment of 2 to 4 months.

Manifestation of SCLC is usually at a later stage; however, initial diagnosis has been made in asymptomatic patients with chest radiographs obtained for unrelated issues. About 50% of patients with limited disease present with a cough. Other symptoms include dyspnea, chest pain, and hoarseness. In patients with distant spread, 50% complain of weight loss followed by weakness, anorexia, paraneoplastic syndromes, and fever.[1] Patients with SCLC frequently have paraneoplastic syndromes. Given the neuroectodermal origin of SCLC, peptide hormones are frequently released. About 15% of patients with SCLC present with the syndrome of inappropriate antidiuretic hormone secretion.[2] Cushing's syndrome is apparent in 2% to 5% of SCLC patients. Neurologic paraneoplastic disease such as the Lambert-Eaton syndrome is caused by cross-reactivity of antibodies to tumor antigens, with native neural tissue resulting in motor weakness.

Viewed radiographically, SCLC usually appears as a centralized lesion with hilar and mediastinal lymphadenopathy. Small cell lung cancer is staged not by the tumor node metastasis (TNM) system but by the two-stage system of limited versus extensive. Limited disease is confined to one hemithorax and/or can be encompassed in one radiotherapy portal. Extensive disease is anything outside the above boundaries.

If SCLC is suspected, the patient should undergo a biopsy of easily accessible material. Usually specimens are obtained by either bronchoscopy or percutaneous needle aspiration. On bronchoscopic examination, these lesions have a classic submucosal infiltrating appearance, which typically causes narrowing of the airway lumen. The infiltrated mucosa has an increased vascular pattern along with a pearly white sheen. Another very common bronchoscopic manifestation is complete bronchial obstruction from extrinsic compression due to a massive hilar and mediastinal lymphadenopathy or tumor burden. The airway mucosa in this situation often appears normal without tumor infiltration.

SCLC is composed of small epithelial tumor cells, which are round, oval, or spindle shaped with scant cytoplasm, ill-defined borders, finely granular nuclear chromatin, and absence of nucleoli.[3] Molecular biologic studies have elucidated some genetic abnormalities in SCLC. About 90% of SCLC has a loss of heterozygosity of the tumor suppressor gene p53 chromosomal locus. Changes in DNA methylation of promotor regions of several genes are present in SCLC. Further molecular defects have been described that are not within the scope of this chapter and can be reviewed elsewhere.[4]

Treatment of limited stage SCLC is with combined chemotherapy and radiation therapy. Two meta-analyses showed that the addition of radiotherapy improved the survival rate at 3 years by 5%.[5,6] The exact timing of radiotherapy whether sequential or concurrent with chemotherapy is controversial, but the use of twice-daily radiotherapy does seems to have an improved survival.[7] Platinum-based chemotherapy is the mainstay for extensive disease. If patients with either extensive or limited stage SCLC undergo complete remission after therapy, they should be offered prophylactic cranial irradiation.

Management of endobronchial small cell lung cancer depends significantly on the severity of symptoms and whether it is life threatening. Because SCLC is very sensitive to radiation and chemotherapy and the endobronchial lesions typically resolve quickly with therapy, many experts reserve the bronchoscopic therapies for treatment failures. The extrinsic airway compression from massive hilar and mediastinal tumor involvement, however, is easily treated by Silastic stent placement through a rigid bronchoscope. This becomes vitally important in maintaining proper pulmonary toilet and preventing the disastrous complication of postobstructive pneumonia while on chemotherapy. There are multiple treatment options available for recurrent endobronchial tumor after maximal radiation has failed. These options include stent placement, photodynamic therapy, Nd:YAG laser therapy, argon plasma coagulation, endobronchial radiotherapy, and cryotherapy.

REFERENCES

1. Chute CG, Greenberg ER, Baron J, et al: Presenting conditions of 1539 population-based lung cancer patients by cell type and stage in New Hampshire and Vermont. Cancer 56:2107-2111, 1985.
2. Johnson BE, Chute JP, Rushin J, et al: A prospective study of patients with lung cancer and hyponatremia of malignancy. Am J Respir Crit Care Med 156:1669-1678, 1997.
3. Hirsch FR, Matthews MJ, Aisner S, et al: Histopathologic classification of small cell lung cancer: Changing concepts and terminology. Cancer 62:973-977, 1988.
4. Wistuba II, Gazdar AF, Minna JD: Molecular genetics of small cell lung carcinoma. Semin Oncol (suppl 4)28:3-13, 2001.
5. Pignon JP, Arriagada R, Ihde DC, et al: A meta-analysis of thoracic radiotherapy for small-cell lung cancer. N Engl J Med 327:1618-1624, 1992.
6. Warde P, Payne D: Does thoracic irradiation improve survival and local control in limited-stage small cell carcinoma of the lung? J Clin Oncol 10:890-895, 1992.
7. Turrisi AT, Kyungmann K, Blum R, et al: Twice-daily compared with once-daily thoracic radiotherapy in limited small-cell lung cancer treated concurrently with cisplatin and etoposide. N Engl J Med 340:265-271, 1999.

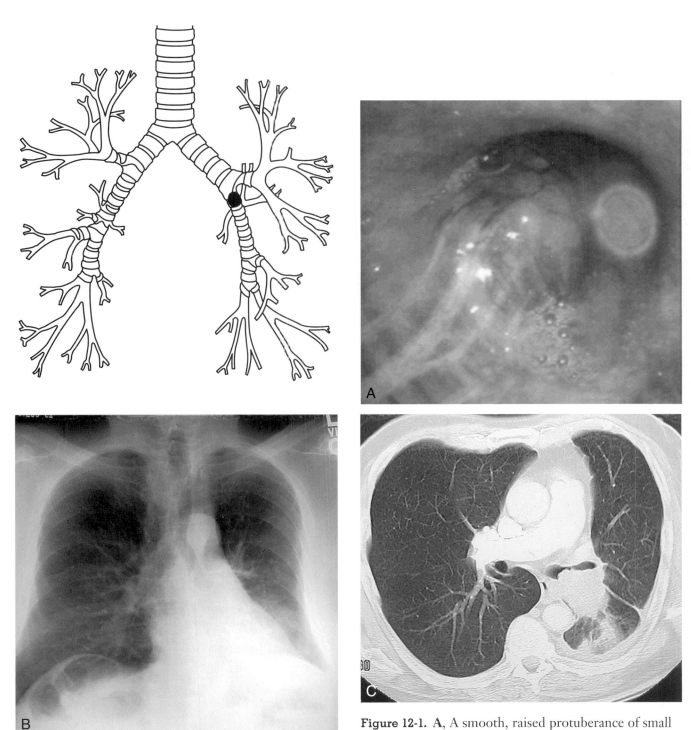

Figure 12-1. A, A smooth, raised protuberance of small cell carcinoma arising in the left lower lobe bronchus. **B,** The frontal radiograph demonstrates left lower lobe collapse. The airway terminates abruptly within the left lower lobe bronchus. **C,** The CT scan demonstrates a large left hilar mass obliterating the left lower lobe bronchus and extending into the left main bronchus.

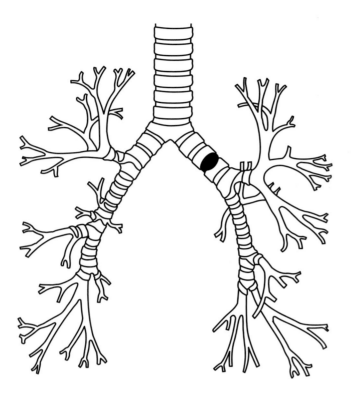

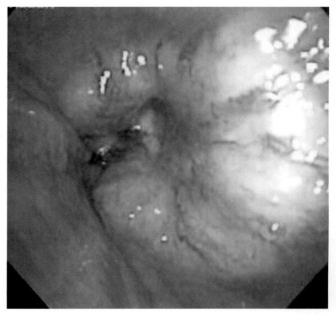

Figure 12-2. A view of the left mainstem bronchus, which is completely occluded from extrinsic compression and mucosal infiltration by small cell carcinoma.

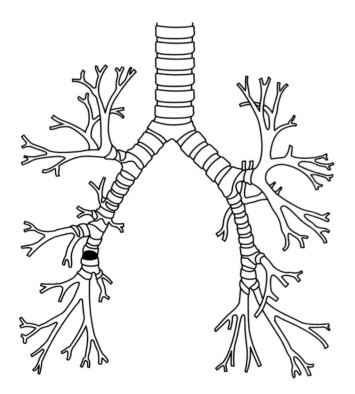

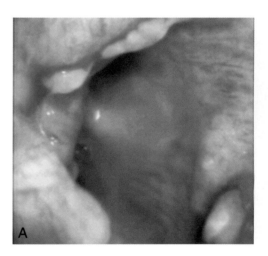

Figure 12-3. **A**, Multiple raised nodules of small cell carcinoma arising in the distal right mainstem bronchus. **B**, Postsurgical changes are noted on the frontal radiograph. Slight enlargement of the left hilum is present. **C**, The CT image demonstrates tumor lying along the aorta. A mass is present within the right lower lobe extending into the right lower lobe bronchus.

Continued

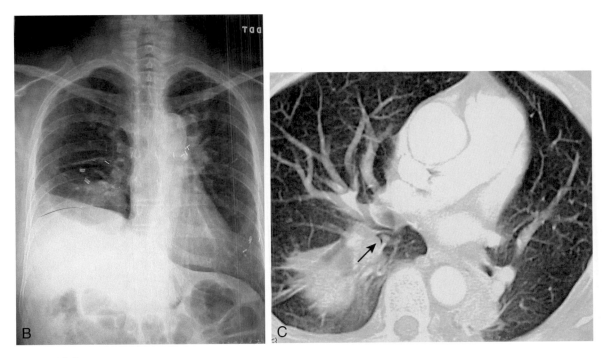

Figure 12-3, *cont'd.*

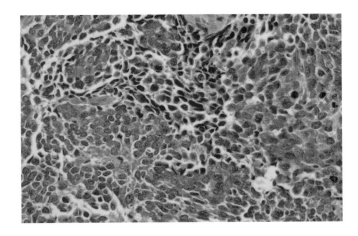

Figure 12-4. The tumor cells are densely packed, small, with scant cytoplasm, and finely granular ("salt and pepper") nuclear chromatin with indistinct nucleoli. Mitoses are frequent (>10/10 high-power fields) (H&E, ×200, original magnification).

CHAPTER 13

Large Cell Carcinoma

Jeffrey S. Prince

Large cell carcinoma of the lung is a relatively uncommon tumor, constituting only 9% of all bronchogenic carcinomas.[1] According to the World Health Organization (WHO) classification, large cell carcinoma is defined as lacking any similarities to small cell carcinoma and lacking histologic evidence of squamous or glandular differentiation by light microscopy. As a result of the exclusionary nature of the pathologic diagnosis, there is some variability in the incidence of this tumor. It is clear that when a large surgical specimen is available for pathologic review, the overall incidence goes down. This is evidenced by a series that reviewed 100 consecutive surgical specimens of lung cancer.[2] Of these 100 specimens, there were no examples of large cell carcinoma. It is an aggressive tumor with 5-year survival rate universally reported below 50%; in some series it is as low as 10%.[3] Survival is felt to be low because most cases manifest at an advanced stage. In a large series of patients with large cell carcinomas, 90% were at stage III or higher at the time of diagnosis.[4]

These tumors are most often found in the lung periphery, although they may be located centrally. Grossly, they appear as large necrotic tumors, with cavitation being seen in about 20% of cases. Most patients have a significant smoking history and are generally older than 60 years. Common presenting symptoms include cough, weight loss, shortness of breath, hemoptysis, bone pain, and superior vena cava syndrome.[3] Rarely does large cell carcinoma manifest as an endobronchial mass. When these masses do appear endobronchially, they have similar symptoms to other endobronchial tumors, including stridor, wheezing, and postobstructive pneumonia.

On bronchoscopy, these lesions are indistinguishable in appearance and behavior from other non–small cell carcinomas. They typically appear as smooth vascular endobronchial masses. On occasion, they extend out of the lung parenchyma through a lobar bronchus to occlude the airway, but in general they arise de novo in the lumen of the bronchus. If the lesions are particularly large, they sometimes appear ulcerated and even necrotic as they outgrow their blood supply. The management of large cell carcinoma involving the airway is similar to that for other types of non–small cell carcinoma. The lesions can be treated and removed with various bronchoscopic techniques including Nd:YAG laser ablation, electrocautery, argon plasma coagulators, photodynamic therapy, airway stenting, and brachytherapy.

In a review of the radiographic findings in bronchogenic carcinoma, obstructive pneumonitis or atelectasis suggest-ing airway involvement was seen in 32 of 97 (33%) large cell carcinomas.[5] Viewed radiographically, these lesions have an appearance similar to that of other masses in the airway. On plain radiographs of the chest, they may be seen as a mass or filling defect in the tracheal or bronchial lumen. Secondary signs include atelectasis or hyperinflation due to air trapping. On CT, these are seen as masses of soft tissue density with either a smooth or an irregular surface. Often the mass has a tip-of-the-iceberg appearance with only a small portion of the mass seen within the lumen and extensive extraluminal component. Differentiation of large cell carcinoma from other malignant or even benign neoplasms based on radiographic characteristics is not reliable. The only significant differentiating characteristic is size. Masses greater than 4 cm are more likely to be malignant, whereas those less than 2 cm are more likely to be benign.[6,7]

Histologically, the tumors usually consist of sheets and nests of large polygonal cells with vesicular nuclear chromatin and prominent nucleoli. Although large cell carcinoma by definition does not exhibit squamous or glandular cell differentiation by light microscopy, ultra-structural features of squamous cell or adenocarcinoma can frequently be seen on electron microscopy.[1] There are several variants of large cell carcinoma recognized in the WHO classification of lung cancer. These variants include large cell neuroendocrine carcinoma, basaloid carcinoma, lymphoepithelial-like carcinoma, and large cell carcinoma with rhabdoid phenotype. There does not appear to be an increased predilection of any of these subtypes of large cell carcinoma for involvement with the airway, although no published review specifically addresses this issue. The diagnosis and management of each of these various subtypes of large cell carcinoma are unique and individualized and probably beyond the scope of this discussion.

REFERENCES

1. Travis WD: Pathology of lung cancer. Clin Chest Med 23:65-81, 2002.
2. McDowell EM, McLaughlin JS, Merenyl DK, et al: The respiratory epithelium. Histogenesis of lung carcinomas in the human. J Natl Cancer Inst 61:587-592, 1978.
3. Mitchell DM, Morgan PGM, Ball JB: Prognostic features of large cell anaplastic carcinoma of the bronchus. Thorax 35:118-122, 1980.
4. Downey RS, Sewell CW, Mansour KA: Large cell carcinoma of the lung: A highly aggressive tumor with dismal prognosis. Ann Thorac Surg 47: 806-808, 1989.
5. Byrd RB, Carr DT, Miller WE, et al: Radiographic abnormalities in carcinoma of the lung as related to histologic cell type. Thorax 24:573-579, 1969.
6. Stark P: Radiology of the Trachea. New York, Thieme Medical Publishers, Inc, 1991.
7. Felson B: Neoplasms of the trachea and main stem bronchi. Semin Roentgenol 18:23-37, 1983.

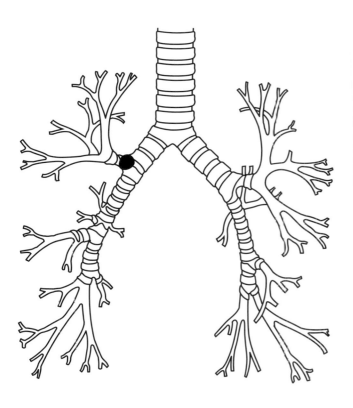

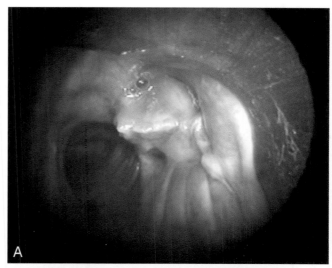

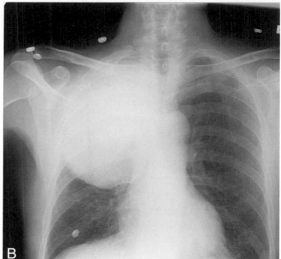

Figure 13-1. A, Large cell carcinoma extending out of the right upper lobe orifice and into the endobronchial lumen. Mucoid secretions have pooled on the lesion. **B,** Frontal radiograph demonstrates a large right upper lobe mass.

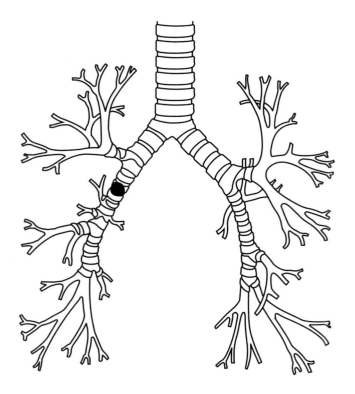

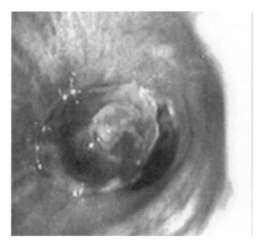

Figure 13-2. Reddish-brown smooth deposit of large cell carcinoma in the right bronchus intermedius.

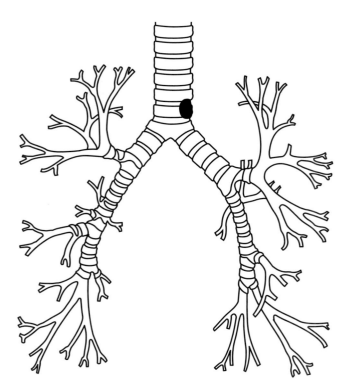

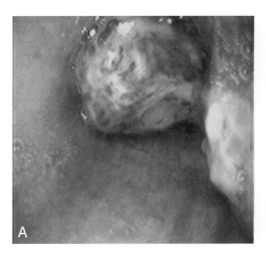

Figure 13-3. A, A friable vascular extension of large cell carcinoma arising from the left lateral tracheal wall. **B,** The frontal radiograph demonstrates a right hilar-suprahilar mass with associated narrowing of the tracheal column.

Continued

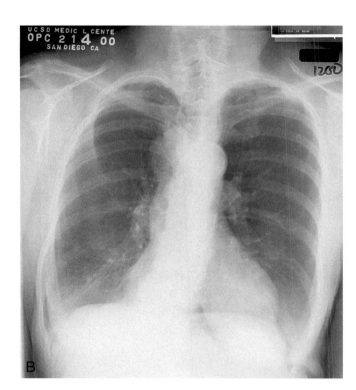

Figure 13-3, *cont'd.*

Figure 13-4. These undifferentiated large cells have abundant cytoplasm with large nuclei, vesicular nuclear chromatin, and prominent nucleoli (H&E, ×200, original magnification).

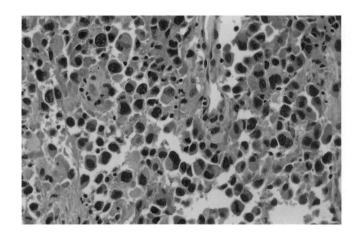

CHAPTER 14

Metastatic Thyroid Cancer

David R. Duhamel

Thyroid cancer is one of the most common malignancies to locally invade the trachea.[1] Tracheal invasion is common in patients with anaplastic thyroid carcinoma and leads to significant mortality from tracheal obstruction.[2] It is due to the close anatomic relationship with the airway and is seen with cancers of the esophagus and larynx. Thyroid cancer has also been reported to metastasize to the airway and manifest as an endobronchial mass. The incidence of endobronchial metastases from extrathoracic malignancy has generally been found to be around 2%.[3] Colt and Dumon reported a similar incidence in thyroid carcinoma, with 2.6% of patients having endobronchial metastases.[4]

Many bronchoscopists recommend a preoperative endoscopic evaluation of the anterior tracheal wall to rule out local invasion in any patient undergoing surgical resection for thyroid malignancy. The endoscopic finding can be subtle, with a slightly increased vascular pattern being the only manifestation. It may also be rather obvious with raised erythematous nodular deposits or plaques of tumor cells arising from the tracheal wall. These are typically located on the proximal anterior tracheal wall.

Viewed radiographically, local invasion of the trachea is very difficult to detect. A CT scan may show thickening of the tracheal wall adjacent to the tumor or loss of the tissue planes separating the trachea and thyroid tissue. An endoluminal mass may also be seen arising from the anterior tracheal wall. Radioactive iodine imaging has also been used in identifying occult pulmonary metastases. Parenchymal pulmonary metastases were noted only in 10% of 1127 patients with a thyroid malignancy seen at the M. D. Anderson Cancer Center over a 30-year period.[5] Papillary carcinoma was the tissue type in 67% of these cases. Papillary carcinoma tends to have a micronodular pattern of metastasis, whereas the follicular cell carcinoma manifests as a larger parenchymal nodule.[6] It is unclear whether either cell type has a greater tendency to involve the airway.

In addition to local invasion, anaplastic thyroid carcinoma also metastasizes to the lung parenchyma and distal airway.

Although local invasion is seen with the papillary and follicular cell types, pulmonary metastases are much less common.[2] Anaplastic thyroid carcinoma is the most likely to invade the trachea of all the histologic tissue types, but this complication has also been described with primary lymphoma, squamous carcinoma, undifferentiated carcinoma, and carcinosarcoma of the thyroid gland.[7]

The treatment and management of endobronchial metastases are variable and are greatly influenced by the histologic tissue type of the primary tumor, its biologic behavior, anatomic location, evidence of other metastases, and the patient's performance status.[8] Therefore, all treatment decisions should be made on a case-by-case basis. Endoluminal therapy in the setting of submucosal tumor infiltration could certainly include brachytherapy or photodynamic therapy. If a tracheal or bronchial obstructing mass has developed, therapy with the Nd:YAG laser is ideal. Survival is dependant to a great degree on the biologic behavior of the particular tumor and its responsiveness to the palliative treatments available.

REFERENCES

1. Kwong JS, Muller NL, Miller RR: Diseases of the trachea and main-stem bronchi: Correlation of CT with pathologic findings. Radiographics 12:645-657, 1992.
2. Tsumori T, Nakao K, Miyata M, et al: Clinicopathologic study of thyroid carcinoma infiltrating the trachea. Cancer 56:2843-2849, 1985.
3. Braman SS, Whitcomb ME: Endobronchial metastases. Arch Intern Med 135:543-547, 1975.
4. Colt HG, Dumon HF: Lasers et endoprotheses en broncholopneumologie. Rev Pneumol Clin 47:65-73, 1991.
5. Massin JP, Savoie JC, Garnier H, et al: Pulmonary metastases in differentiated thyroid carcinoma. Cancer 53:982-987, 1984.
6. Nemec J, Pohunkova D, Zamrazil V, et al: Pulmonary metastases of thyroid carcinoma. Czech Med 2:78-81, 1979.
7. Stark P: Radiology of the Trachea. New York, Thieme Medical Publishers, 1991.
8. Kiryu T, Hoshi H, Matsui E, et al: Endotracheal/endobronchial metastases: Clinicopathologic study with special reference to developmental modes. Chest 119:768-775, 2001.

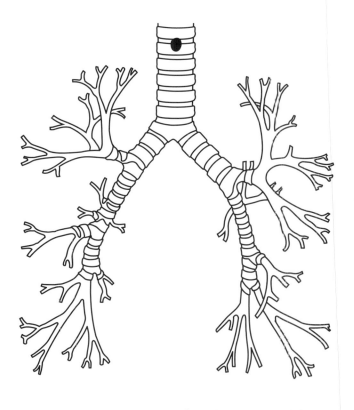

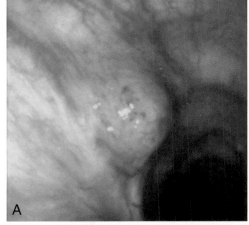

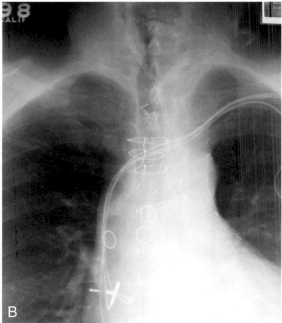

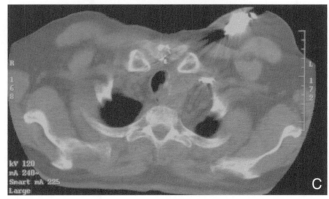

Figure 14-1. A, A yellowish-pink extension of thyroid carcinoma through the tracheal wall from the adjacent thyroid gland. **B,** The frontal radiograph demonstrates marked narrowing of the trachea at the level of the thoracic inlet. **C,** The CT image demonstrates a thyroid mass with extension into the trachea.

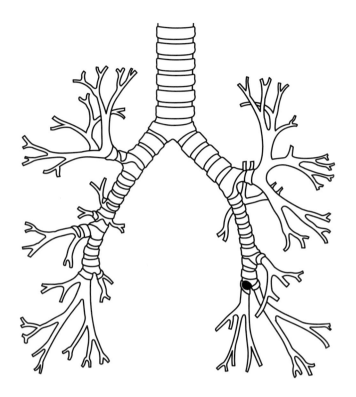

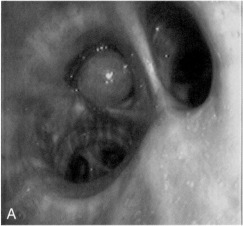

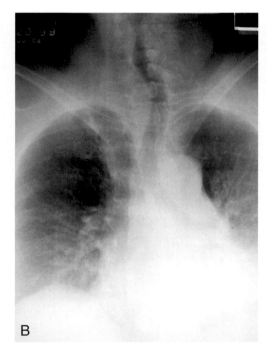

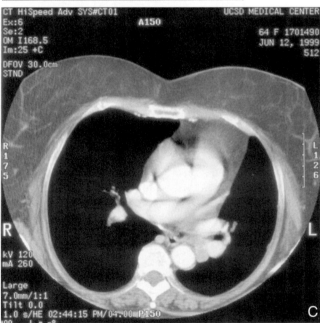

Figure 14-2. A, Smooth, pink, metastatic deposit of thyroid carcinoma in the left lower basilar subsegments. **B,** Frontal radiograph demonstrates deviation of the trachea to the left at the thoracic inlet. **C,** A CT image demonstrates soft tissue within the left lower lobe bronchus. **D,** A CT image demonstrates marked enlargement of the thyroid with deviation of the trachea to the left.

Continued

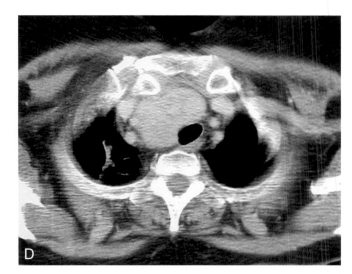

Figure 14-2, *cont'd.*

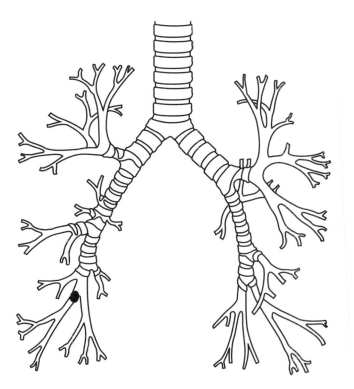

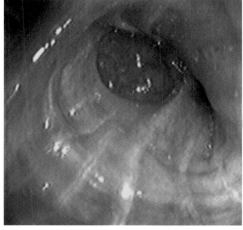

Figure 14-3. A smooth, red, vascular, metastatic thyroid carcinoma lesion in the right lower lobe.

Figure 14-4. Thyroglobulin immunostain confirms the thyroid origin of these metastatic tumor cells to the bronchus (antithyroglobulin antibody, ×200, original magnification).

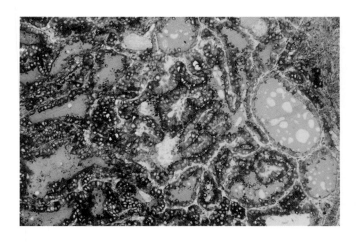

CHAPTER 15

Metastatic Esophageal Cancer

David R. Duhamel

In the United States, cancer of the esophagus is a relatively uncommon but extremely lethal malignant disease. The incidence worldwide is highly variable, with a significant increase in frequency in the so-called Asian esophageal cancer belt.[1] Certain etiologic factors are believed to be associated with esophageal cancer including excessive alcohol consumption, tobacco smoke, nitrates, lye ingestion, Barrett's esophagus, and the fungal toxins in pickled vegetables. Esophageal cancer is a frequent cause of malignant invasion of the trachea. This is due to its anatomic proximity to the trachea and is seen with cancers of the thyroid and larynx. Esophageal cancer is especially infamous for its tendency to form a fistula between the esophagus and the trachea. The midesophageal tumors are particularly prone to this complication.[2] Approximately 50% of esophageal cancers occur in the middle third of the esophagus, 15% in the upper third, and 35% in the lower third.

Progressive dysphagia and weight loss of short duration are the usual presenting symptoms in the vast majority of patients. Once the symptoms of dysphagia have developed, the disease is often incurable because difficulty with swallowing often does not manifest until 60% of the esophageal circumference is infiltrated with cancer.[3] The development of a cough following the ingestion of liquid can mean one of two things. The patient may be aspirating liquid via the larynx due to high-grade obstruction in the esophagus or a tracheoesophageal fistula may have developed. These fistulas can develop spontaneously but are frequently seen after radiation therapy. The radiation causes necrosis of the infiltrating malignant tissue, and a fistulous track can develop between the two structures.

The bronchoscopic findings in esophageal cancer can be impressive. It is not uncommon to find small fistulous tracts to the esophagus in a mass of edematous and erythematous tissue. These are classically located in the posterior membrane of the proximal left mainstem bronchus, because the two structures are in close contact at that point. The opening of the fistula may range from a pinhole to a gaping orifice but can usually be identified by the bubbling up of secretions at that location. The oral ingestion of methylene blue has been used on occasion to help localize a fistula, but this technique quickly becomes confusing when all the secretions turn blue. Local tissue invasion of the airway does occur without the formation of a fistula. These findings can range from a subtle hypervascular pattern with erythema and tissue edema to raised nodular plaques of tumor cell to a blatant endobronchial mass. Once again all these findings tend to arise from the posterior membrane, especially in the left mainstem bronchus.

Conventional radiography can provide some valuable clues, which should raise the suspicion of esophageal cancer. In a study of 103 patients, radiographic abnormalities were found in 47%.[4] These included a widened mediastinum, a posterior tracheal indentation, widened retrotracheal stripe, esophageal fluid level, and tracheal deviation. The CT scan manifestations of esophageal cancer include esophageal wall thickening, proximal dilation, obscuration of the periesophageal fat planes, and periesophageal lymphadenopathy.[5] The findings on CT scan with esophageal cancer may also include a prominent fistula tract connecting the esophagus to the trachea. Free air in the mediastinum is a frequent finding with a fistula tract, which may be seen on plain radiograph. If the concern for a fistula tract persists after a bronchoscopy and CT scan are nondiagnostic, then a barium swallow should be performed. The more common findings with neoplastic invasion of the airway include the loss of a tissue plane separating the esophagus and trachea and a posterior indentation of the airway lumen. The reported sensitivity of CT scan in the detection of tracheobronchial involvement ranges from 31% to 100% in various studies.

More than 85% of esophageal tumors are squamous cell carcinomas, arising from the squamous epithelium that lines the lumen of the esophagus.[6] Adenocarcinomas, although far less frequent, arise from the columnar epithelium, which may appear dysplastic in the distal esophagus in association with chronic gastric reflux or Barrett's esophagus. The prognosis for patients with esophageal cancer is extremely poor. Less than 5% of patients are alive 5 years after the initial diagnosis.[6] Surgical resection is an option in only 40% of cases, and of those patients that undergo surgery, many have margins that are positive.[7] The therapeutic outcome following radiation is similar to that of surgery but less efficacious at treating the symptoms of obstruction. Owing to these dismal statistics, many physicians focus their management efforts solely on relieving symptoms. The symptoms of tracheoesophageal fistula are extremely difficult to palliate, and most patients die miserably from overwhelming infection. There has been some minimal success with stenting of both the esophagus and the trachea to help inhibit aspiration through the fistula. It is important to stent the airway before the esophagus because a large tumor burden can sometimes cause compression of the airway lumen with deployment of the stent.

REFERENCES

1. Lightdale CJ, Winawer SJ: Screening, diagnosis and staging of esophageal cancer. Semin Oncol 11:101-109, 1984.
2. Stark P: Radiology of the Trachea. New York, Thieme Medical Publishers, 1991.
3. Boyce HW: Palliation of advanced esophageal cancer. Semin Oncol 11:186-195, 1984.
4. Lindell MM, Hill CA, Libshitz HI: Esophageal cancer: Radiographic chest findings and their prognostic significance. Am J Roentgenol 133:461-464, 1979.
5. Quint LE, Glazer GM, Orringer MB, et al: Esophageal carcinoma: CT findings. Radiology 155:171-176, 1985.
6. Schottenfeld D: Epidemiology of cancer of the esophagus. Semin Oncol 11:92-100, 1984.
7. Skinner DB: Surgical treatment of esophageal carcinoma. Semin Oncol 11:136-143, 1984.

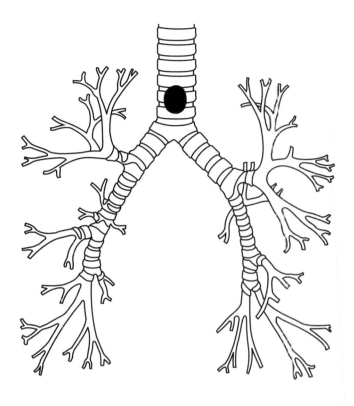

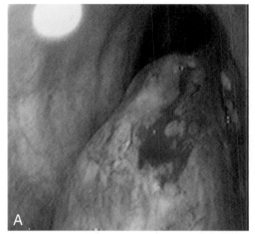

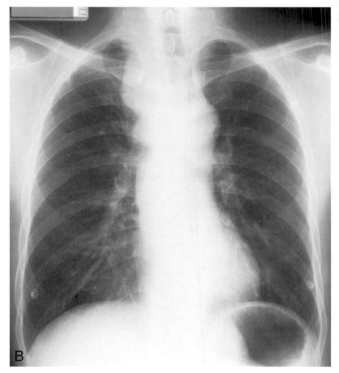

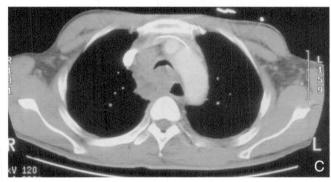

Figure 15-1. A, A view of the posterior membrane of the trachea being extrinsically compressed by a large esophageal carcinoma. Note the friable hemorrhagic mucosa due to infiltrating carcinoma. **B,** A frontal radiograph demonstrates a large, predominantly right mediastinal mass with deviation of the trachea to the left. **C,** A CT image demonstrates an extensive soft tissue mass within the mediastinum. The mass extends between the trachea and the esophagus and narrows the posterior trachea.

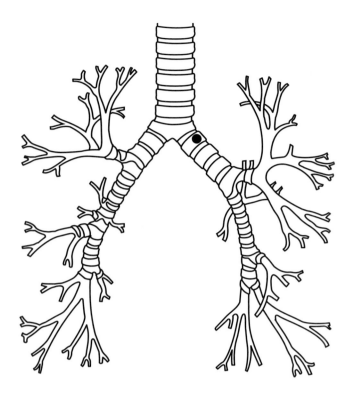

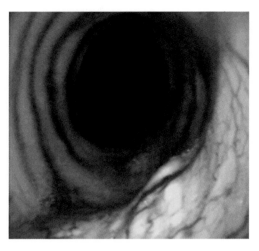

Figure 15-2. A raised papule of infiltrating carcinoma in the left mainstem bronchus due to an adjacent esophageal carcinoma. Note the prominent overlying vascular pattern.

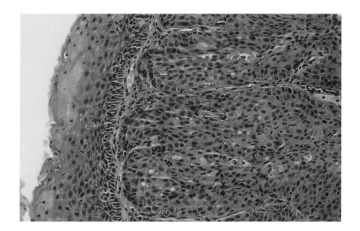

Figure 15-3. Benign bronchial epithelium with squamous metaplasia and the underlying submucosal squamous cell carcinoma in a patient who had advanced esophageal carcinoma (H&E, ×200, original magnification).

CHAPTER 16

Metastatic Ovarian Cancer

David R. Duhamel

Ovarian carcinoma is third in frequency among the gynecologic cancers, yet it accounts for the greatest number of fatalities from gynecologic malignancy and is the fifth leading cause of cancer fatalities in women.[1] Although pleural and parenchymal lung metastases are common with ovarian carcinomas,[1] tracheobronchial metastases are extremely rare. The world literature reports only six cases to date of metastatic ovarian cancer to the airway.[2-7]

Clinically significant tracheobronchial metastases are symptomatic in more than 80% of cases diagnosed antemortem, with cough and hemoptysis being seen most frequently.[2] The remainder are identified only by radiographic studies. The clinical picture and radiographic findings are usually indistinguishable from primary bronchogenic tumors.[7] Segmental or lobar atelectasis is the most frequent radiographic finding of bronchial metastases. The majority of metastatic ovarian carcinoma involves either the right or left mainstem bronchus, although there is a single case report of a distal tracheal lesion.[8]

The bronchoscopic findings should appear similar to those of most other metastatic endobronchial lesions; however, the data are limited. The example presented here appears to be a partially obstructing mass growing from the medial wall of the left mainstem bronchus. It was smooth and glistening but very friable and bled easily. The adjacent bronchial wall had a prominent vascular pattern, raising the concern for lymphangitic disease. It is unclear whether this lesion represented a hematogenous metastasis to the bronchial wall or, more likely, the erosion of a mediastinal lymph node into the airway.

The pathology of these lesions appears slightly variable. Studies suggest that the majority of primary ovarian carcinomas are of epithelial origin. The two most common cell types are papillary mucinous adenocarcinoma and serous cystadenocarcinoma. There has been a case report of a metastatic lesion from a granulosa cell tumor. In an autopsy series of 100 patients with ovarian cancer, 49% had evidence of pulmonary metastasis.[9] A parenchymal lesion was seen in 39%, a visceral pleural lesion in 39%, and pleural effusion in 48%. Despite this high incidence of metastatic lung involvement, there was no mention of any endobronchial lesions in this study. Therefore, the rate of metastatic endobronchial involvement in ovarian carcinoma appears to be relatively minuscule. The high rate of pleural involvement is believed related to the very high incidence of peritoneal involvement and the formation of malignant ascites. The malignant cells are shed from the ovary and seed the entire peritoneal space. As malignant ascites develops, some of the cells are carried into the pleural space through small rents in the diaphragm and seed the pleural surface.

Parenchymal lung lesions are thought to develop from contiguous local invasion at the site of a pleural metastasis rather than hematogenous spread. This unusual mode of metastasis helps to explain why airway lesions from ovarian carcinoma are such a unique occurrence.

Tracheobronchial metastases frequently develop late in a patient's clinical course. In Baumgartner's series, the mean duration from diagnosis of the primary lesion to discovery of the metastasis was 5 years.[3] Metastatic lesions to the bronchus have been discovered as late as 14 years after initial diagnosis, and in one case of ovarian carcinoma, 12 years. This relatively indolent course generally supports a more aggressive and optimistic therapeutic approach. The metastatic lesions are typically amenable to laser resection with an Nd:YAG laser. A Silastic stent can then be placed to maintain airway patency while further therapy including chemotherapy and radiation are given. The case presented here was treated successfully with laser resection and Silastic stenting, as was one other case presented in the world literature. Survival after diagnosis appears to be prolonged as well. Five of the six cases in the literature lived longer than 22 months and in one case that was treated with a combined laser and surgical resection, survival has exceeded 2 years.[9] The case presented here is doing well 6 months after laser resection. In general, if a patient's malignant airway lesion is successfully resected with bronchoscopic laser therapy, the patient typically improves symptomatically and goes on to expire from other causes besides asphyxiation or airway compromise.[8]

REFERENCES

1. Kerr VE, Cadman E: Pulmonary metastases in ovarian cancer: Analysis of 357 patients. Cancer 56:1209-1213, 1985.
2. Freedlander SS, Greenfield J: Hemoptysis in metastatic tumors of the lung simulating bronchogenic cancer. J Thorac Surg 12:109-116, 1942.
3. Seiler HH, Clagett DT, McDonald JR: Pulmonary resection for metastatic malignant lesions. J Thorac Surg 19:655-675, 1950.
4. Merrill CR, Hopkirk JC: Late endobronchial metastases from ovarian tumor. Br J Dis Chest 76:253-254, 1982.
5. Mateo F, Serur E, Smith PR: Bronchial metastases from ovarian carcinoma. Gyn Onc 46:235-238, 1992.
6. Asamura H, Goya T, Hirata K, et al: Esophageal and pulmonary metastases from ovarian carcinoma: A case report of long-term survival following metastatic resections. Jpn J Clin Oncol 21:211-217, 1991.
7. Westerman DE, Urbanetti JS, Rudders RA, Fanburg BL: Metastatic endotracheal tumor from ovarian carcinoma. Chest 77:798-800, 1980.
8. Dumon JF, Rebard E, Garbe L, et al: Treatment of tracheobronchial lesions by laser photoresection. Chest 81:278-284, 1982.
9. Dvoretsky PM, Richards KA, Angel C, et al: Distribution of disease at autopsy in 100 women with ovarian cancer. Human Pathol 19:57-63, 1988.

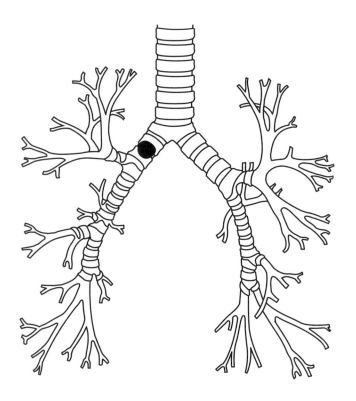

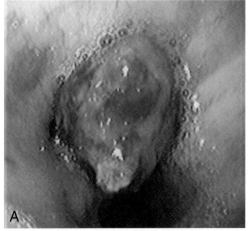

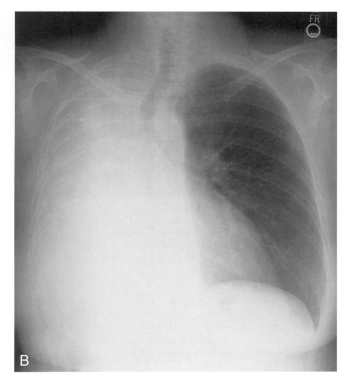

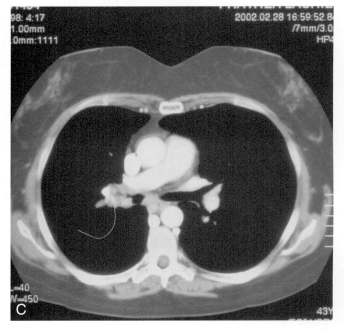

Figure 16-1. A, A smooth pink nodule of metastatic ovarian carcinoma obstructing the right mainstem bronchus. **B,** A frontal radiograph demonstrates complete opacification of the right hemithorax. A slight narrowing of the distal tracheal air column is present. **C,** A CT scan obtained after therapy demonstrates re-expansion of the right lung.

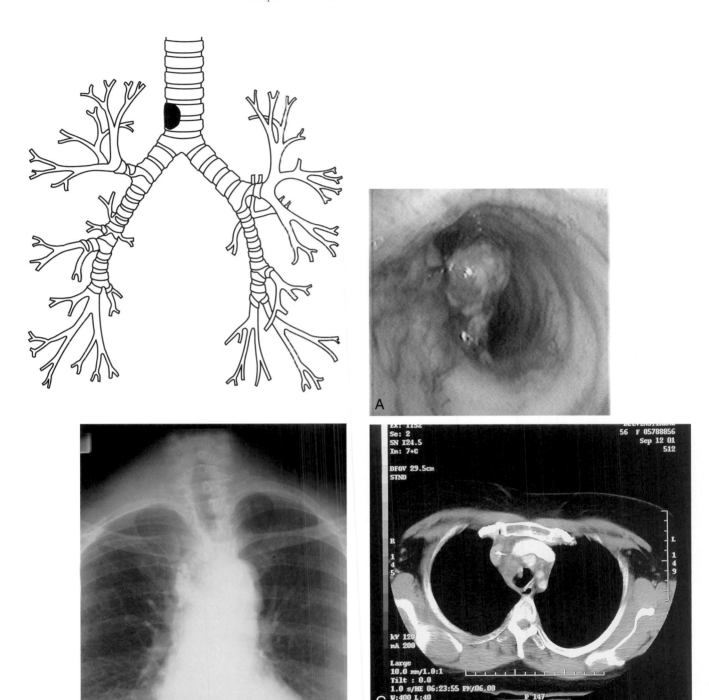

Figure 16-2. A, A friable vascular growth of ovarian carcinoma extending out of the right lateral tracheal wall. **B**, The frontal radiograph demonstrates a right paratracheal mass with narrowing of the trachea and slight deviation to the left. **C**, The CT image demonstrates a mass extending within the right paratracheal space with invasion of the superior vena cava and innominate artery. A small portion of the mass extends into the trachea.

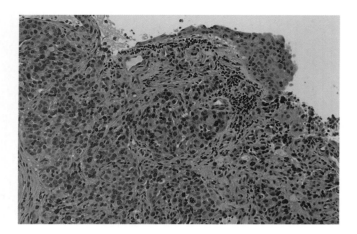

Figure 16-3. Submucosal infiltration of adenocarcinoma with the features similar to the patient's previously diagnosed papillary serous cystadenocarcinoma of the ovaries (H&E, ×200, original magnification).

CHAPTER 17

Metastatic Renal Cell Cancer

David R. Duhamel

The lung is an extremely common site of metastasis and is involved in 50% to 60% of all cases of metastatic renal cell cancer.[1] Although renal cell cancer is a rare type of tumor, representing 2% of all malignancies, it is the second most common cause of endobronchial metastasis. In an autopsy study of endobronchial metastatic disease, 30% of lesions were due to renal cell cancer. It is a common mode of presentation as shown by Gerle and Felson, who found that in 7 of 17 patients with renal cell carcinoma the metastasis was diagnosed before the primary tumor was identified.[2] In patients with tumor involvement of the central airways, dyspnea is a major clinical symptom. This is in contrast to patients with metastatic involvement of the lung parenchyma, who are frequently asymptomatic. Hemoptysis is another common presenting symptom. A bizarre form of presentation unique to metastatic renal cell carcinoma is the expectoration of tumor fragments, which has been reported with some prevalence in the literature.[2,3]

Matthay and Arroliga point out the necessity of bronchoscopy before planning metastasis surgery in order not to overlook an endobronchial tumor.[4] Thirty percent of all interventional bronchoscopic procedures to relieve metastatic endobronchial obstruction were for renal cell carcinoma. Three unique bronchoscopic characteristics have been reported by Dobbertin and colleagues: a thrombus-like pattern of growth resembling a luminal blood clot, a strong incidence of significant hemorrhage with manipulation, and a tendency for the tumor to obstruct adjacent bronchial

orifices.[5] In other case reports, the lesion was found to be pedunculated. The most frequently involved region of the airway was the right mainstem bronchus and the bronchus intermedius. The majority of endobronchial metastases are located distal to the carina, but endotracheal metastases have been reported.[6]

Chest radiographs are not very sensitive at distinguishing between primary bronchogenic lung cancer and endobronchial metastasis, because they often manifest in a similar fashion. The CT scan, however, may show multiple lesions supporting the diagnosis of metastasis even if the chest film shows a single nodule. In a series by Ikezoe and co-workers, endobronchial metastases were diagnosed in 4% of patients with known pulmonary metastasis who underwent CT examination.[7] In a review of 24 patients with known endobronchial metastasis from renal cell cancer, 54% had evidence of diffuse metastatic parenchymal disease (of interest, 25% had no evidence of parenchymal involvement), 50% had enlarged hilar or mediastinal lymphadenopathy, 25% had atelectasis or lobar pneumonia, and 8% had a tumor mass with extension into the hilar region.[5]

There are five potential routes for metastatic tumor cells to reach the bronchial lumen: (1) centripetal growth of adjacent parenchymal tumor, (2) penetration of tumor lymph nodes, (3) endoluminal growth from smaller bronchi, (4) lymphangitic, and (5) hematogenous spread to the bronchial mucosa. In the setting of renal cell carcinoma, it is fairly well accepted that metastases occur hematogenously after invading the renal vein.[8] As a result, widespread dissemination of tumor emboli occurs, some of which reaches the bronchial mucosa. Histologically, the tumors typically contain the large clear cells characteristic of renal cell carcinoma. However, making the diagnosis can be difficult because the tumor cells on occasion appear spindle shaped, suggesting a sarcomatous pattern.

Because the treatment of endobronchial metastasis

is often palliative, surgical therapy has a limited role. Bronchoscopic therapy with Nd:YAG laser is the treatment of choice. Bronchoscopic resection is indicated only if functional lung is present distal to the obstruction as evidenced by aerated lung on chest radiograph. Endoscopic resection of renal cell cancer is often made difficult by significant hemorrhage, and multiple procedures are often required. In particularly difficult cases, preoperative bronchial artery embolization has proven beneficial. Endoluminal brachytherapy can be used to inhibit tumor growth and increase the interval between tumor resections. Silastic stents have also been used after bronchoscopic therapy to help maintain luminal patency. The overall prognosis in metastatic renal cell carcinoma is poor, but the tumor is well known for its tendency to develop late metastasis. The average time between nephrectomy and detection of endobronchial metastasis is about 4.8 years,[2] but metastasis has been reported as much as 12 years later. This emphasizes the point that a high index of suspicion must be maintained in anyone with pulmonary complaints and a remote history of renal cell carcinoma.

REFERENCES

1. Motzer RJ, Bander NH, Nanus DM: Renal cell carcinoma. N Engl J Med 335:865-875, 1996.
2. Gerle R, Felson B: Metastatic endobronchial hypernephroma. Chest 44:225-233, 1963.
3. Jariwalla AG, Seaton A, McCormack RJM, et al: Intrabronchial metastases from renal carcinoma with recurrent tumour expectoration. Thorax 36:179-182, 1981.
4. Matthay RA, Arroliga AC: Resection of pulmonary metastases. Am Rev Respir Dis 148:1691-1696, 1993.
5. Dobbertin I, Dierkesmann R, Kwiatkowski J, Reichardt W: Bronchoscopic aspects of renal cell carcinoma. Anticanc Res 19:1567-1572, 1999.
6. MacMahon H, O'Connell DJ, Cimochowski GE: Pedunculated endotracheal metastasis. Am J Roentgenol 131:713-714, 1978.
7. Ikezoe J, Johkoh T, Takeuchi N, et al: CT findings of endobronchial metastasis 32:455-460, 1991.
8. Patel NP, Lavengood RW: Renal carcinoma: natural history and results of treatment. J Urol 119:722-726, 1978.

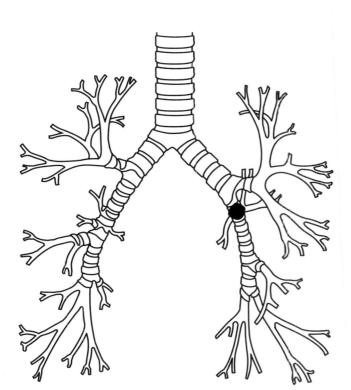

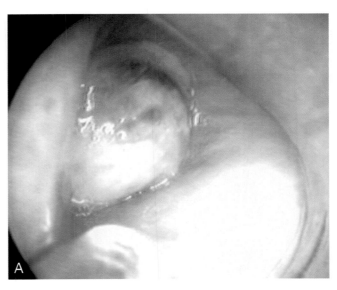

Figure 17-1. A, A smooth, fleshy hyperpigmented tumor completely obstructing the left lower lobe orifice. On endoscopic removal, the lesion was found to be pathologically identical to a renal cell carcinoma resected 8 years earlier. *Continued*

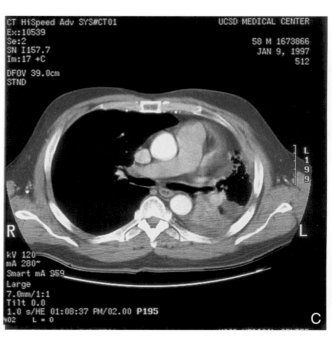

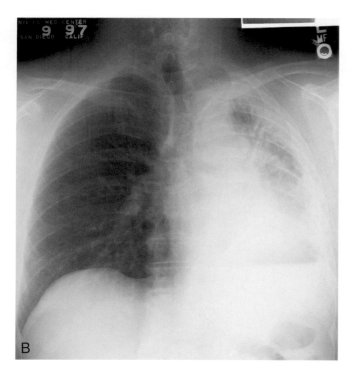

Figure 17-1, *cont'd.* **B,** The frontal radiograph demonstrates left lower lobe collapse with left pleural effusion and thickening. The left lower lobe bronchus cannot be identified. **C,** The CT scan demonstrates a mass obstructing the left lower lobe bronchus with collapse of the left lower lobe.

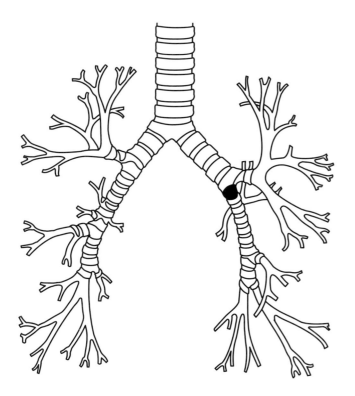

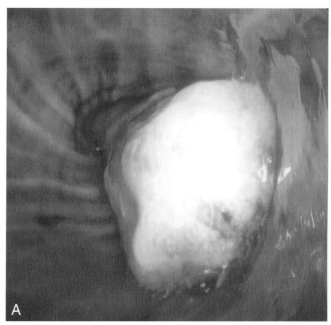

Figure 17-2. A, A white, fibrous, pedunculated tumor arising from the left lower lobe that manifested with intermittent left upper lobe, left lower lobe, and complete left lung atelectasis. **B,** The frontal radiograph demonstrates left lower lobe collapse. **C,** The CT image demonstrates a mass within the distal left main bronchus at the bifurcation of the lower and upper lobe bronchi.

Continued

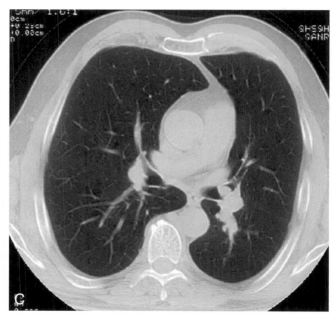

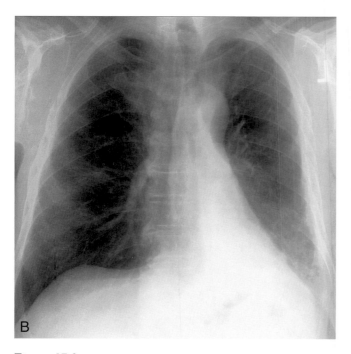

Figure 17-2, *cont'd.*

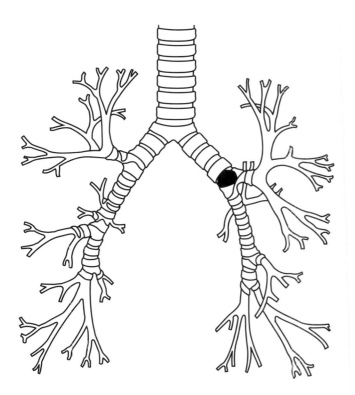

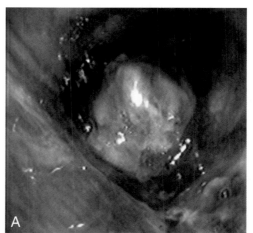

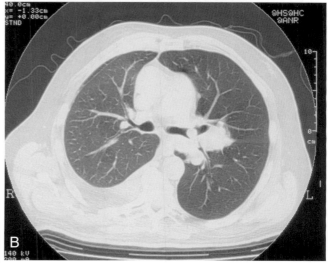

Figure 17-3. A, A large deposit of very vascular metastatic renal cell carcinoma at the bifurcation between the left upper and lower lobes. **B,** The CT scan demonstrates a mass within the distal left main bronchus.

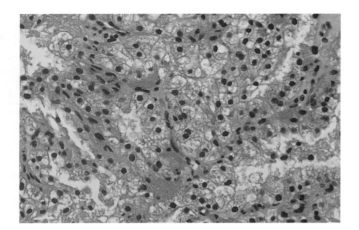

Figure 17-4. Renal cell carcinoma composed of tumor cells with clear cytoplasm and highly vascular stroma (H&E, ×400).

CHAPTER 18

Metastatic Melanoma

David R. Duhamel

Malignant melanoma is capable of metastasizing to any organ in the body, with lung, liver, brain, and bone being the most frequent locations. Pulmonary involvement occurs in nearly all cases of disseminated disease.[1] There are well-documented reports of primary melanoma of the lung occurring in an endobronchial location as well.[2] Metastatic disease is known to affect both the trachea and bronchi. Expectoration of tumor fragments is a reported complication and has even resulted in complete resolution of symptoms and clearing of atelectasis on chest radiograph.[1] Melanoma is well known to be a very vascular tumor, and therefore hemoptysis is a frequent presenting sign.

Viewed bronchoscopically, the tumor may appear darkly pigmented or melanotic. Grossly amelanotic lesions have been reported as well, which may be easily confused with other endobronchial lesions, including bronchogenic carcinoma. In one case report of a patient with widely disseminated melanoma, diffuse melanosis of the airway was seen without specific endobronchial lesion.[1]

Intrathoracic metastases in patients with melanoma are very common. In one series of 65 patients, 57 had radiographic evidence of metastasis consisting of solitary nodules in 14, multiple nodules in 41, a miliary pattern in 8, and lymphangitic carcinomatosis in 5. Radiographic evidence of endobronchial obstruction includes atelectasis, volume loss, and luminal filling defects. These airway findings are typically seen in combination with the more common parenchymal findings.

The diagnosis of metastatic melanoma is fairly easy to establish with a good tissue specimen. The tumor cells typically show a strong immunohistochemical reaction for S-100 protein and HMB-45.

Bronchoscopic therapy to relieve endobronchial obstruction from melanoma is not a new concept. In 1934, Clerff reported that bronchoscopic resection was useful in relieving symptoms from an obstructing endobronchial melanoma.[3] Today the therapeutic armamentarium is diverse and includes laser therapy, brachytherapy, electrocautery, cryotherapy, and photodynamic therapy. Nd:YAG laser therapy with a rigid bronchoscope has been used with success in the majority of case reports. The prognosis is very poor in metastatic melanoma. In general, the 5-year survival rates even after resection of a metastasis range from 5% to 25%.[4,5]

REFERENCES

1. Sutton FD, Vestal RE, Creagh CE: Varied presentations of metastatic pulmonary melanoma. Chest 65:415-419, 1974.
2. Salm R: A primary malignant melanoma of the bronchus. J Pathol 85:121-126, 1963.
3. Clerff LH: Metastasis simulating bronchogenic neoplasm. Ann Otol Rhinol Laryngol 43:887-891, 1934.
4. Karakousis CP, Velez A, Driscoll DL, et al: Metastasectomy in malignant melanoma. Surgery 115:295-298, 1994.
5. Wong JH, Euhus DM, Morton DL: Surgical resection for metastatic melanoma of the lung. Arch Surg 123:1091-1094, 1988.

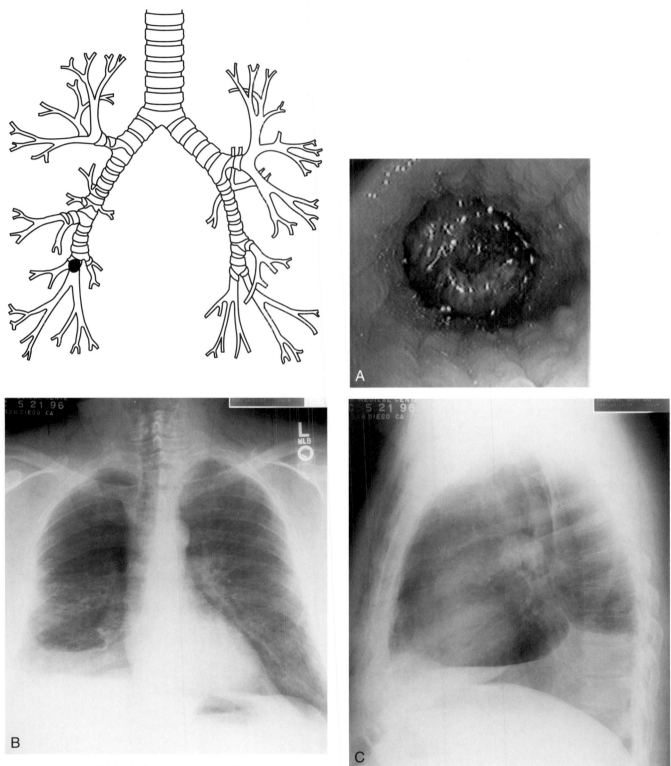

Figure 18-1. **A**, A black, hyperpigmented, metastatic melanoma lesion that is obstructing the right lower basilar subsegments. Frontal (**B**) and lateral (**C**) radiographs demonstrate right lower lobe collapse.

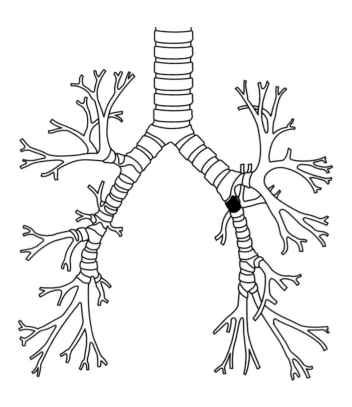

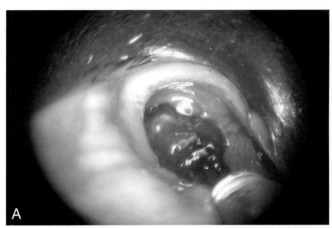

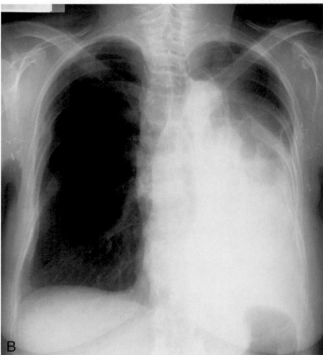

Figure 18-2. A, A hemorrhagic, vascular, endobronchial lesion obstructing the left lower lobe bronchus. The pathology was found to be consistent with a previously diagnosed melanoma. **B,** The frontal radiograph demonstrates left lower lobe collapse and left effusion. The air column within the left lower lobe terminates abruptly near the origin of the upper lobe.

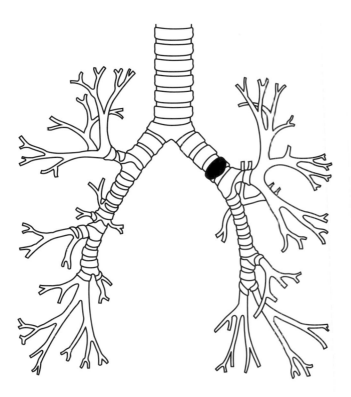

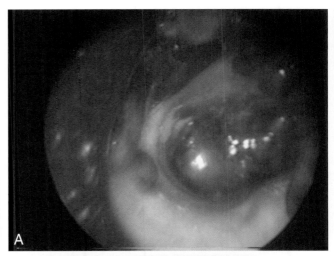

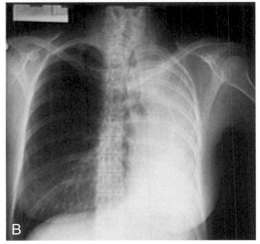

Figure 18-3. A, A darkly pigmented, obstructing metastatic melanoma lesion in the left mainstem bronchus. **B,** The frontal radiograph demonstrates complete collapse of the left lung with marked hyperinflation of the right lung. The left mainstem bronchus terminates abruptly.

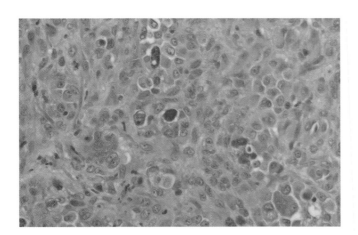

Figure 18-4. Malignant melanoma cells with intracytoplasmic melanin pigments that are appreciated at high magnification (H&E, ×400, original magnification).

CHAPTER 19

Metastatic Breast Cancer

David R. Duhamel

It was reported in a classic article in 1975 by Braman and Whitcomb that the incidence of metastatic endobronchial disease is about 2%.[1] Since then, multiple case series have shown that breast cancer is the most frequent cause of endobronchial metastasis, not renal cell carcinoma as was previously thought.[2,3] Some case series of endobronchial metastatic disease report that as many as 35% of all lesions are due to breast carcinoma.[2] It is an unusual presenting feature and more commonly heralds recurrent disease. Manifestations can be indolent, with some patients developing pulmonary symptoms 5 years after the primary diagnosis has been made. According to one study, the time from diagnosis of primary nonpulmonary malignancy to the diagnosis of endobronchial metastasis averages about 60 months for most tumors.[4] However, it was found that, on average, endobronchial breast cancer tends to develop late, at 92 months. Hemoptysis was seen in up to 41% of patients at presentation. Other presenting symptoms include cough, pneumonia, and wheeze.

Bronchoscopy should be performed early in anyone with pulmonary symptoms and a recent or remote history of breast cancer. Bronchoscopy is very sensitive for detecting occult airway metastases. The bronchoscopic appearance in general is one of mucosal edema and thickening. The tumor cells are present in the submucosal lymphatics and have a layer of airway epithelium covering them. This explains the relatively low diagnostic yield of bronchial brush specimens and emphasizes the need for a deep biopsy specimen to make the diagnosis.[5] Albertini and Ekberg[5] reported a diagnostic yield rate of about 70% with endobronchial biopsy. They continue to recommend cytologic brushings as well, because a diagnosis was made with a negative biopsy in two cases. Multiple metachronous lesions have also been reported on occasion.

In general, endobronchial metastases are incidental findings seen by the pathologist at autopsy or by the bronchoscopist. Metastatic breast carcinoma has the tendency to grow rather slowly, such that a lesion may be of considerable size before it manifests clinically or radiographically. If a tumor were large enough to cause radiographic findings, the findings would be typical of bronchial obstruction. Bronchial obstruction can be partial (causing oligemia and expiratory air trapping) or complete (with atelectasis and obstructive pneumonitis).[6] In a series of 42 patients with known endobronchial breast cancer, 24 (57%) had atelectasis or obstructive pneumonitis.[7]

Histologically, the vast majority of metastatic tumors are of the infiltrating ductal carcinoma cell type, more than 80% in some series.[5] This cell type, however, is the most common of all primary breast carcinomas. Metastases can occur both hematogenously and by lymphatic spread, but the latter seems more common with breast cancer.

Therapy for endobronchial metastases in general is palliative, but in certain individualized situations the patient may be a suitable candidate for surgical resection. Endoluminal therapies can be extremely effective at relieving the obstruction and eliminating the associated morbidities. Laser ablation with the Nd:YAG laser and rigid bronchoscope has a successful clinical track record. Other therapies including cryotherapy, electrocautery, photodynamic therapy, and brachytherapy have been used with some success. Silastic stents are also beneficial for maintaining luminal patency. Mean survival time from the diagnosis of endobronchial metastases to death is on the order of 12 months for most tumors[4]; however, in breast cancer, long-term survival has been reported. Ettensohn and colleagues[7] reported a 21-month mean survival, whereas Baumgartner and associates[8] reported an overall 32-month survival and made the recommendation that aggressive treatment should be considered in these patients.

REFERENCES

1. Braman SS, Whitcomb ME: Endobronchial metastasis. Arch Intern Med 135:543-547, 1975.
2. Fitzgerald RH: Endobronchial metastasis. South Med J 70:440-441, 1977.
3. Citroni GA, DiGuglielimo L: Neoplasmie metastatiche dei grossibronchi con sintomatologia di tumore primitivo: Osservazioni bronchografiche. Minerva Med 2:924-930, 1956.
4. Heitmiller RF, Marasco WJ, Hruban RH, Marsh BR: Endobronchial metastasis. J Thorac Cardiovasc Surg 106:537-542, 1993.
5. Albertini RE, Ekberg NL: Endobronchial metastasis in breast cancer. Thorax 35:435-440, 1980.
6. Fraser RS, Muller NL, Colman N, Paré PD: Diagnosis of Disease of the Chest. Philadelphia, WB Saunders, 1999.
7. Ettensohn DB, Bennet JM, Hyde RW: Endobronchial metastases from carcinoma of the breast. Med Pediatr Oncol 13:9-14, 1985.
8. Baumgartner WA, Mark JBD: Metastatic malignancies from distant sites to the tracheobronchial tree. Thorac Cardiovasc Surg 79:499-503, 1980.

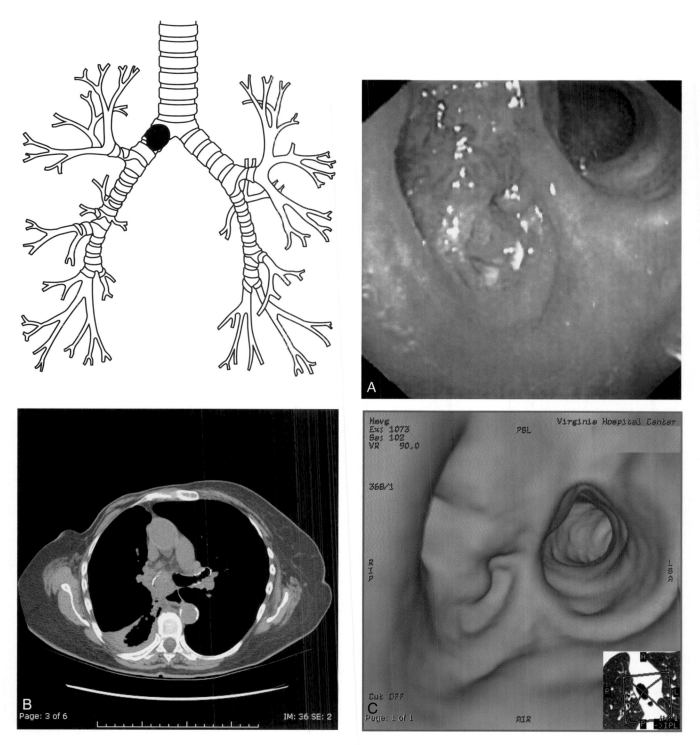

Figure 19-1. A, Complete obstruction of the right mainstem bronchus at the level of the carina by metastatic breast cancer. The irregular surface is very vascular and appears to be arising from the medial wall of the bronchus. **B,** A CT scan showing complete obstruction of the right mainstem bronchus at the level of the carina by a mass of metastatic breast cancer. Other than some lower lobe segmental atelectasis, the lung is surprisingly well aerated. **C,** A virtual bronchoscopic image reconstructed from the CT scan data showing complete obstruction of the right mainstem bronchus and a fully patent left mainstem bronchus. The image is nearly identical to the true bronchoscopic image. A great benefit of this technology is the ability to visualize the airway beyond the obstruction.

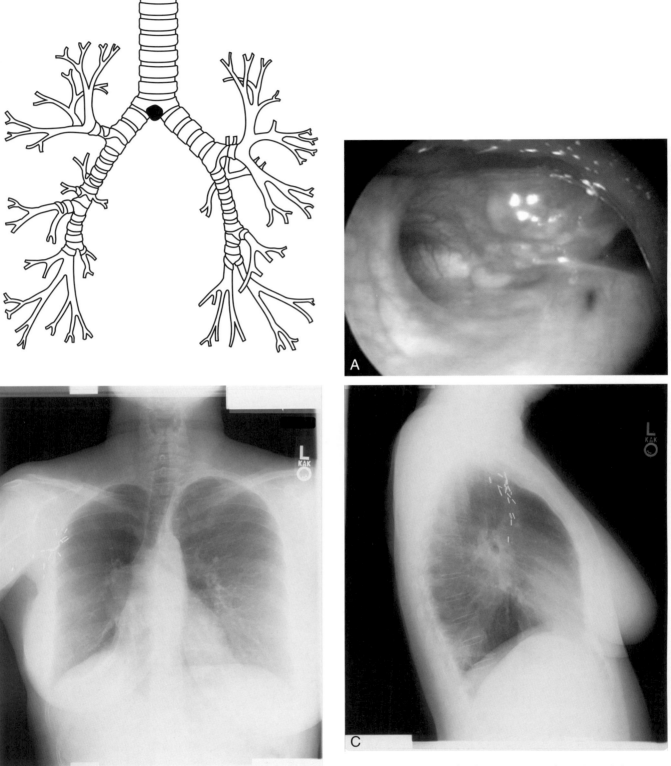

Figure 19-2. A, Multiple metastatic deposits arising from the carina in a woman with known breast cancer. These lesions were estrogen and progesterone receptor positive, as was her primary carcinoma. Frontal (**B**) and lateral (**C**) radiographs demonstrate a right hilar and subcarinal mass with right lower lobe atelectasis. A nodular density projects within the bronchus intermedius just distal to the right upper lobe takeoff.

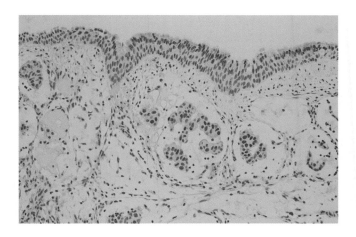

Figure 19-3. Metastatic mucinous (colloid) carcinoma of the breast. Tumor cell nuclei are positive for estrogen receptor immunostain (antiestrogen receptor antibody, ×200, original magnification).

CHAPTER 20

Metastatic Colorectal Cancer

David R. Duhamel

Metastatic colon cancer to the lung is characteristically peripheral in location but does on occasion manifest as an endobronchial lesion. Necroscopy studies have shown a 2% to 5% incidence of endobronchial metastases in patients with solid tumors, with colorectal, breast, and renal cell being the most common cell types.[1,2] Colorectal cancer is the cause of 10.9% to 26% of all endobronchial and endo-tracheal metastatic lesions. Most patients with a pulmonary parenchymal metastasis are asymptomatic at the time of diagnosis, whereas the vast majority of patients with endo-bronchial metastasis are symptomatic.[3] The most common presenting symptoms include cough and hemoptysis, followed by fever, dyspnea, pneumonia, or chest pain.[2] An endobronchial metastasis may be the initial clinical manifestation of a neoplasm but more commonly is a late complication in the setting of a widely disseminated disease. This is evidenced by the observation that 87% of patients diagnosed with endobronchial metastasis also have extra-bronchial involvement.[4] In the setting of colorectal carcinoma, this almost always includes the liver. The diagnosis of endobronchial metastases may occur at any time after the diagnosis of the primary colorectal cancer. The time interval ranges from 8 to 188 months, with a mean of 45 months.

Endobronchial metastasis is a manifestation of widely disseminated disease and carries a very poor prognosis; therefore, all treatment should be considered palliative. Survival has been reported to range from 1 to 24 months, with a mean of 13 months.[5] Survival seems to be related to the behavior of the primary tumor and to a certain extent the palliative therapy. Palliation has been obtained with Nd:YAG laser tumor ablation, external beam radiation, brachytherapy, and photodynamic therapy. Silastic stents have also been used to help maintain luminal patency. In selected cases, a lobectomy or pneumonectomy may improve survival.

It is interesting that colorectal cancer, when compared with all extrathoracic malignancies, is the most common cause of a solitary metastatic neoplasm to the lung. It accounts for 30% to 40% of all solitary pulmonary metastases. However, even in the setting of a known cancer in the gastrointestinal tract, there is only a 50% chance of a solitary lesion on a chest radiograph being malignant.[6] The radiographic manifestations of colon cancer involving the airway are similar to those of other neoplastic lesions. These findings include volume loss, atelectasis, post-obstructive pneumonitis, and luminal filling defects.

From a pathologic standpoint, metastatic involvement of the lung in colorectal cancer almost always affects the liver first. It is often very difficult to distinguish histologically between metastatic colorectal cancer and primary broncho-genic adenocarcinoma, especially if the tumor cells are poorly differentiated. A careful comparison of the primary and metastatic tissue is necessary to search for similarities. Electron microscopy, immunohistochemistry, phospholipid analysis, and mucin histochemistry may aid in making a distinction. In those cases in which the histologic differentiation is still unclear, the demonstration of carcinoma in situ in adjacent bronchial mucosa is strong evidence for primary bronchogenic lung cancer.[7]

REFERENCES

1. Braman SS, Whitcomb ME: Endobronchial metastasis. Arch Intern Med 135:543-547, 1975.

2. Carlin BW, Harrell JH, Olson LK, Moser KM: Endobronchial metastases due to colorectal carcinoma. Chest 96:1110-1114, 1989.
3. McCormack PM, Martini N: The changing role of surgery for pulmonary metastases. Ann Thorac Surg 28:139-145, 1979.
4. Heitmiller RF, Marasco WJ, Hruban RH, Marsh BR: Endobronchial metastasis. J Thorac Cardiovasc Surg 106:537-542, 1993.
5. Casino AR, Bellmunt J, Salud A, et al: Endobronchial metastasis in colorectal adenocarcinoma. Tumori 78:270-273, 1992.
6. Cahan WG, Castro EB: Significance of a solitary lung shadow in patients with breast cancer. Ann Surg 181:137-143, 1975.
7. Baumgartner WA, Mark JBD: Metastatic malignancies from distal sites to the tracheobronchial tree. J Thorac Cardiovasc Surg 79:499-503, 1980.

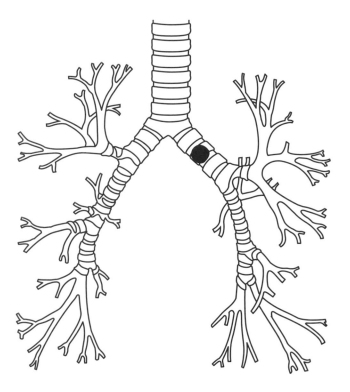

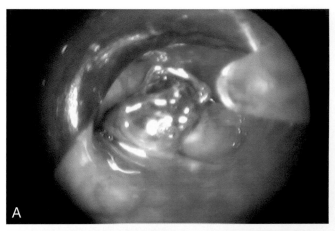

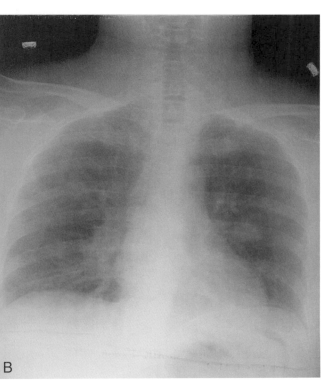

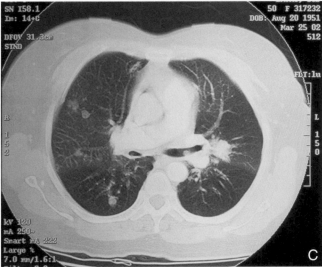

Figure 20-1. A, A smooth black growth of metastatic colon cancer partially obstructs the left mainstem bronchus. **B**, The frontal radiograph demonstrates bilateral parenchymal metastases. **C**, The CT image demonstrates multiple parenchymal metastases as well as an endobronchial metastasis within the left main bronchus.

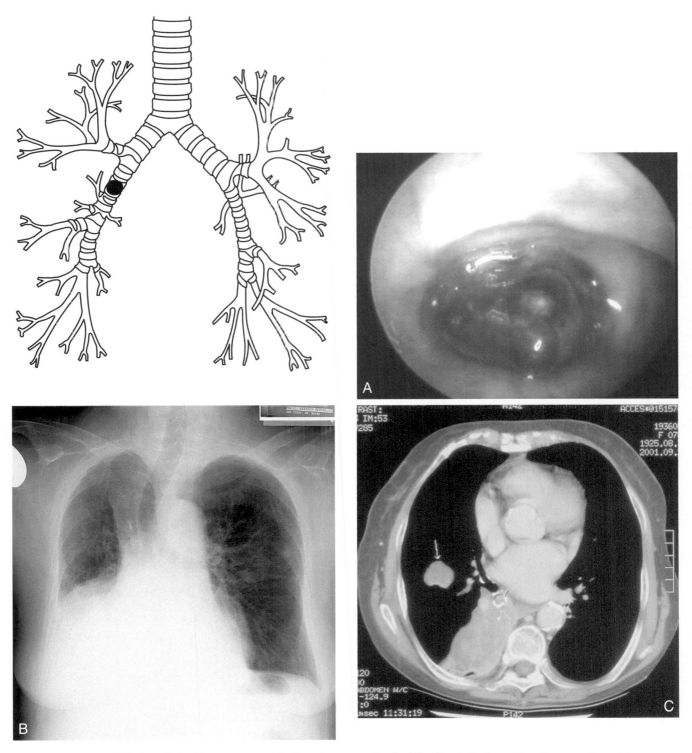

Figure 20-2. A, A lobulated, darkly pigmented lesion that completely fills the right bronchus intermedius. After bronchoscopic resection, the lesion was found to be very similar to a colon carcinoma that had been resected 4 years earlier. **B,** The frontal radiograph demonstrates right middle and lower collapse The air column within the bronchus intermedius terminates abruptly. A parenchymal metastasis is seen within the peripheral left midlung. **C,** The CT image demonstrates occlusion of a right lower lobe stent with right lower lobe collapse. A right middle lobe metastasis is present.

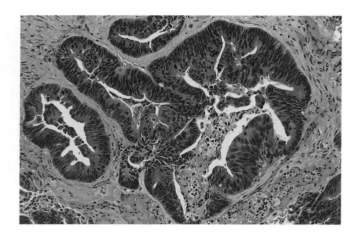

Figure 20-3. Well-formed glands with tall columnar lining cells are typical of metastatic colonic adenocarcinoma (H&E, ×200, original magnification).

CHAPTER 21

Sarcomas

David R. Duhamel

Sarcomas are a family of malignant neoplasms having mesenchymal phenotypes. They are classified according to the mesenchymal cell type most prevalent within the tumor. The cell types are varied and may include smooth muscle cells, striated muscle cells, lipocytes, chondrocytes, and even osteocytes. Primary sarcomas of the lung are extremely rare and constitute 0.01% to 0.2% of all lung tumors.[1] The precise histologic classification of these tumors has been difficult, but with the development of newer diagnostic tools, including electron microscopy, immunohistochemistry, genetic typing, and molecular studies, a higher level of accuracy can be achieved. It is also important to remember that certain carcinomas (carcinosarcomas and spindle cell carcinomas), by definition, have sarcomatous differentiation. Other epithelial tumors, especially renal cell carcinoma and melanoma, may have a sarcomatoid appearance on biopsy. Therefore, a large biopsy specimen is frequently necessary to make an accurate diagnosis, and typically the final diagnosis is not made until a surgical resection has been performed.

Because smooth muscle is widely present in the airways and vasculature of the lung, it is not surprising that leiomyosarcomas are among the most common primary sarcomas of the lung.[2,3] It is important to remember that primary pulmonary leiomyosarcomas remain exceedingly rare, with only 92 reported in the world literature at last review, 7 of which were localized to the trachea.[3] Leiomyomas, the benign smooth muscle tumor counterpart, are seen much more commonly in the airway. Viewed bronchoscopically, leiomyosarcomas appear fleshy and are often pedunculated. They partially or completely occlude the airway, but extension into the adjacent tracheobronchial wall is unusual.[4] The radiographic manifestations include atelectasis and obstructive pneumonitis. Leiomyosarcomas that affect the lung parenchyma are sharply defined, smooth and lobulated in contour, and homogeneous in density. On occasion they demonstrate cavitation or calcification. Histologically, smooth muscle tumors are characterized by bundles of spindle cells intersecting one another at wide angles. There are areas of high cellularity with large, clefted irregular nuclei. The diagnosis can be supported by Masson trichrome stain or by the immunostain for myosin and desmin. The prognosis is good if the tumor can be adequately excised, because local recurrence and metastases are unusual.[4]

Although primary bronchopulmonary fibrosarcoma is probably the second most common intrathoracic sarcoma after leiomyosarcoma, fewer than 100 cases have been reported.[5] The incidence of this tumor appears to be dropping off in recent years, which most certainly reflects the development of newer diagnostic technologies that greatly enhance our histologic accuracy. This raises questions about the pathologic classification of some of the earlier reported cases. Fibrosarcomas have been reported to arise in the trachea and bronchi, with the vast majority developing in the lobar or main bronchi of children and young adults.[6] The bronchoscopic appearance is highly varied, with descriptions ranging from a pedunculated lesion, to a circumferential polypoid mass, to even a cherry-red polyp.[6,7] The histologic appearance is that of highly cellular sheets and bundles of spindle cells arranged in the classic herringbone pattern. The tumors exhibit strongly positive staining for vimentin, and reticulin fibers are seen on silver stain. Interestingly, parenchymal fibrosarcomas tend to develop in middle-aged and elderly adults. They are typically asymptomatic and appear as smooth, lobulated masses on radiograph; they carry a poor prognosis, however, with death occurring within 2.5 years.[4,5] In general, endobronchial fibrosarcomas carry a much better prognosis over their parenchymal counterparts. Metastases are unusual, and long-term survival is the rule if a complete excision can be obtained. Lobectomy or sleeve resection is preferred over endobronchial resection because adequate margins cannot be guaranteed with the latter.

The fact that skeletal muscle is not normally found in the lung makes the concept of primary pulmonary rhabdomyosarcomas somewhat difficult to explain. It is no surprise that these are extremely rare tumors, with only 18 cases reported to have lower airway involvement. Of the 18 cases, 5 were purely endobronchial and 2 originated in the trachea.[8,9] The lesions are typically described as broad-based sessile neoplasms arising from the bronchial wall with partial or complete occlusion of the airway lumen. However, there is a case report of a pedunculated lesion arising from the right mainstem bronchus, which was found to pendulate and cause intermittent asphyxia by obstructing the trachea.[9] The tumors are known to be locally invasive, and mediastinal infiltration has been reported. Distant metastatic sites have been described as well, including the heart and small intestine.[10,11] Histologically, the tumors consist of fascicles of spindle-shaped mesenchymal cells. The usual histologic classification is pleomorphic rhabdomyosarcoma; however, occasional subtypes of embryonal and alveolar rhabdomyosarcoma have been reported. A defining characteristic of a rhabdomyosarcoma is the presence of the cross-striations of skeletal muscle within the cytoplasm on light microscopy. The diagnosis can be confirmed by the demonstration of myofibrillar elements on electron microscopy or positive immunostains for myoglobin and myogenin. The presence of skeletal tissue in the airway is difficult to explain. One theory proposes that the tumor arises from primitive mesenchyme, which has the capability for rhabdomyoblastic differentiation. An alternative hypothesis is that the tumors arise from displaced skeletal muscle derived from the pharynx during embryonic development.[8]

Angiosarcomas of the lung typically represent metastatic disease, with the common primary site being the right atrium. Primary angiosarcomas of the lung are extremely rare with only eight cases known in the literature, all of which were located in the lung parenchyma.[12] The most common presenting symptom appears to be hemoptysis. A primary angiosarcoma of the trachea or bronchus has never been described, and only one example of endobronchial involvement from parenchymal extension has been reported.[13] The lesion presented by the authors does not represent a primary angiosarcoma of the bronchus but rather sarcomatous differentiation of primitive endothelial mesenchymal cells found in a germ cell tumor. Nevertheless, the tumor did manifest the characteristics of an angiosarcoma, which includes positive staining for factor VIII–related antigen and CD34.[14] The presence of vasoformative structures with malignant cells lining the vascular spaces is also necessary to make the histologic diagnosis. The bronchoscopic appearance was that of a very vascular, grainy-appearing lesion growing out of the lobar bronchus and completely filling the right mainstem bronchus. In general, the prognosis of angiosarcoma involving the lung is extremely poor, with survival being measured in months.

On occasion, the cartilaginous tissues of the trachea and bronchi gives rise to a form of mesenchymal tumor called a *chondrosarcoma*. These tumors are extremely rare, with only 16 cases being reported in a 1993 review.[15] These tumors are believed to arise from normal tracheobronchial cartilage, although malignant degeneration of a benign chondroma or chondromatous hamartoma is an alternative possibility. Chondrosarcomas of the distal extremities are known to metastasize to the lung as well. Grossly, the tumor may manifest as a hard, white, polypoid, intraluminal growth filling the lumen of the trachea or bronchus.[16] The histologic appearance is that of foci of myxoid and cartilaginous tissue containing chondrocytes with pleomorphic nuclei and variable mitotic rates. Calcification and ossification are not uncommon findings. Complete surgical excision can be curative, especially in low-grade lesions.

Primary osteosarcoma of the lung is extremely rare, whereas metastatic involvement of the lung from a bone primary is very common. A classic presentation of a metastatic osteosarcoma to the lung is a spontaneous pneumothorax.[17] Surprisingly, primary osteosarcomas manifest as noncalcified masses seen on radiograph.[18] Speckled calcifications may be seen on CT scan, even if not present on plain radiograph. They have also been reported to have intense uptake on technetium-labeled bone scans.[18] A primary osteosarcoma of the tracheobronchial tree has never been reported in the world literature. Histologically, the tumors contain variable amounts of cytologically malignant myxomatous, chondroid, and osteoid tissue. Very little is known about the clinical course and prognosis of these extremely rare lung tumors.

REFERENCES

1. Martini N: Invited commentary. Ann Thorac Surg 58:1155-1156, 1994.
2. Ramanathan T: Primary leiomyosarcoma of the lung. Thorax 29:482-485, 1974.
3. Yellin A, Rosenman Y, Lieberman Y: Review of smooth muscle tumors of the lower respiratory tract. Br J Dis Chest 78:337-351, 1984.
4. Guccion JG, Rosen SH: Bronchopulmonary leiomyosarcoma and fibrosarcoma: A study of 32 cases and review of the literature. Cancer 30:836-843, 1972.
5. Ono N, Sato K, Yokomise H, et al: Primary bronchopulmonary fibrosarcoma: Report of a case. Surg Today 28:1313-1315, 1998.
6. Pettinato G, Manivel JC, Saldana MJ, et al: Primary bronchopulmonary fibrosarcoma of childhood and adolescence: Reassessment of a low-grade malignancy. Hum Pathol 20:463-471, 1989.
7. Kunst PWA, Sutedja G, Golding RP, et al: Diagnosis in oncology. Case 1. A juvenile bronchopulmonary fibrosarcoma. J Clin Oncol 20:2745-2746, 2002.
8. Ho KL, Rassekh ZS: Rhabdomyosarcoma of the trachea: First reported case. Hum Pathol 11:572-574, 1980.
9. Eriksson A. Thunell M, Lundqvist G: Pendulating endobronchial rhabdomyosarcoma with fatal asphyxia. Thorax 37:390-391, 1982.
10. Przygodzki RM, Moran CA, Suster S, et al: Primary pulmonary rhabdomyosarcomas: A clinicopathologic and immunohistochemical study of three cases. Mod Pathol 8:658-662, 1995.
11. Avagnina A, Elsner B, De Marco L, et al: Pulmonary rhabdomyosarcoma with isolated small bowel metastasis: A report of a case with immunohistochemical ultrastructural studies. Cancer 53:1948-1953, 1984.
12. Patel AM, Ryu JH: Angiosarcoma of the lung. Chest 103:1531-1535, 1993.

13. Ali MY, Lee GS: Sarcoma of the pulmonary artery. Cancer 17:1220-1224, 1964.
14. Mullick SS, Mody DR, Schwartz MR: Angiosarcoma at unusual sites. A report of two cases with aspiration cytology and diagnostic pitfalls. Acta Cytologica 41:839-844, 1997.
15. Hayashi T, Tsuda N, Iseki M, et al: Primary chondrosarcoma of the lung: A clinicopathologic study. Cancer 72:69-75, 1993.
16. Yellin A, Schwartz L, Hersho E, et al: Chondrosarcoma of the bronchus: Report of a case with resection and review of the literature. Chest 84:224-230, 1983.
17. Dines DE, Cortese DA, Brennan MD, et al: Malignant pulmonary neoplasms predisposing to spontaneous pneumothorax. Mayo Clin Proc 48:541-545, 1973.
18. Petersen M: Radionucleotide detection of primary pulmonary osteogenic sarcoma: A case report and review of the literature. J Nucl Med 31: 1110-1115, 1990.

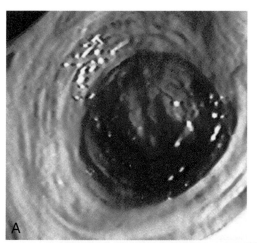

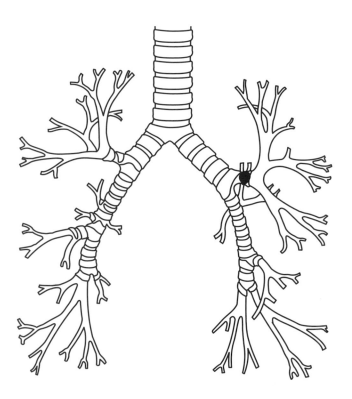

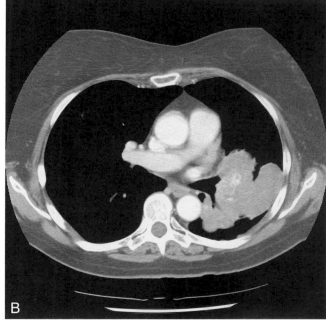

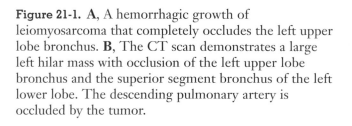

Figure 21-1. A, A hemorrhagic growth of leiomyosarcoma that completely occludes the left upper lobe bronchus. **B,** The CT scan demonstrates a large left hilar mass with occlusion of the left upper lobe bronchus and the superior segment bronchus of the left lower lobe. The descending pulmonary artery is occluded by the tumor.

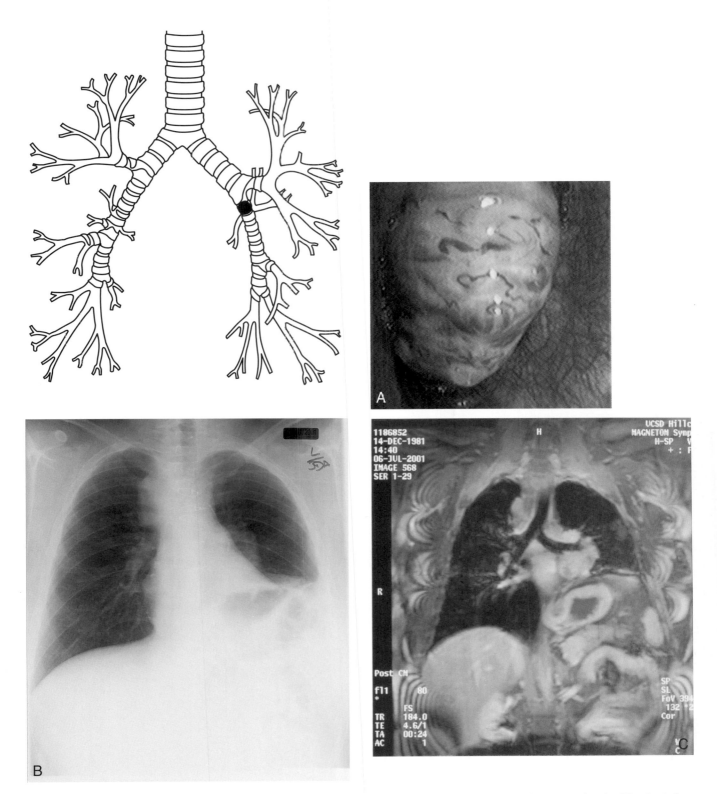

Figure 21-2. A, A grayish-white and very vascular mass of endobronchial angiosarcoma that completely fills the left lower lobe bronchus. **B,** The frontal radiograph demonstrates right superior mediastinal and left hilar masses. There is partial left lower lobe collapse. **C,** A T1-weighted coronal MR image demonstrates occlusion of the left lower lobe bronchus by the left hilar mass. Additional abnormal soft tissue is seen within the anteroposterior window and right paratracheal space. A parenchymal nodule is present in the left midlung.

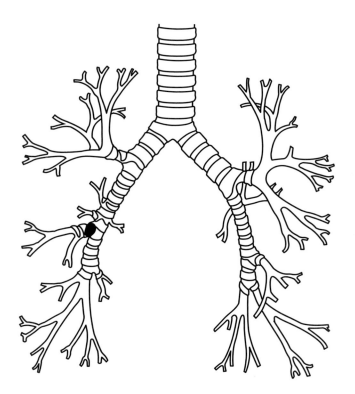

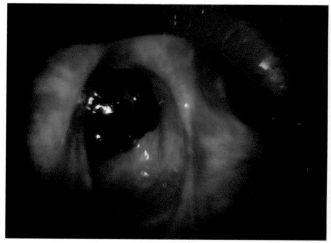

Figure 21-3. A black smooth mass of sarcomatous tissue obstructs the superior segment of the right lower lobe.

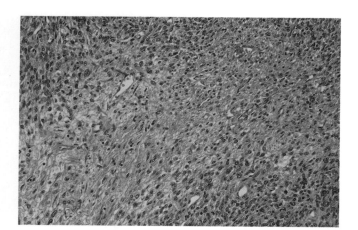

Figure 21-4. Pulmonary artery sarcoma manifesting as an endobronchial lesion; a subsequent pneumonectomy revealed extensive pulmonary parenchymal involvement (H&E, ×40, original magnification).

CHAPTER 22

Endobronchial Lymphoma

David R. Duhamel

Endobronchial involvement by primary bronchogenic tumor or metastatic solid tumor is a well-described occurrence. Lymphomatous involvement of the airways, however, is much less commonly described. The first description of any type of endobronchial involvement occurred in 1934, when Moolten described malignant plaques and ulcerations of the airways in two patients with Hodgkin's disease.[1] Subsequently, there have been multiple case reports in the literature of endobronchial involvement with both Hodgkin's[2,3] and non-Hodgkin's lymphoma.[4,5] However, it should be pointed out that from reviewing the world literature there appears to be a much higher incidence of endobronchial involvement with Hodgkin's disease versus non-Hodgkin's lymphoma. Endobronchial lymphoma has also been reported as the presenting manifestation of disease.[6] The most common pulmonary manifestations of endobronchial lymphoma are cough, dyspnea, and hemoptysis. In one case report wheezing was the only presenting symptom.[7]

Two bronchoscopic patterns have been described with lymphoma: an isolated endobronchial mass or diffuse submucosal nodules that may ulcerate.[8] In a small study of patients undergoing bronchoscopy for initial staging, 25% of Hodgkin's disease cases and 38% of non-Hodgkin's lymphoma cases had histologic evidence of endobronchial involvement.[9] The more common pattern is the diffuse whitish submucosal nodules lining the airway. This pattern is typically associated with systemic disease. The nodules are between 2 and 5 mm in diameter and are scattered diffusely through the airway. The other pattern of involvement, a localized endobronchial mass, invariably manifests with signs and symptoms of airway obstruction. The majority of these tumors appear to arise at a point of bifurcation in the airway. It is also typically associated with disease confined to the thoracic cavity. It is important to remember, however, that narrowing or displacement of the tracheobronchial tree by external compression of enlarged lymph nodes remains the most common airway finding.

In an analysis by Filly and colleagues of 300 previously untreated lymphoma patients, only 1 had radiographic evidence of endobronchial involvment.[10] In the setting of submucosal nodular involvement, a radiographic pattern of regional lymphadenopathy and parenchymal infiltrates is typically seen. Signs of endobronchial obstruction are rare in this pattern. The radiographic findings associated with a localized endobronchial mass are the classic lobar atelectasis and volume loss. Regional lymphadenopathy is also seen invariably.

The infrequency with which lymphoma occurs endobronchially was documented in an autopsy study by Vieta and Craver.[11] They found no evidence of pathologic involvement of the trachea or bronchi in 106 autopsies. The pattern of histologic involvement in endobronchial lymphoma could certainly be explained by hematogenous and/or lymphangitic spread of tumor. The diffuse submucosal nodular pattern could be a result of the centripetal spread of lymphoma cells from the parenchymal tissue to the central bronchi via lymphatics. It could also be explained by the hematogenous spread of lymphoma to the bronchial-associated lymphoid tissue, or BALT. It does seem certain that in the localized endobronchial tumor pattern the lesion arises from this BALT tissue. Evidence for this comes from immunoperoxidase stains of the obstructing lesion, which show surface expression of IgA, the major immunoglobulin class synthesized by BALT.[12] This also explains why the obstructing tumor arises at the bifurcation in the airway where the BALT tissue is most concentrated.

The clinical and prognostic impact of endobronchial involvement with lymphoma is unclear at this point. In a review of the literature by Rose and colleagues, it was found that 7 of 11 cases of non-Hodgkin's lymphoma had an initial complete response with radiation or chemotherapy or both. Unfortunately, no long-term follow-up information was available. The treatment of diffuse submucosal nodular involvement is no different from the treatment for routine thoracic lymphoma and should include radiation and chemotherapy. This disease pattern should respond to brachytherapy very well, although it has yet to be reported. A localized endobronchial tumor can be managed with any of the available interventional bronchoscopic techniques including Nd:YAG laser ablation, but should certainly be followed up by chemotherapy and radiation.

REFERENCES

1. Moolten SW: Hodgkin's disease of the lung. Am J Cancer Med 21:253-294, 1934.
2. Harper PG, Fisher C, McLennan K, Souhami RL: Presentation of Hodgkin's as an endobronchial lesion. Cancer 53:147-150, 1984.
3. Seward CW, Safdar SH: Endobronchial Hodgkin's disease presenting as a primary pulmonary lesion. Chest 62:649-651, 1972.
4. Pradham DJ, Rabuzzi D, Meyer JA: Primary solitary lymphoma of the trachea. J Thorac Cardiovasc Surg 70:938-940, 1975.
5. Kilgore TL, Chasen MH: Endobronchial non-Hodgkin's lymphoma. Chest 84:58-61, 1983.
6. Higginson JF, Grismer JT: Obstructing intrabronchial Hodgkin's disease. J Thorac Cardiovasc Surg 20:961-963, 1950.
7. Scully RE, Mark EJ, McNeely BU: Case 25-1984. Case records of the Massachusetts General Hospital. N Engl J Med 310:1653-1661, 1984.
8. Rose RM, Grigas D, Strattemeir E, et al: Endobronchial involvement with non-Hodgkin's lymphoma. A clinical radiologic analysis. Cancer 57:1750-1755, 1986.
9. Gallagher CJ, Knowles GK, Habeshaw JA, et al: Early involvement of the bronchi in patients with malignant lymphoma. Br J Cancer 48:777-781, 1983.
10. Filly R, Blank N, Catellino RA: Radiographic distribution of intrathoracic disease in previously untreated

patients with Hodgkin's disease and non-Hodgkin's lymphoma. Radiology 120:277-281, 1976.

11. Vieta JO, Craver LF: Intrathoracic manifestations of lymphomatoid diseases. Radiology 37:138-159, 1941.

12. Rudzik O, Clancy R, Perey D, et al: The distribution of a rabbit thymic antigen and membrane immunoglobulins in lymphoid tissue with special reference to mucosal lymphocytes. J Immunol 114:1-4, 1975.

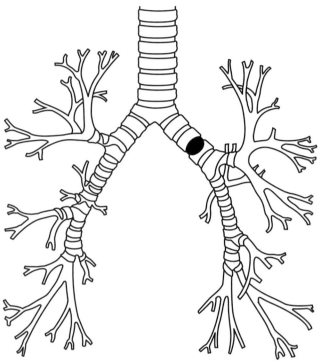

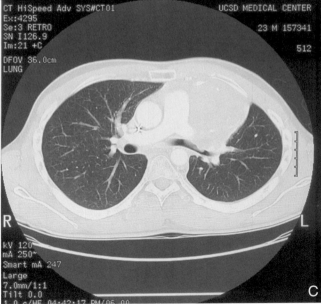

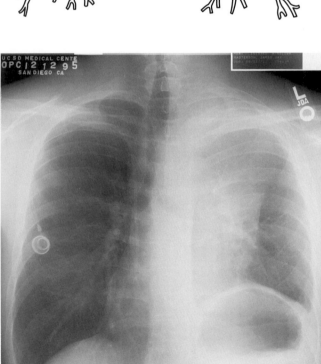

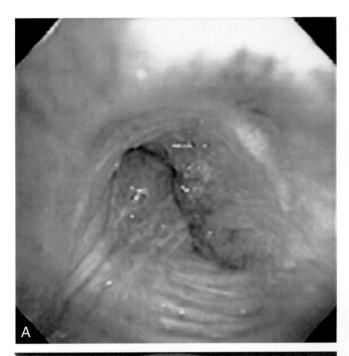

Figure 22-1. A, Complete obstruction of the left mainstem bronchus due to extrinsic compression and mucosal infiltration by lymphoma. **B,** A frontal radiograph demonstrating a large left hilar mass with an elevated left hemidiaphragm and volume loss. **C,** A CT scan demonstrating a large mediastinal mass with extension into the left mainstem bronchus.

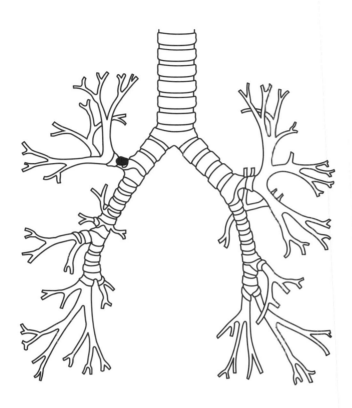

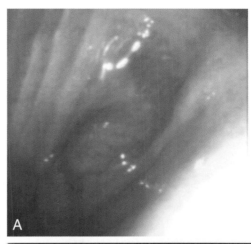

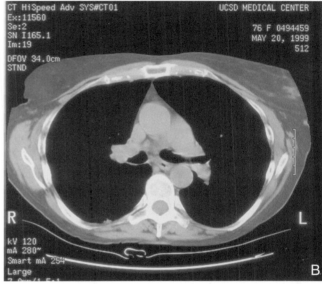

Figure 22-2. A, A smooth pink vascular lesion in the right upper lobe orifice that was found to be a lymphoma on biopsy. **B**, A CT scan demonstrating a right suprahilar tissue mass with involvement of the right upper lobe orifice.

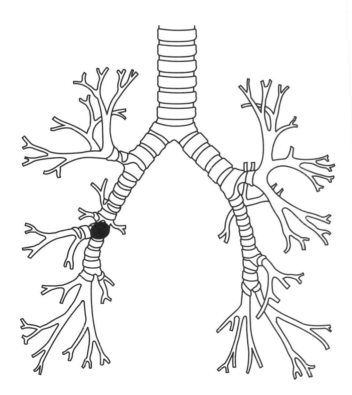

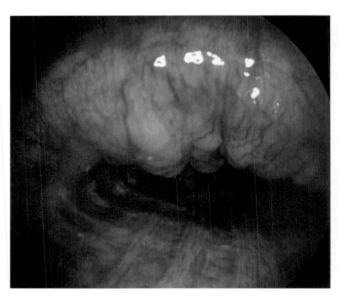

Figure 22-3. Partial obstruction of the right mainstem bronchus by an extensive lobulated growth of lymphoma tissue arising from the anterior bronchial surface.

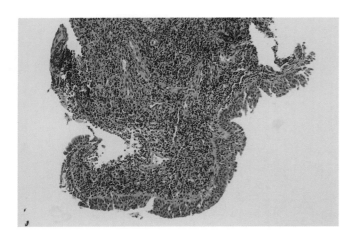

Figure 22-4. Submucosal infiltration of monotonous lymphoid cells (H&E, ×100, original magnification).

CHAPTER 23

Lipoma

David R. Duhamel

Although lipomas are the most common benign neoplasm throughout the body, thoracic lipomas remain relatively rare. Thoracic lipomas can appear within the tracheobronchial walls, lung parenchyma, pleura, or mediastinum. Endobronchial lipomas are estimated to be 0.1% of all pulmonary tumors[1] and 13% of benign lung tumors.[2] Despite their rarity, they can be clinically significant by simulating malignancy and causing lung destruction from recurrent postobstructive pneumonias. Unlike subcutaneous lipomas, which can be numerous, endobronchial lipomas are typically single lesions. They arise from the submucosal fat of the tracheobronchial tree and grow into the lumen of the bronchus. They typically manifest with symptoms of endobronchial obstruction, but this is variable and dependent on the size and location of the lesion. The average age of the patient is the mid-50s, and there is a definite male predominance.

The bronchoscopic appearance is that of a pedunculated tumor with a narrow stalk, composed of mature fat cells and covered with normal respiratory mucosa. They are firm, smooth, rounded, and freely movable. They are located most frequently in the lobar or segmental bronchi. On occasion, the lipoma extends in an hourglass-shaped fashion between cartilaginous rings and into the peribronchial tissue or even into the lung parenchyma.[3] The tissue coloration ranges from gray to pale pink. The mucosa is usually intact without ulcerations. The tumor often has a rubbery elastic texture that is due to the pliable capsule. As a result of this capsule, the tumor is resistant to "biting" with the biopsy forceps, and endobronchial biopsy specimens are frequently nondiagnostic.[4]

Viewed radiographically, the tumor can manifest with a normal chest film or with evidence of atelectasis, lobar collapse, postobstructive pneumonia, or even bronchiectasis from endobronchial obstruction. On CT scan, these lesions sometimes can be identified definitively based on the low attenuation values of fatty tissue. This is more easily seen in the lung parenchyma than the air-filled trachea. Nonetheless, the CT findings of a homogeneous mass with fatty density and no tumor contrast enhancement are considered diagnostic for lipoma.[5]

Endobronchial lipomas arise from histologically normal fat cells found in the peribronchial and submucosal tissue of the large bronchi. The tumor typically contains lobules of adipose tissue separated by fibrous septa. These tumor cells are indistinguishable from fat cells found elsewhere in the body, but do not appear to be metabolically active or utilized with starvation.[6] The tumors may be encapsulated and on occasion may exhibit squamous metaplasia of the overlying epithelium from recurrent infectious irritation.[7] There have been no reports of aggressive malignant behavior or metastatic complications seen with endobronchial lipomas. However, these tumors are not to be confused with their much more malignant relative, the liposarcoma.

Once the diagnosis has been made, there are a few treatment options. Endoscopic management has been very successful with a very low incidence of recurrence.[4] This technique includes devascularization with the Nd:YAG laser followed by mechanical débridement with the rigid bronchoscope. If the lesion is too distal to reach with the rigid bronchoscope, or if the distal lung parenchyma has been destroyed by recurrent infection, then thoracotomy with lobar resection is a better option. The role of bronchotomy with sleeve resection is limited because the majority of these patients can be treated safely and completely with a much less invasive endoscopic technique.

REFERENCES

1. Politis J, Funahashi A, Gehlsen JA, et al: Intrathoracic lipomas: Report of three cases and a review of the literature with emphasis on endobronchial lipoma. J Thorac Cardiovasc Surg 77:550-556, 1979.
2. Schraufnagel DE, Morin JE, Wang NS: Endobronchial lipoma. Chest 75:97-99, 1979.
3. Touroff ASW, Seley GP: Lipoma of the bronchus and the lung. A report of two unusual cases. Ann Surg 134:244-248, 1951.
4. Shah H, Garbe L, Nussbaum E, Dumon JF, et al: Benign tumors of the tracheobronchial tree, endoscopic characteristics and the role of laser resection. Chest 107:1744-1751, 1995.
5. Meta J, Caceres J, Ferrer J, et al: Endobronchial lipoma. J Comput Assist Tomogr 15:750-751, 1991.
6. Ten Eyck EA: Subpleural lipoma. Radiology 74:295-297, 1960.
7. Hakimi M, Font-Soto D, Gonzalez-Lavin L, et al: Endobronchial lipoma associated with squamous metaplasia of bronchial mucosa. Mich Med 3:129-131, 1975.

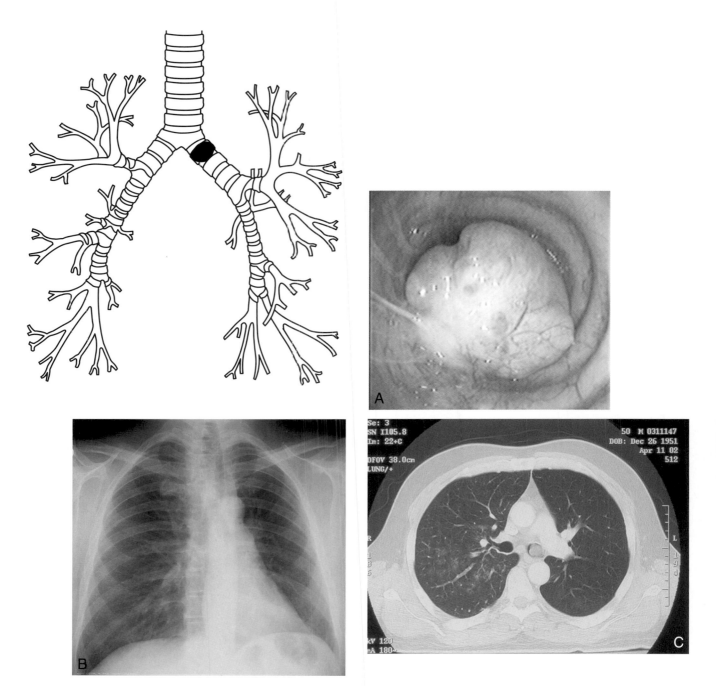

Figure 23-1. A, A pedunculated, smooth, yellow endobronchial lipoma that almost completely obstructs the proximal left mainstem bronchus. **B,** The frontal radiograph demonstrates a subtle soft tissue density that is present within the proximal left mainstem bronchus. No significant volume loss is present. **C,** A single CT image demonstrates a soft tissue mass within the left mainstem bronchus, nearly occluding the bronchus. The left lung remains well aerated.

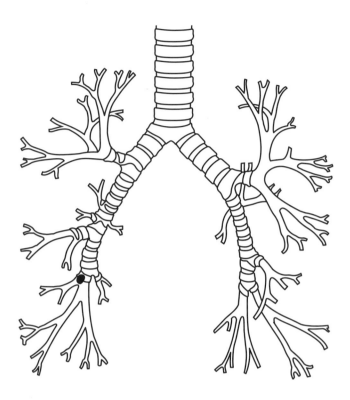

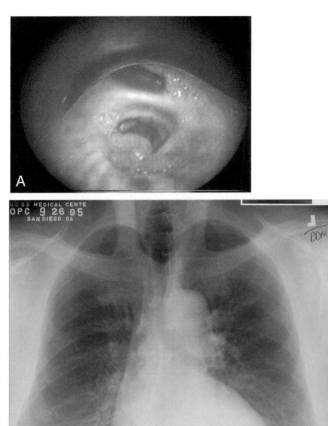

Figure 23-2. A, A soft gelatinous growth of endobronchial lipoma partially occludes the opening to the right lower lobe basilar subsegments. **B**, The frontal radiograph demonstrates a slight narrowing of the airway within the distal bronchus intermedius. No discrete mass is seen.

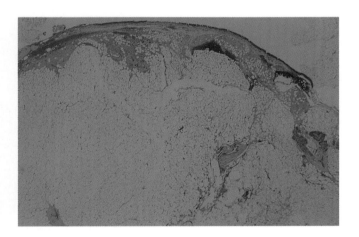

Figure 23-3. An endobronchial lipoma shows the same histologic features as seen in lipomas at other sites that are composed of mature fat and variable amounts of fibrous tissue (H&E, ×100, original magnification).

CHAPTER 24

Hamartoma

Jeffrey S. Prince

The term *hamartoma* refers to a tumor-like structure within an organ composed of an abnormal arrangement of tissue components normally found in that organ.[1] Pulmonary hamartomas are the second most common benign neoplasm of the pulmonary system.[2] However, they are rare within the central airways, accounting for 1.5%[3] and 8%[4] of all pulmonary hamartomas in the two large series. Airway hamartomas are of mesenchymal tissue origin and typically contain a predominance of adipose tissue. They have also been found to contain cartilage, myxomatous connective tissue, and smooth muscle epithelial structures.[5-7] Most hamartomas are discovered during adulthood with a peak incidence in the fifth decade. There is a 2 to 3:1 male prevalence. The majority of endobronchial hamartomas are isolated lesions, but they do arise in combination with parenchymal hamartomas. In the unusual occurrence of multiple hamartomas, the lesions often exhibit a predominance of leiomyomatous tissue. There is also a female predominance in this setting with an association with uterine leiomyomas.[8,9]

Clinical presentation in reported cases has varied depending on both the size of the lesion and the location within the tissue layers of the airway. In general, symptoms of airway obstruction with wheezing, stridor, and eventual respiratory compromise are common. Many cases have been misdiagnosed as asthma until the lesions were identified on either chest radiograph or at bronchoscopy. One case of a paratracheal mass without airway compromise was reported.[4] In the case of both airway and parenchymal lesions, the patients showed no symptoms of airway compromise. One had a history of recurrent pneumonia that was postulated to be secondary to focal obstruction resulting from the airway lesion.[6] The other patient had the endobronchial lesion discovered in the course of the workup for a pulmonary nodule that was also eventually diagnosed as a hamartoma.[5]

Bronchoscopically, the lesions are smooth, fleshy, pedunculated masses that may be tan to pink. The lesion is usually attached to the bronchial wall by a narrow fibrous stalk arising from the endobronchial mucosa. Rarely does the stalk arise from a cartilaginous ring. In the cases in which severe respiratory distress was encountered, the mass obscured 70% to 75% of the tracheal lumen.[3,5] Endobronchial hamartomas have been successfully removed both endoscopically and surgically without significant complication. One episode of recurrence after bronchoscopic removal is described.[5]

Radiographic findings include soft tissue masses within the central airways, which may have calcification. Secondary signs of lung hyperinflation, recurrent pneumonia, and bronchiectasis due to airway obstruction have also been described.[3,6] On CT scan, these lesions are described as rounded soft tissue masses that frequently exhibit calcifications. Because most endobronchial hamartomas exhibit a large proportion of adipose tissue, they can be recognized easily by their unique tissue density on CT scan. Lesions have also been described in both the parabronchial and paratracheal locations.[4,5]

From a histologic standpoint, the mesenchymal components of the endobronchial hamartomas are highly varied. There is a definite predominance of adipose tissue over other mesenchymal components.[10] This is probably related to the increased quantities of mural adipose tissue normally present in the larger airways. Cartilage is often absent or present in small amounts. There is also a paucity of epithelial clefts found in the hamartomas of the central airway compared with those found in the lung parenchyma. This probably reflects outward expansion, rather than an infolding growth process. The external surface is often lined by normal respiratory epithelium or metaplastic squamous epithelium. Most experts agree that the pathogenesis of a hamartoma can be explained by the pluripotent nature of the mesenchymal cell. In other words, a single mesenchymal cell has the ability to aberrantly differentiate into a host of mesenchymal tissue cell types. Some experts, however, would argue that the term *hamartoma* is defunct and should no longer be used to identify these lesions. Instead they should be named according the mesenchymal cell type or cell types that are most prevalent. I agree with this newer nomenclature but have opted to include this chapter for historical purposes because so much of the world literature makes use of the term *hamartoma*.

REFERENCES

1. Albrecht E: Ueber hamartome. Verh Dtsch Ges Pathol 7:153, 1904.
2. Hurt R: Benign tumours of the bronchus and trachea, 1951-1981. Ann R Coll Surg Engl 66:22-26; 1984.
3. Gjevre JA, Myers JL, Prakash UB: Pulmonary hamartomas. Mayo Clin Proc 71:14-19, 1996.
4. Van Den Bosch JMM, Wagenaar SS, Corrin B, et al: Mesenchymoma of the lung (so-called hamartoma): A review of 154 parenchymal and endobronchial cases. Thorax 42:790-797, 1987.
5. Carilli AD, Locurto J, Conoscenti C, et al: Tracheal hamartoma. Am J Med 81:1113-1114, 1986.
6. Gross E, Chen MK, Hollabaugh RS, Joyner RE: Tracheal hamartoma: Report of a child with a neck mass. J Ped Surg 31:1584-1585; 1996.
7. Reittner P, Mueller NL: Tracheal hamartoma: CT findings in two patients. J Comput Assist Tomogr 23(6):957-958, 1999.
8. Suzuki N, Ohno S, Ishii Y, Kitamura S: Peripheral intrapulmonary hamartoma accompanied by a similar endotracheal lesion. Chest 106(4):291-293, 1994.
9. Dominguez H, Hariri J, Pless S: Multiple pulmonary chondrohamartomas in trachea, bronchi, and lung parenchyma. Review of the literature. Respir Med 90:111-114, 1996.
10. Tomashefski JF: Benign endobronchial mesenchymal tumors. Their relationship to parenchymal pulmonary hamartomas. Am J Surg Path 6:531-540, 1982.

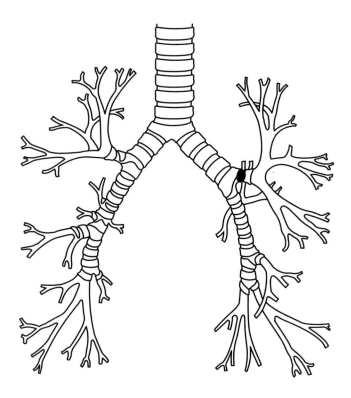

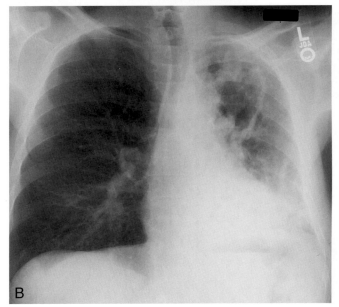

Figure 24-1. A, A chondromatous hamartoma that completely obstructs the left upper lobe orifice. **B,** The frontal radiograph demonstrates volume loss within the left lung with patchy air-space opacities within the left upper and lower lobes. No discrete mass is seen.

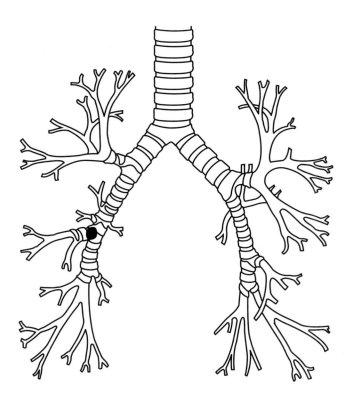

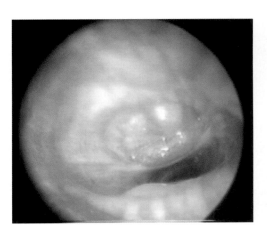

Figure 24-2. A smooth, pinkish, rubbery endobronchial hamartoma growing out of the right middle lobe orifice.

CHAPTER 25

Papillomatosis

Jeffrey S. Prince
David R. Duhamel

Papillomatosis is an uncommon disease entity caused by infection of the upper respiratory tract by the human papillomavirus (HPV). This disease entity is most common in children but may also occur in adults. Two thirds of patients are diagnosed before 5 years of age and most between 2 and 4 years of age, and symptoms at birth are not rare.[1] Infection may occur at the time of birth by passage of the child through an infected birth canal or later in life by oral contact with infected external genitalia. Laryngeal papillomas are the most common manifestation. Multifocal infection or aspiration of infected tissue from laryngeal papillomas may lead to infection of the trachea, bronchi, or even alveoli. However, this is a very rare manifestation of the disease. Involvement of the central airways occurs in 5% of patients with laryngeal papillomas. Small airway and alveolar involvement occur in less than 1%. Papillomas may be present singularly or multiply.[2] Presenting symptoms are hoarseness secondary to laryngeal papillomas and stridor.

Viewed bronchoscopically, these lesions appear white or pink and have a polypoid or lobulated appearance. The lesions have been described as fimbriated, or having the appearance of a cluster of "fish eggs." They are most frequently seen in the larynx but have been found in the trachea and bronchi as well. Near total obstruction of the airway is not an uncommon occurrence, especially in diffusely involved cases. In particularly severe cases, distal spread along the airway is the usual clinical course, with eventual involvement of the lung parenchyma.

The chest radiograph shows nodular narrowing of the airway, which may be focal or diffuse. Diffuse nodules are more common in children, whereas solitary nodules are more common in adults. If the papillomas have grown to adequate size, they may result in obstruction of the airways leading to atelectasis, air trapping, postobstructive infection, or bronchiectasis.[3] On CT scans, noncalcified intraluminal nodules may be seen. These affect only the mucosa and are therefore limited by the tracheal cartilaginous rings.[4] Parenchymal nodules may also be seen if there is alveolar involvement. These nodules commonly cavitate and are centrilobular on high-resolution CT of the chest.[2]

Pathologically, the nodules are limited to the mucosa. The lesion represents a proliferation of stratified squamous epithelium growing in a papillary or sessile fashion around a core of fibrovascular tissue.[5] Mitoses are rare but are not atypical. Malignant degeneration to squamous cell carcinoma occurs in approximately 10% of adult cases.[3] Of the greater than 46 types of HPV, two have been specifically associated with papillomatosis, HPV-11 and HPV-6.

These lesions are typically treated with endoscopic therapies including Nd:YAG laser and photodynamic therapy. Laser ablation seems to work very well, but recurrence is definitely a problem. The virus has been cultured out of the laser smoke plume, so proper respiratory precautions should be taken during laser therapy. Caution should also be taken during bronchoscopy not to macerate or traumatize the surrounding normal mucosa. Some bronchoscopists feel this contributes significantly to the spread of the disease into the distal airways. One promising new endoscopic therapy is called photodynamic therapy. The therapy is based on the concept that hematoporphyrin derivatives can be injected into the peripheral vein and disseminated throughout the entire body. It is cleared rapidly by normal cells but remains longer in neoplastic tissue. Because it is a dye, it preferentially absorbs light of a certain wavelength. The absorption of light activates a photochemical reaction and releases free radicals that cause cell death. Because the neoplastic cells concentrate the dye, they are the only ones affected by the reaction.[6] Topical application of cidofovir and other antiviral medications to the lesions is tedious and has been found to be of limited benefit. Our anecdotal experience has demonstrated a significant reduction in the extent of papillomatosis when the patient underwent external beam radiation for a concombinant squamous cell carcinoma. This finding suggests the possibility of using brachytherapy as a treatment option, but it needs to be evaluated further before it can be recommended.

REFERENCES

1. McCarthy MJ, Rosado-de-Christenson ML: Tumors of the trachea. J Thorac Imaging 10:180-198, 1995.
2. Gruden JF, Webb WR, Sides DM: Adult-onset disseminated tracheobronchial papillomatosis: CT features. J Comput Assist Tomogr 18(4):640-642, 1994.
3. Stark P: Radiology of the Trachea. New York, Thieme Medical Publishers, 1991.
4. Kwong JS, Müller NL, Miller RR: Diseases of the trachea and main-stem bronchi: Correlation of CT with pathologic findings. Radiographics 12:645-657, 1992.
5. Naka Y, Nakao K, Hamajii Y, et al: Solitary squamous cell papilloma of the trachea. Ann Thorac Surg 55:189-193, 1993.
6. McCaughan JS, Williams TE, Bethel B: Photodynamic therapy of endobronchial tumors. Lasers Surg Med 6:336-345, 1986.

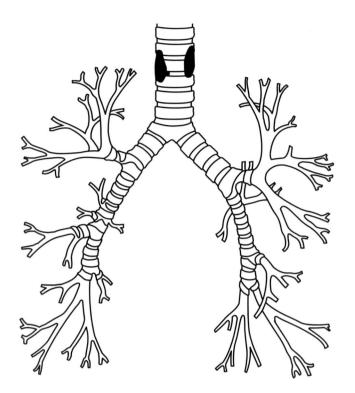

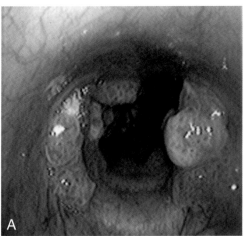

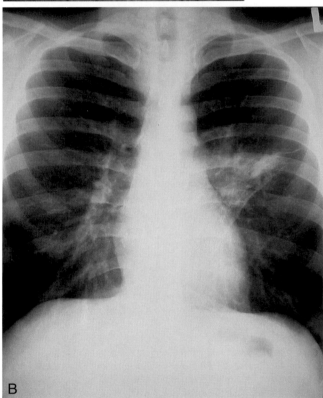

Figure 25-1. A, Multiple raised pinkish nodules in the trachea of a young man with congenital papillomatosis. This patient later succumbed from complications of squamous cell carcinoma. **B,** The frontal chest radiograph demonstrates partial left upper lobe collapse. A nodular focus is also present within the left midlung.

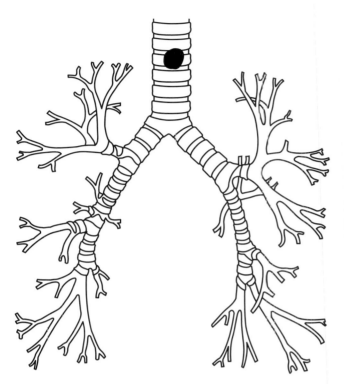

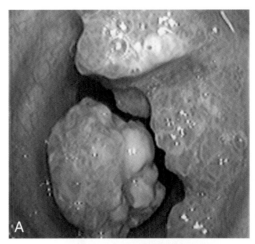

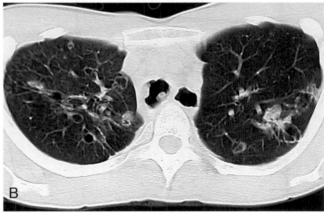

Figure 25-2. A, These partially obstructing papillomas in the trachea have the classic lobulated pattern on their surface. **B,** A single CT image demonstrates multiple nodules within the trachea and lung parenchyma. Several of the parenchymal nodules demonstrate cavitation.

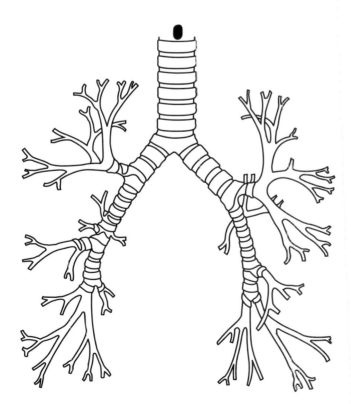

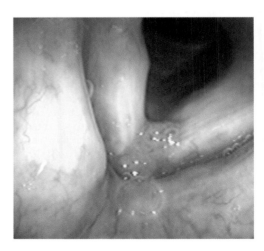

Figure 25-3. The typical "fish egg" appearance of papillomatosis seen on the anterior commissure of the vocal cords.

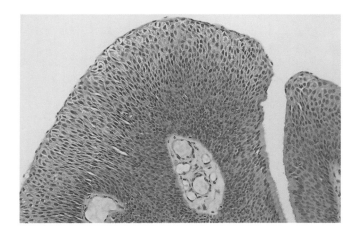

Figure 25-4. Squamous cell papillomatosis affecting the larynx and trachea. Some areas show cytologic changes reminiscent of cervical condyloma (H&E, ×20).

CHAPTER 26

Tumors of Nerve Sheath Origin

Jeffrey S. Prince
David R. Duhamel

Although neurogenic tumors are the most common primary tumor of the posterior mediastinum, they are exceedingly rare within the airway.[1] Benign neurogenic tumors arise from the Schwann cells of the peripheral nerve sheath and essentially occur in two forms: the neurofibroma and the neurilemoma. The neurofibroma is seen most frequently in association with neurofibromatosis or von Recklinghausen's disease. Neurofibromas are multiple, unencapsulated, occur within the nerve sheath, and are prone to malignant degeneration.[2] The neurilemoma is less common and is better known as a schwannoma. Neurilemomas are typically single, unencapsulated, attached to the nerve, and rarely undergo malignant degeneration.[2] Neurogenic tumors of the airway occur most frequently in the distal third of the trachea. In general, they are slow growing and can manifest at any age. Overall they represent approximately 0.2% of all lung tumors, with only 50 cases having been reported by 1983.[3]

Unger and associates[4] described 30 cases of primary neurogenic tumors and found that they could not be distinguished by their endoscopic appearance alone. Typically, they appear as smooth, rubbery, encapsulated lesions and are a pale tan-yellow. Sometimes the tumor manifests as a mass extruding into the tracheal lumen and other times as a submucosal bulge occluding the airway.[3] Neurofibromas of the vagus nerve have been reported to cause bronchial obstruction by extrinsic compression.[5] In addition, malignant

transformation of a neurofibroma to a neurofibrosarcoma can occur endobronchially or at a distant site, with subsequent metastasis to the airway.[6,7] Extensive submucosal infiltration and luminal obstruction due to multiple tracheal neurofibromas have been described in a human immuno-deficiency virus (HIV)–positive patient.[8] A prominent network of vasculature can sometimes be seen on the tumor surface, although an increased risk of bleeding has not been reported with biopsy or removal of these lesions.

Radiography may demonstrate a mass outlined against the tracheal air column. This is better demonstrated with a 30-degree left anterior oblique chest film to separate the trachea and vertebral column.[9] Less commonly, atelectasis or obstructive pneumonia is present due to bronchial obstruction. Neurilemomas typically show heterogeneous enhancement on CT scan with contrast enhancement due to the presence of lipid within myelin and areas of hypo-cellularity, cystic degeneration, or hemorrhage. Punctate foci of calcification are seen in about 10% of cases.[10] The characterization of a "dumbbell"-shaped tumor is sometimes used to describe the lesion's appearance on CT scan. This is because schwannomas arise from intramural neurogenic tissue. As the tumor grows, it is compressed by the cartilaginous rings and forced to expand into both the tracheal lumen and paratracheal space. The radiographic presentation of neurofibromatosis can be puzzling if a cutaneous truncal lesion appears to be a masslike density on chest radiograph, mimicking an intraparenchymal process. Bullae and pulmonary fibrosis are also seen. Neurofibromas of the phrenic nerve may manifest as mediastinal widening. Tumors of the intercostal nerves manifest with rib destruction and a chest wall mass. Rarely, pulmonary hypertension can develop from the interstitial fibrosis or neurofibromas impinging on the pulmonary arteries.

The pathologic diagnosis of a schwannoma can be difficult to make with only a bronchoscopic biopsy, and a definitive diagnosis is often only made upon resection. The distinguishing characteristics include a cellular Antoni A area with Verocay bodies; a loose, myxoid Antoni B area; and a uniformly intense staining for S-100 protein.[11] The majority of schwannomas are benign, but on occasion one exhibits malignant characteristics and is therefore considered a malignant schwannoma. Features suggestive of a malignant diagnosis include irregular wavy nuclei, nuclear palisading, tactoid differentiation, perineural and intraneural spread, and the presence of heterologous elements such as bone, cartilage, and muscle.[12] Histologically, neurofibromas are somewhat variable in appearance and consist of a mixture of spindle cells, myxoid stroma, and mature collagen.

The prognosis of patients with benign schwannomas or neurofibromas removed endoscopically or surgically is usually excellent. The tumors are amenable to resection with the Nd:YAG laser, but close follow-up is necessary owing to their tendency to recur.[13] The malignant neurogenic tumors including neurofibrosarcoma and malignant schwannoma carry a much worse prognosis. In one review of 40 malignant schwannomas, more than 75% of the patients died, with an average survival from the time of diagnosis being only 2 years.[14] The preferred treatment in these situations is surgery, if possible. Tracheal resection with end-to-end anastomosis is the ideal procedure and typically yields excellent results if the margins are free of disease.

REFERENCES

1. Bartley TD, Arean VM: Intrapulmonary neurogenic tumors. J Thorac Cardiovasc Surg 50:114-123, 1965.
2. Horovitz AG, Khalil KG, Verani RR, et al: Primary intratracheal neurilemoma. J Thorac Cardiovasc Surg 85:313-320, 1983.
3. Roviaro G, Montorsi M, Varoli F, et al: Primary pulmonary tumors of neurogenic origin. Thorax 38:942-945, 1983.
4. Unger PD, Geller SA, Anderson PJ: Pulmonary lesions in a patient with neurofibromatosis. Arch Pathol Lab Med 108:654-657, 1984.
5. Ross CR, McCauley DI, Naidlich DP: Intrathoracic neurofibroma of the vagus nerve associated with bronchial obstruction. J Comput Assist Tomogr 6(2):406-408, 1982.
6. Kodama K, Doi O, Higashiyama M, et al: Bronchial neurofibrosarcoma. Ann Thorac Surg 52(4):855-857, 1991.
7. Urrutia A, Guarga A, Tor J, et al: Endobronchial metastasis of a fibrosarcoma in multiple neurofibromatosis. Med Clin (Barc) 80(13):600, 1983.
8. Gillissen A, Kotterba S, Rasche K, et al: A rare manifestation of von Recklinghausen neurofibromatosis: Advanced neurofibromatous infiltration in lung of a HIV-positive patient. Respiration 61(5):292-294, 1994.
9. Weber AL, Grillo HC: Tracheal tumors. A radiological, clinical, and pathological evaluation of 84 cases. Radiol Clin North Am 16:227-246, 1978.
10. Ko SF, Lee TY, Lin JW, et al: Thoracic neurilemomas: An analysis of computed tomography findings in 36 patients. J Thorac Imaging 13:21-28, 1998.
11. McCluggage WG, Bharucha H: Primary pulmonary tumours of nerve sheath origin. Histopathology 26:247-254, 1995.
12. Enzinger FM, Weiss SW: Soft Tissue Tumors, 2nd ed. St Louis, CV Mosby, 1988, p 781.
13. Abudallo K, Romanoff H, Stern J, et al: Primary tumors of the thoracic trachea with special emphasis on surgical management. Int Surg 61:347-349, 1976.
14. Ingels GW, Campbell DC, Giampetro AM, et al: Malignant schwannomas of the mediastinum. Cancer 27:1190-1194, 1971.

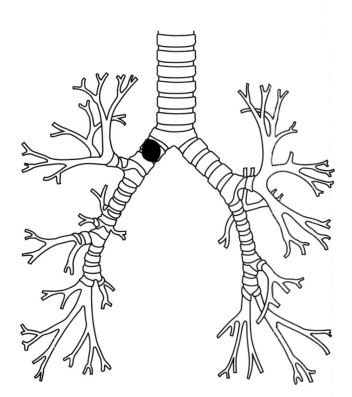

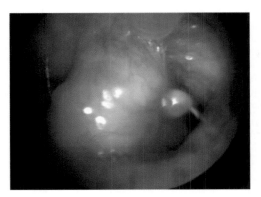

Figure 26-1. A smooth, pink, rubbery neurofibroma filling the proximal right mainstem bronchus. Note the nodular protuberance on the surface of the neurofibroma.

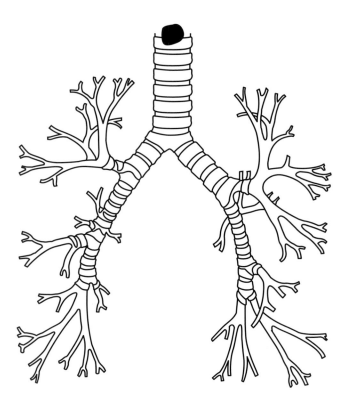

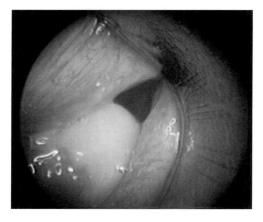

Figure 26-2. A smooth white schwannoma seen through the vocal cords in the subglottic space.

CHAPTER 27

Kaposi's Sarcoma

Gehan Devendra

Moritz Kaposi first described the skin malignancy that bears his name in 1872. He discovered these lesions among older men of eastern European, Mediterranean, or Jewish descent. Kaposi's sarcoma (KS) now is the most frequent neoplasm in the acquired immunodeficiency syndrome (AIDS) patient. The prevalence of KS varies from 1% of hemophiliacs to 21% of homosexuals.[1] The incidence of KS is declining, which is thought to be related to the increase in heterosexual AIDS patients. The difference in prevalence between groups is not known but may be related to infection with human herpesvirus 8 (HHV-8). The etiology of KS is believed to be related to, and possibly even caused by, HHV-8. HHV-8 can be extracted from a KS lesion, and the viral load has been correlated to extent of disease.[2]

KS in AIDS patients is usually located in the skin and oral mucosa. In decreasing frequency, the larynx, tracheo-bronchial tree, lung parenchyma, and the pleura are affected. Bronchopulmonary manifestations range between 3% and 13% in AIDS patients; up to 49% of AIDS patients have cutaneous KS. Pulmonary KS rarely occurs without lesions already diagnosed in another site. Naidich and colleagues found that of 114 patients with pulmonary manifestations of KS, about 28% had endobronchial disease.[3] Symptoms of endobronchial KS include dyspnea, cough, and hemoptysis. Stridor can also be a presenting symptom owing to a KS mass lesion in the trachea.[4] Caution must be applied because some patients have both KS and an infectious source, leading to the dyspnea. In these patients, there is usually a sign of mucocutaneous KS.

Radiographic studies of KS are nonspecific and do not correlate with the bronchoscopic findings. Chest CT features demonstrate thickening of the interlobular septa, ill-defined nodules with or without ground glass opacity, mediastinal adenopathy, and pleural and pericardial effusions.[5]

Bronchoscopic findings, for the most part, are classic in appearance. Usually the lesions are erythematous or violaceous and flat or slightly raised. These are discrete findings in the trachea and main bronchi, but they become more confluent in the distal airways and can be mistaken for bronchoscope trauma.[6] As described above, life-threatening airway obstruction has been documented. Biopsy of the lesions usually fails to yield a diagnosis. However, one report describes a technique for successfully obtaining a diagnostic specimen by biopsy of the minor carina subdividing the segmental orifices. The routine technique for biopsy of airway mucosa is frequently unsuccessful because the angle of the forceps with the bronchial wall is too oblique.[6] However, the numbers in this study were too small to make a definitive conclusion. The risk of bleeding after bronchoscopic biopsy has been controversial, with some studies reporting significant bleeding.[7] Therefore, if a biopsy cannot be obtained from an easily accessible location and the bronchoscopic findings are characteristic, a biopsy is probably not necessary.

Pathologically, KS lesions demonstrate neoformation of atypical lymphatics. Spindle cells in KS lesions express endothelial markers including CD31 and CD34. Factor VIII is expressed but in a small amount of cells. The spindle cells are latently infected with HHV-8. The KS spindle cells also express matrix metalloproteinase (MMP), which lyses extracellular matrix proteins.[8]

Therapy for AIDS-KS is directed toward palliation because no cure exists. The disease, however, responds to therapy. Intensification of highly active antiretroviral therapy (HAART) is first line. Pulmonary KS has shown regression with HAART.[9] Given the HHV-8 connection to KS, treatments directed against HHV-8 have been performed, with foscarnet and cidofovir showing some effect. Local therapy is not practical in disseminated disease such as pulmonary KS. Systemic therapies include interferon-alfa, liposomal daunorubicin, and paclitaxel, all of which have shown a clinical response. Experimental therapies include thalidomide, antiangiogenesis factors, and inhibition of MMP.[10]

REFERENCES

1. Beral V, Peterman TA, Berkleman RL, Jaffe HW: Kaposi's sarcoma among persons with AIDS: A sexually transmitted infection? Lancet 335:123-128, 1990.
2. Lucht E, Brytting M, Bjerregaard L, et al: Shedding of cytomegalovirus and herpesviruses 6, 7, and 8 in saliva of human immunodeficiency virus type 1–infected patients and healthy controls. Clin Infect Dis 27:137-141, 1998.
3. Naidich DP, Tarras M, Garay SM, et al: Kaposi sarcoma: CT-radiographic correlation. Chest 96:723-728, 1989.
4. Belda J, Canalis E, Gimferrer JM, et al: Subglottic stenosis in an HIV positive patient and exceptional form of clinical presentation in Kaposi's sarcoma. Eur J Cardiothorac Surg 11:191-193, 1997.
5. Traill ZC, Miller RF, Shaw PJ: CT appearances of intrathoracic Kaposi's sarcoma in patients with AIDS. Br J Radiol 69:1104-1107, 1996.
6. Hamm PG, Judson MA, Aranda CP: Diagnosis of pulmonary Kaposi's sarcoma with fiberoptic bronchoscopy and endobronchial biopsy. Cancer 59:807-810, 1987.
7. Pitchenik AE, Fischl MA, Saldana MJ: Kaposi's sarcoma of the tracheobronchial tree. Clinical, bronchoscopic, and pathologic features. Chest 87(1):122-124, 1985.
8. Meade-Tollin LC, Way D, Witte MH: Expression of multiple matrix metalloproteinases and urokinase type plasminogen activator in cultured Kaposi sarcoma cells. Acta Histochem 101:305-316, 1999.
9. Aboulfia DM: Regression of acquired immunodeficiency syndrome–related pulmonary Kaposi's sarcoma after highly active antiretroviral therapy. Mayo Clin Proc 73:439-443, 1998.
10. Hengge UR, Ruzicka T, Tyring SK, et al: Update on Kaposi's sarcoma and other HHV-8 associated diseases. Part 1: Epidemiology, environmental predispositions, clinical manifestations, and therapy. Lancet Infect Dis 2:281-292, 2002.

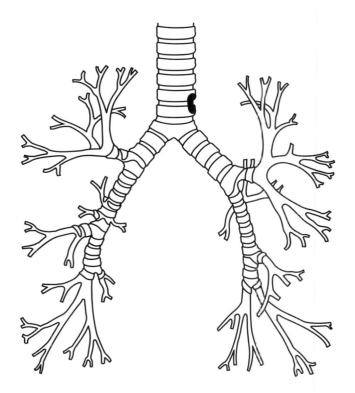

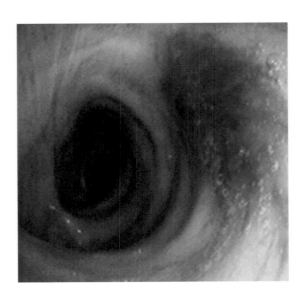

Figure 27-1. A, A classic, raised, reddish macular lesion on the distal left trachea of an AIDS patient with disseminated Kaposi's sarcoma.

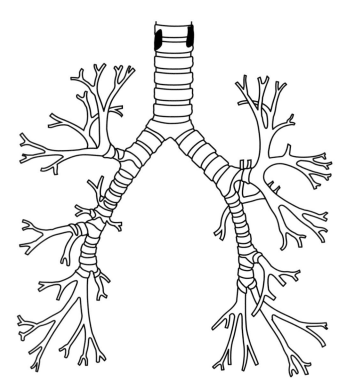

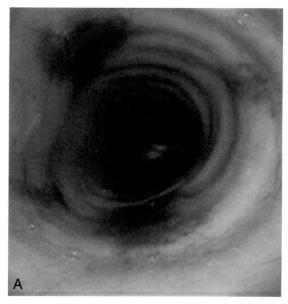

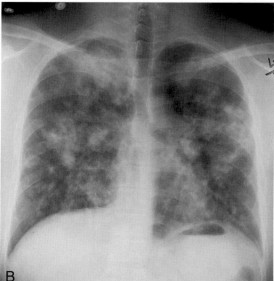

Figure 27-2. A, Multiple raised reddish patches in the trachea of a patient with AIDS. **B,** The frontal radiograph demonstrates multiple, ill-defined parenchymal nodules and masses.

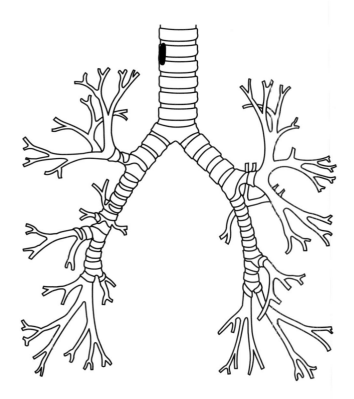

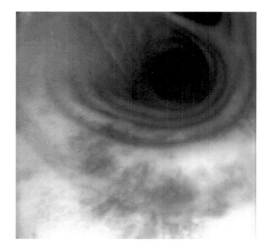

Figure 27-3. A reddish infiltrating lesion in the right lateral tracheal wall consistent with Kaposi's sarcoma.

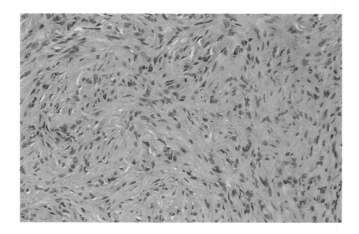

Figure 27-4. Atypical spindle cells forming slitlike spaces, interspersed red blood cells, and hemosiderin pigments in Kaposi's sarcoma (H&E, ×200).

CHAPTER 28

Leiomyoma

Jeffrey S. Prince

Leiomyomas of the tracheobronchial tree are extremely rare tumors. They make up 2% of all benign lesions of the airways. The first case report of a pulmonary leiomyoma was by Forkel in 1910. Leiomyomas manifest in a fashion very similar to other masses of the trachea with cough, hemoptysis, and shortness of breath, although many are asymptomatic at the time of presentation. A few case reports document positional dyspnea, which is increased with recumbency. This is probably related to a pendulating pedunculated lesion that intermittently obstructs the airway. These tumors generally occur in the fourth decade of life, but there are a significant number that occur in the pediatric age group. Tumors are generally solitary and may occur in the lung parenchyma, bronchi, or trachea. Parenchymal masses are twice as common in females as males. Tracheal occurrence is more common in males. The tumors are more common in the distal tracheobronchial tree and generally arise from the posterior membrane, where the majority of the smooth muscle is present.[1]

Histologically, smooth muscle tumors are characterized by bundles of spindle cells intersecting each other at wide angles. Masses found in the trachea and bronchi generally have little associated connective tissue stroma. Those found in the lung parenchyma have more vascular and fibrous stroma. Histologically, the parenchymal leiomyomas have an appearance very similar to uterine leiomyomas.[1] The smooth muscle origin of the cells is confirmed by Masson trichrome or lissamine fast red stains. Increased diagnostic accuracy may be obtained by using immunocytochemical staining or enzyme assays. These specialized techniques include the immunoperoxidase-myosin antibody test and the creatine phosphokinase isoenzyme assay, although the diagnosis of endobronchial smooth muscle tumor is made by light microscopy alone in more than 90% of cases.[2]

Viewed radiographically, these masses appear as smooth masses within the airway or hila on plain film. Larger masses may cause obstruction resulting in atelectasis, air-trapping, or postobstructive pneumonia.[1] In cases in which dysphagia is present, an esophagogram may be performed as part of the workup. A leiomyoma arising from the posterior membrane of the trachea may cause dysphagia by extrinsic compression of the esophagus.[3] CT findings include a smooth endotracheal, endobronchial, or hilar mass without invasion of adjacent structures.[4]

Bronchoscopic findings are that of a smooth endobronchial mass that may or may not cause obstruction. The lesions are more often pedunculated and rarely extend into the adjacent tracheobronchial wall. Ulceration of the mass is uncommon.[3-5] A prominent meshlike pattern of vascularity is often present on the tumor surface. Therapy for leiomyomas of the respiratory tract is most commonly surgical resection. The lesions have little or no response to chemotherapy or radiation. Resection may be performed via a thoracotomy or neck incision depending on the location of the mass. Segmental bronchial or tracheal resection with reanastomosis is the preferred operation. Bronchoscopic excision has been attempted but is not used as commonly as surgical resection unless the patient is a poor surgical candidate. Treatment of postobstructive sequelae may require lobectomy or alternatively bronchoscopic resection followed by surgery after the infection has resolved.[1,3] Provided that the tumors can be adequately excised, the prognosis is good even in histologically malignant forms; both local recurrence and metastases are exceptional.[6]

REFERENCES

1. White SH, Ibrahim NB, Forrester-Wood CP, Jeyansingham K: Leiomyomas of the lower respiratory tract. Thorax 40(4):234-237, 1985.
2. Yellin A, Rosenman Y, Lieberman Y: Review of smooth muscle tumors of the lower respiratory tract. Br J Dis Chest 78:337-351, 1984.
3. Borski TG, Stucker FJ, Grafton WD, Nathan CA: Leiomyoma of the trachea: A case report and a novel surgical approach. Am J Otolaryngol 21(2):119-121, 2000.
4. Allen HA, Angell F, Hankins J, Whitley NO: Leiomyoma of the trachea. AJR Am J Roentgenol 141(4):683-684, 1983.
5. Paludetti G, Rosignobi M: Leiomyoma of trachea: Report of case and review of the literature. J Laryngol Otol 98(9):947-951, 1984.
6. Guccion JG, Rosen SH: Bronchopulmonary leiomyosarcoma and fibrosarcoma: A study of 32 cases and review of the literature. Cancer 30:836-841, 1972.

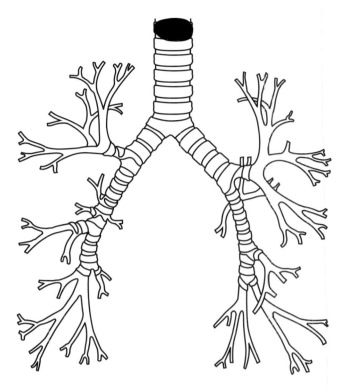

Figure 28-1. A, A smooth vascular leiomyoma arising from the right lateral trachea that is touching but not infiltrating the left tracheal wall. **B,** The frontal radiograph demonstrates irregularity of the proximal tracheal air column with a soft tissue density arising from the right lateral aspect of the tracheal wall.

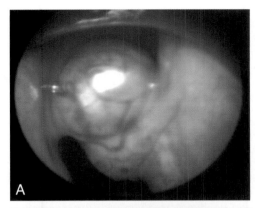

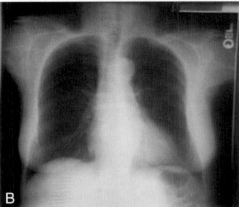

CHAPTER 29

Plasma Cell Granuloma

David R. Duhamel

Plasma cell granuloma of the lung is a slow-growing, localized, benign lesion of lung parenchyma, airways, and, rarely, pleura. It is characterized by a connective tissue stroma infiltrated by many plasma cells along with a few lymphocytes, histiocytes, and mast cells.[1] There is considerable variation in nomenclature, and the lesion has been called inflammatory pseudotumor, histiocytoma, xanthoma, xanthogranuloma, and mast cell granuloma, which makes understanding the incidence, natural history, pathology, and clinical course very difficult.[2] The typical patient is younger than 30, with men and women being affected equally.

Golbert and Pletnev noted an incidence of 0.7% in a large series of tumors of the lung and bronchi.[3] The majority of patients with plasma cell granuloma are asymptomatic owing to its more frequent presentation as a solitary parenchymal lung nodule. Endobronchial lesions can occur rarely, and typically manifest with shortness of breath, cough, hemoptysis, and postobstructive pneumonia. In various case series, endobronchial involvement was seen from 5.5% to 12% of the time.[4] The etiology is unclear, but localized injury with subsequent chronic inflammation is believed to play a role.[2] A significant proportion of patients give a recent history of pneumonia or upper respiratory tract infection, but a specific etiologic agent has rarely been isolated. There are two reported cases of inflammatory pseudotumor of the lung in association with *Coxiella burnetii*[5,6] as well as with actinomyces and mycoplasma.

There are a few different radiologic presentations for this disease, but none is very specific for the diagnosis. Cox and colleagues described the most common presentation as a well-circumscribed round or oval homogeneous mass lesion of the lung parenchyma without surrounding tissue reaction.[7] These lesions range in size from 1 cm in diameter to those that affect the entire hemithorax. In a recent review of the radiologic manifestations of plasma cell granuloma, calcifications were seen in 15%, cavitation in 5%, and pleural effusions in less than 1%.[8] A second manifestation is that of pneumonic consolidation along with atelectasis and air bronchograms.[9] An endobronchial lesion can be seen, with airway obstruction leading to atelectasis, hyperinflation, or postobstructive pneumonia.

The bronchoscopic appearance of these lesions is highly variable. Depending on the amount of fibrosis and the degree of histiocytic, lymphocytic, and plasmacytic infiltration, the color can be gray, tan, or yellow. Endobronchial and transbronchial biopsies are unfortunately infrequently diagnostic due to inadequate size and tissue architecture of the specimen. For the same reasons, fine-needle aspiration is often not helpful. The diagnosis is usually made from the resected surgical specimen.

Microscopically, plasma cell granulomas are a localized proliferation of mature plasma cells, histiocytes, and lymphocytes supported by a stroma of granulation tissue. Cytologic features are bland and mitotic features are rare. Russell bodies are often seen within the plasma cell representing an accumulation of immunoglobulins. Immunoperoxidase staining reveals the polyclonal nature of the plasma cell proliferation, which supports a non-neoplastic nature of the plasma cells. However, clonal abnormalities in the spindle cells have been reported.[10] Subsequently, fusion oncogenes were reported in these lesions, thus indicating that at least a subset represents a mesenchymal neoplasm currently known as inflammatory myofibroblastic tumor.[11] There are no reported cases of metastasis, but the lesions have been shown to invade various structures including the spine, chest wall, diaphragm, great vessels, and mediastinum.

Complete surgical resection with adequate tissue margins is the treatment of choice. In the setting of isolated endobronchial disease, a sleeve resection is sometimes curative, but due to concomitant parenchymal involvement a lobectomy or even pneumonectomy is often required. Unfortunately, the diagnosis is often made on the surgical specimen, but if the diagnosis is made before surgery, a lung-sparing operation is recommended. There have been rare case reports of successful endobronchial resection with a rigid bronchoscope and Nd:YAG laser. In surgically unresectable cases, radiation therapy has been reported to exhibit both good and bad responses.[2,12] The role of steroids is uncertain at this point. Recurrence rate is almost zero if the lesion is completely removed. However, long-term follow-up is required because recurrent tumors have developed many years after resection.

REFERENCES

1. Bahadori M, Liebow A: Plasma cell granulomas of the lung. Cancer 31:191-208, 1973.
2. Mehta J, Desphande S, Stauffer JL, et al: Plasma cell granuloma of the lung: Endobronchial presentation and absence of response to radiation therapy. South Med J 73:1198-1201, 1980.
3. Golbert ZV, Pletnev SV: On pulmonary "pseudotumors." Neoplasma 14:189-198, 1967.
4. Berardi RS, Lee SS, Chen HP, Stines GJ: Inflammatory pseudotumors of the lung. Surg Gyn Obstet 156:89-96, 1983.
5. Janigan DT, Marrie TJ: An inflammatory pseudotumor of the lung in Q fever pneumonia. N Engl J Med 308:86-88, 1983.
6. Lipton JH, Fong TC, Gill MJ, et al: Q fever inflammatory pseudotumor of the lung. Chest 92:756-757, 1987.
7. Cox IL, Chang CHJ, Mantz F: Pseudotumor of the lung: A case report and review stressing radiographic criteria. Chest 67:723-725, 1975.
8. Agrons GA, Rosado-de-Christenson ML, Kirejczyk WM, et al: Pulmonary inflammatory pseudotumor: Radiologic features. Radiology 206:511-518, 1998.
9. McCall IW, Woo-Ming W: The radiologic appearances of plasma cell granuloma of the lung. Clin Radiol 29:145-150, 1978.
10. Snyder CS, Dell'Aquila M, Haghighi P, et al: Clonal changes in inflammatory pseudotumor of the lung. Cancer 76:1545-1549, 1995.
11. Lawrence B, Perez-Alayde A, Hibbard MK, et al: TPM 3-ALK and TPM 4-ALK oncogenes in inflammatory myofibroblastic tumors. Am J Pathol 157:377-384, 2000.
12. Imperato JP, Folkman J, Sagerman RH, et al: Treatment of plasma cell granuloma of the lung with radiation therapy: A report of two cases and review of the literature. Cancer 57:2127-2129, 1986.

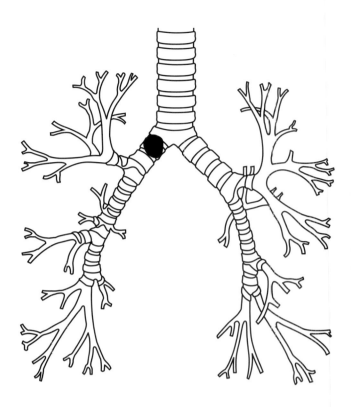

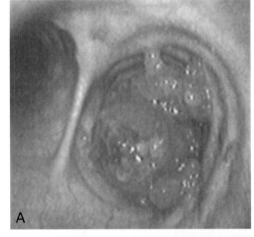

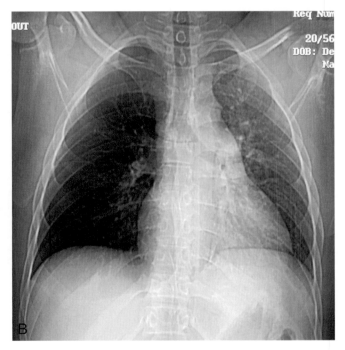

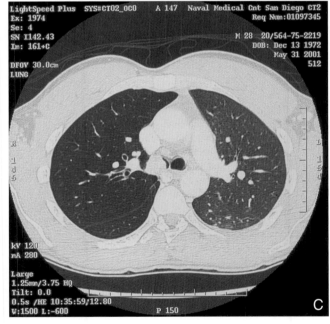

Figure 29-1. A, A reddish-brown lobulated growth arising from the right mainstem bronchus and found to be a plasma cell granuloma on bronchoscopic resection. There is no mucosal infiltration seen, which is consistent with a benign process. **B,** A scout image from a CT study demonstrates a soft tissue mass arising from the proximal right main bronchus. **C,** The CT image demonstrates near complete occlusion of the right main bronchus. There is hyperinflation of the right lung secondary to air trapping.

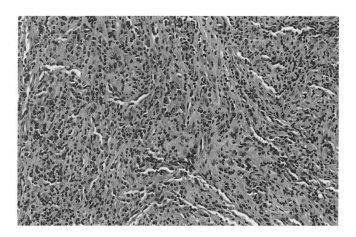

Figure 29-2. The tumor shows a mixture of bland spindle cell (myofibroblastic) proliferation and heavy inflammatory infiltrates (H&E, ×100, original magnification).

CHAPTER 30

Granular Cell Tumor

David R. Duhamel

Granular cell tumors, or granular cell myoblastomas as they were originally called, are fairly common benign neoplasms found predominantly in the skin, tongue, breast, and subcutaneous tissue. Originally described in 1926 by Abrikossoff,[1] who thought that they originated from embryonic muscle cells, they are now believed to be neuronal in origin, derived from the Schwann cell.[2] They occur in the lung as endobronchial tumors, predominantly affecting the larynx and main bronchi. Tracheal involvement is much less common. The tumors are more common in women and in the black population, with the majority of patients between ages 30 and 50. Patients typically present with cough, hemoptysis, localized wheezing, chest pain, and recurrent infections.

The diagnosis is typically made at bronchoscopy. Tumors appear as a yellowish-white, irregular, polypoid protuberance into the airway lumen or, less commonly, as a raised sessile plaque on the bronchial wall. The lesions are typically small, ranging from 1 to 2 cm in size up to 8 cm. The classic bronchial location is at a bifurcation in the airway. A significant number of granular cell tumors of the airway are multicentric, with percentages ranging from 8% to 15%.[3,4]

Due to the small size and endobronchial location, the tumor is rarely evident on chest roentgenogram. The radiographic manifestations, when they occur, are due to endobronchial obstruction and include segmental or lobar consolidation, atelectasis, bronchiectasis, and hilar or parenchymal mass.[5]

Histologically, the tumors consist of large polyhedral cells with abundant granular eosinophilic cytoplasm and relatively small round or oval nuclei. There is no significant nuclear atypia, pleomorphism, or increased mitotic figures.

Grossly, they are not encapsulated, and extension into the submucosa and peribronchial interstitial tissue is frequent. However, involvement of the adjacent pulmonary parenchyma and distant metastasis are extremely rare. A frequent finding is pseudoepitheliomatous hyperplasia of the overlying epithelium, which can easily be confused with squamous cell carcinoma.[3]

Treatment of these benign lesions has been debated widely. The treatment of choice is surgical excision, which is successful in 99% of cases. Daniel and colleagues,[6] after reviewing the literature and their own experience, made some recommendations. They believed that endobronchial therapy, including laser, was indicated for lesions smaller than 8 mm and lung-sparing surgical resection was needed for lesions larger than 8 mm. Their recommendations were based on the observation that full-thickness bronchial extension of the tumor had occurred in all lesions larger than 8 mm and that this was associated with a high incidence of recurrence after endobronchial therapy. It should be pointed out that the majority of endobronchial resections in this study were done with a CO_2 laser, which in general is far inferior to the Nd:YAG laser when treating endobronchial neoplasms. Multiple case reports of successful endobronchial therapy using Nd:YAG laser[7] and bipolar cautery[8] have been published recently, which are strong evidence for the rethinking of Daniel's recommendations. Neither chemotherapy nor radiation has a role in the treatment of this disease entity. Overall, the prognosis is excellent after successful surgical or bronchoscopic treatment.

REFERENCES

1. Abrikossoff AJ: Über myome, ausgehend von der guergestreiften willkürlichen Muskulatur. Arch Pathol Anat 260:215-233, 1926.
2. Sobel HJ, Marguet E, Avrin E, Schwarz R: Granular cell myoblastoma: An electron microscopic and cytochemical study illustrating the genesis of granules and aging of myoblastoma cells. Am J Pathol 65:59-71, 1971.

3. Mikaelian DO, Cohn H, Israel H, Jabourian Z: Granular cell tumor of the trachea. Ann Otol Rhinol Laryngol, 93:457-459, 1984.

4. Ivatury R, Shah D, Ascer E, et al: Granular cell tumor of the larynx and bronchus. Ann Thorac Surg 33:69-73, 1982.

5. Redjaee B, Rohatgi PK, Herman MA: Multicentric endobronchial granular cell myoblastoma. Chest 98:945-948, 1990.

6. Daniel TM, Smith RH, Faunce HF, Sylvest VM: Transbronchial versus surgical resection of tracheobronchial granular cell myoblastomas: Suggested approach based on follow up of all treated cases. J Thorac Cardiovasc Surg 80:898-903, 1980.

7. Epstein LJ, Mohsenifar Z: Use of Nd:YAG laser in endobronchial granular cell myoblastoma. Chest 104:958-960, 1993.

8. Cunningham L, Wendell G, Berkowitz L, et al: Treatment of tracheobronchial granular cell myoblastomas with endoscopic bipolar cautery. Chest 96:427-429, 1989.

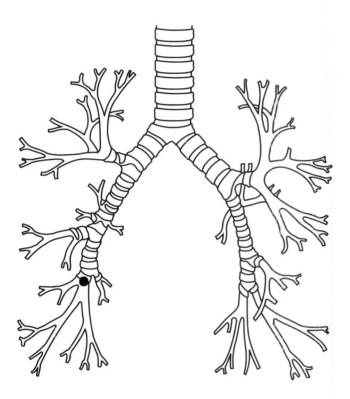

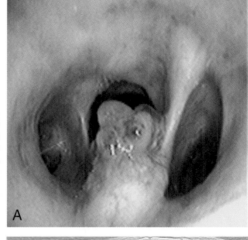

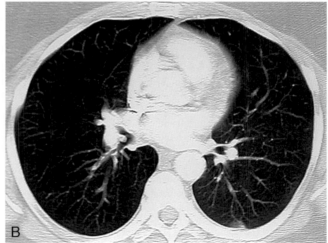

Figure 30-1. A, A tan polypoid pedicle of granular cell tumor growth at the level of the right basilar segment orifices. **B,** A CT image demonstrates a small endobronchial mass within the right lower lobe bronchus.

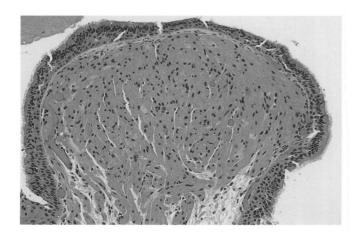

Figure 30-2. Granular cell tumor covered with intact endobronchial mucosa (H&E, ×20).

CHAPTER 31

Smooth Muscle Tumors Related to the Human Immunodeficiency Virus

David R. Duhamel

Tumors of smooth muscle origin such as leiomyomas and leiomyosarcomas are extremely unusual in the lung. It is well known that the human immunodeficiency virus (HIV) predisposes an individual to certain neoplasms, and it has recently been recognized that leiomyomas and leiomyosarcomas are included among these tumors. These tumors have been reported to arise in the skin, liver, adrenal glands, gastrointestinal tract, and the airway of HIV-positive children and adults. More recently, McClain and coworkers[1] reported an association between the Epstein-Barr virus and smooth muscle tumors occurring in patients with acquired immunodeficiency syndrome (AIDS). They demonstrated the presence of the Epstein-Barr virus genome within tumor cell nuclei. Similar tumors have been reported in patients with various immunocompromising conditions, such as liver and kidney transplants and following chemotherapy for cancer and leukemia.[2]

Tumors of smooth muscle origin involving the airway are rare in HIV-positive patients. The world literature contains reports of six cases of endobronchial leiomyomas and leiomyosarcomas.[2-4] The majority of these lesions are reported in the pediatric and young adult population. These tumors have been reported to be multicentric in at least two patients.[3,4] In one patient both a leiomyoma and a leiomyosarcoma were discovered, suggesting the possibility of malignant degeneration. These lesions are known to develop more commonly in the bronchi rather than the trachea and have been reported to completely obstruct a lobar bronchus, resulting in atelectasis. The most common presenting symptom appears to be wheezing that fails to respond to bronchodilator therapy.

The smooth muscle tumors appear smooth and rounded on bronchoscopic inspection. They appear to have an intact mucosal surface and can grow large enough to completely fill the endobronchial lumen. Smaller satellite lesions have been noted in proximity to the primary lesion. The lesion can be biopsied easily without increased bleeding risk. These tumors tend to have subtle, if any, radiographic findings on presentation. Unexplained air trapping due to complete endobronchial obstruction was seen in a few patients. One lesion was reported to be partially calcified on CT scan.

The histopathology of these endobronchial tumors revealed a proliferation of spindle cells with cigar-shaped nuclei and eosinophilic fibrillar cytoplasms that were arranged in bundles and fascicles characteristic of smooth tissue tumors.[4] The tumors appeared poorly circumscribed and were partially covered with reactive bronchial epithelium and without evidence of necrosis. The leiomyomas lacked any overtly sarcomatous regions and had low mitotic indexes with fewer than five mitotic figures per 50 high-power fields. The tumor cells are typically strongly reactive for smooth muscle markers such as actin and desmin. The association between these tumors and the Epstein-Barr virus (EBV) can be confirmed by in situ hybridization using an oligonucleotide against EBV-encoded ribonucleic acid (RNA)-1.[4] The absence of EBV in smooth muscle tumors of nonimmunocompromised patients[1] and the monoclonality of EBV in tumor tissue[5] strongly suggest that EBV infection may contribute to the pathogenesis of these tumors in the HIV-positive patient.[1] HIV probably does not play a direct role in the tumorigenesis of these lesions, as evidenced by the extremely low levels of virus in the tumor tissue.[1]

The treatment of many of these airway lesions has not been an issue because they were found at autopsy. In two cases, attempts were made to endoscopically resect the lesions using laser therapy.[3,4] This effort was found to be partially successful, but the lesions tended to recur or develop at other sites. There are no reports of chemotherapy, radiation, or surgery being used to treat these lesions. The overall life expectancy of patients who develop these tumors is limited. However, they typically succumb to complications of HIV disease rather than airway obstruction. As a result of new antiretroviral therapies being developed, patients are living much longer with AIDS and HIV. One should therefore anticipate a rising number of clinically symptomatic smooth muscle tumors of the airway in the future. Unexplained wheezing or volume loss seen on a radiograph in an HIV-positive patient should raise a clinician's suspicion for a leiomyoma or leiomyosarcoma of the airway.

REFERENCES

1. McClain KL, Leach CT, Jensen HB, et al: Association of Epstein-Barr virus with leiomyosarcomas in young people with AIDS. N Engl J Med 332:12-18, 1995.
2. de Chadarevian JP, Wolk JH, Iniss S, et al: A newly recognized cause of wheezing: AIDS-related bronchial leiomyomas. Pediatr Pulmonol 24:106-110, 1997.
3. Balsam D, Segal S: Two smooth muscle tumors in the airway of an HIV-infected child. Pediatr Radiol 22:552-553, 1992.
4. Bluhm JM, Yi ES, Diaz G, et al: Multicentric endobronchial smooth muscle tumors associated with the Epstein-Barr virus in an adult with acquired immunodeficiency syndrome. Cancer 80:1910-1913, 1997.
5. Lee ES, Locker J, Nalesnik M, et al: The association of Epstein-Barr virus with smooth-muscle tumors occurring after organ transplant. N Engl J Med 332:19-25, 1995.

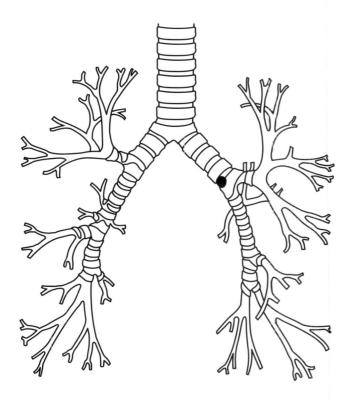

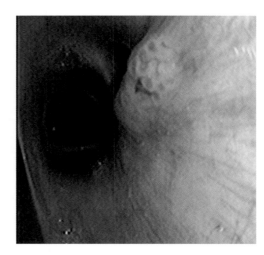

Figure 31-1. A small raised deposit of smooth muscle tumor arising from the wall of the left mainstem bronchus in a patient with AIDS. Note the appearance is similar to that of a papilloma.

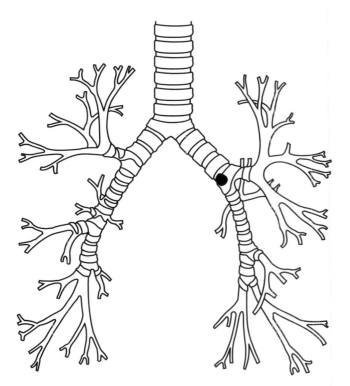

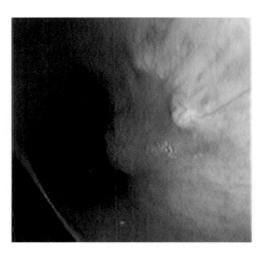

Figure 31-2. Three months later the same lesion appears to have developed satellite lesions.

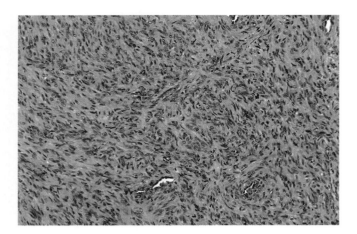

Figure 31-3. The smooth muscle tumor cells (H&E, ×100) contain Epstein-Barr virus RNA as shown by an in situ hybridization study.

CHAPTER 32

Pleomorphic Adenoma

David R. Duhamel

Pleomorphic adenomas, also commonly referred to as mixed tumors, are the most common histologic form of salivary gland neoplasm.[1] Tumors of salivary gland origin are known to occur in the lung and typically arise from the tracheal and bronchial seromucous glands. This family of tumors forms less than 0.5% of all lung cancers. The more common tumors of the bronchial mucous glands include muco-epidermoid carcinoma and adenoid cystic carcinoma. Other rare variants include acinic cell carcinoma and pulmonary oncocytoma, with the pleomorphic adenoma being reported least commonly. These tumors are extremely uncommon, with approximately 20 verifiable cases documented in the literature by 1995.[1] The age of patients affected ranges from 27 to 74 years, with equal distribution between men and women. These tumors tend to have an indolent course with one third of cases being discovered incidentally. The remainder manifest with the typical symptoms of obstructive pneumonitis, which include cough, hemoptysis, inspiratory wheezing, and dyspnea.

These tumors may grow significantly and in so doing occupy a large portion of lung parenchyma, making their bronchial origin difficult to appreciate. Other lesions have been noted to arise solely from lung parenchyma without any bronchial component.[1] Viewed bronchoscopically, these tumors are described as polypoid lesions typically arising in the trachea but also are known to develop in the mainstem bronchi. The lesions classically arise from the posterolateral surface of the trachea or bronchus where the glandular elements are most densely concentrated. The lesions have been described as anything from grayish white to pale pink.

Occasionally, the tumor surface contains a prominent vascular pattern but always an epithelial lining. Because the histologic pattern is highly variable within a particular tumor, it may prove difficult to establish a diagnosis with small biopsy fragments obtained bronchoscopically.[2]

Viewed radiographically, there may be evidence of volume loss, atelectasis, or obstructive pneumonitis seen with a large endobronchial lesion. A significant infiltration of the lung parenchyma by the tumor mass is sometimes seen with the pleomorphic adenomas. This behavior is unique compared with other types of salivary gland tumors such as adenoid cystics and mucoepidermoids. CT scan plays a vital role in the initial detection of endobronchial disease, as well as the depth and extent of mediastinal and parenchymal involvement.

By light microscopy, the tumors are seen to be biphasic, consisting of epithelial and myoepithelial structures. The epithelial component consists of sheets or glandular structures. The myoepithelial component consists of myxomatous and chondroid stroma.[1] The pleomorphic adenoma is not infrequently confused with a bronchial carcinoid. The stroma of the carcinoid may on occasion undergo osseous, cartilaginous, or amyloid changes similar to what is seen histologically with the pleomorphic adenoma.[3] The presence of adipose tissue has been noted within the tumor stroma as well.[4] Mitotic figures are an unusual finding with most pleomorphic adenomas, but some tumors display more malignant characteristics including frequent mitoses and nuclear atypia. The immunohistochemical stains S-100 and glial fibrillary acidic protein (GFAP) also appear to be helpful tools in making the diagnosis of pleomorphic adenoma.[5]

Because so few cases of pleomorphic adenoma of the airways have been documented, it is difficult to assess their prognosis. In the salivary gland, pleomorphic adenomas are noted for their tendency to recur, mostly owing to their gross morphology and difficulty in obtaining clear surgical margins. However, recurrence of a pleomorphic adenoma of the bronchus has been documented only once, and in that instance it was unclear whether adequate surgical margins were obtained.[6] Metastases in general are absent. There has been no published experience of endobronchial therapy used to treat this type of lesion; however, both examples noted here were successfully treated by Nd:YAG laser resection. Each patient remains disease free 10 years later.

REFERENCES

1. Moran CA, Suster S, Askin FB, Koss MN: Benign and malignant salivary gland-type mixed tumors of the lung. Clinicopathologic and immunohistochemical study of eight cases. Cancer 73:2481-2490, 1994.
2. Clarke PJ, Dunnill MS, Gunning AJ: Mixed tumours of the lung: A report of three cases. Br J Dis Chest 80:80-87, 1986.
3. Spencer H: Bronchial mucous gland tumors. Virchows Arch 383:101-115, 1979.
4. Sweeney EC, McDermott M: Pleomorphic adenoma of the bronchus. J Clin Pathol 49:87-89, 1996.
5. Hemmi A, Hiraoka H, Mori Y, et al: Malignant pleomorphic adenoma (malignant mixed tumor) of the trachea. Report of a case. Acta Pathol Jpn 38:1215-1226, 1988.
6. Payne W, Schier J, Woolner I: Mixed tumors of the bronchus, salivary gland type. J Thorac Cardiovasc Surg 49:663-668, 1965.

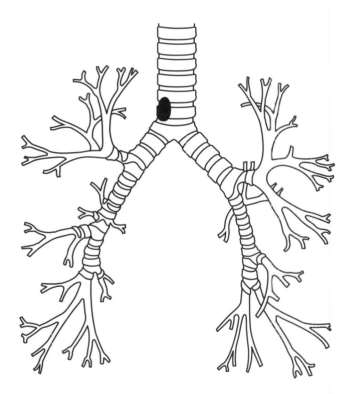

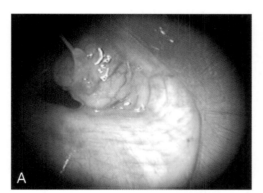

Figure 32-1. A, A firm, pinkish, vascular lesion arising from the right lateral wall of the distal trachea. On biopsy, the lesion was found to be a pleomorphic adenoma. *Continued*

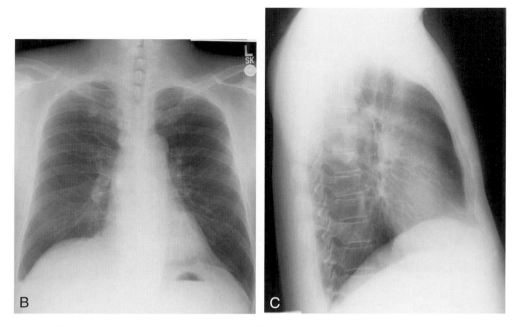

Figure 32-1, *cont'd.* Frontal (**B**) and lateral (**C**) radiographs demonstrate a subtle soft tissue mass projecting over the distal tracheal air column.

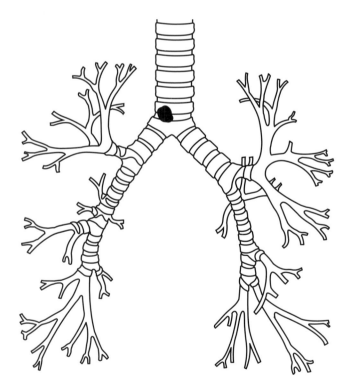

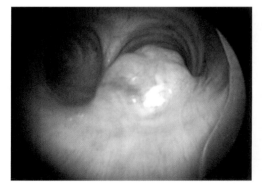

Figure 32-2. A smooth, pink, sessile, pleomorphic adenoma grows on the posterior membrane of the distal trachea.

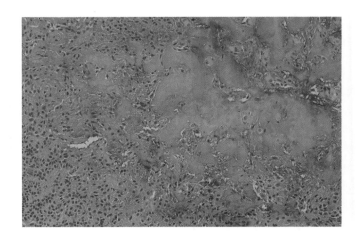

Figure 32-3. The tumor shows a combination of myxochondroid stroma and benign glandular components (H&E, ×100, original magnification).

CHAPTER 33

Chondroma

David R. Duhamel

Chondromas of the lung and tracheobronchial tree are rare occurrences. The lesions are considered benign cartilaginous tumors, but their etiology remains unclear. Some experts feel that a chondroma results from the one-sided neoplastic development of a bronchial mesenchymal cell. Following this criterion, these tumors should then be subclassified in the family of hamartomas and referred to as a chondromatous hamartoma.[1,2] Other experts believe that the entity of a true chondroma does exist and should be defined as a tumor composed of pure cartilage in continuity; apparently, it arises from underlying tracheobronchial cartilage.[3,4] It is more than likely that both types of tumor do exist; however, these lesions are so extremely rare that no large series of endobronchial lesions has been collected to help clarify this question. Regardless of the etiology, chondromas are known to develop in both parenchymal and endobronchial locations. In a subset of 60 chondromas analyzed by Tomashefski, only 3 (5%) were endobronchial in location.[3]

Chondromas have also been described as part of a unique syndrome called *Carney's triad*. First described in 1977, this syndrome consists of the development of pulmonary chondromas, gastric epithelioid leiomyosarcomas, and extra-adrenal paragangliomas.[5] The patients are almost all females between the ages of 10 and 30, and all three tumors need not be present to be diagnosed with the syndrome. As of 1994 there were 66 reported cases in the world literature.[6] The lesions are frequently multiple and can develop synchronously or metachronously.[7] Unfortunately, the benign pulmonary chondromas seen on chest radiograph are often assumed to be metastatic leiomyosarcomas or paragangliomas. However, the presence of calcification is a distinguishing characteristic unique to chondromas.

Endoscopically, the lesions are grayish white with a bosselated appearance and are almost always encapsulated. According to the strict definition, the tumor needs to arise from a portion of tracheobronchial cartilage that may be apparent bronchoscopically. Some lesions have been reported to be a pedunculated growth stemming from a cartilaginous ring, whereas others appear sessile on the cartilaginous tracheal wall. These lesions are truly cartilaginous in texture, making them difficult to biopsy using a flexible bronchoscope. The calcifications within the tissue may give it a gritty consistency.

On chest roentgenography, they appear well circumscribed with a lobulated or smooth margin. Approximately 30% of chondromas show evidence of calcification. The calcifications may have a nodular pattern within the tumor or, more commonly, a peripheral rim distribution. The tumors may be single or multiple and may show no preferential localization. They essentially remain stable for years radiographically, without evidence of growth or change. A CT scan may be helpful in differentiating chondromas from gastric metastases in Carney's syndrome, because it is very sensitive for peripheral rim calcification.[6]

Microscopically, focal areas of calcification are often present. A variable cellular pattern is seen that ranges from mature cartilage to scattered stellate cells surrounded by myxomatous stroma. The distinction between a chondromatous hamartoma and a true chondroma can often be made histologically because true chondromas are devoid of any epithelial or lipid elements.[7]

Chondromas are considered benign lesions without reported tissue invasion, mitosis, or metastasis. If any of these findings are noted, the possibility of the more malignant chondrosarcoma needs to be considered. Most lesions are diagnosed at surgical resection because bronchoscopic and needle biopsies are typically nondiagnostic. In the setting of Carney's triad, most experts feel surgical resection is not necessary if the lesion is calcified and metastasis is of low concern. All endobronchial chondromas reported in the literature were treated successfully with lobectomy or sleeve resection. The example noted here was successfully treated with Nd:YAG laser resection.

REFERENCES

1. Davidson M: A case of primary chondroma of the bronchus. Br J Surg 28:571-574, 1941.
2. Kaufman J: Endobronchial chondroma: Clinical and physiologic improvement following excision. Am Rev Respir Dis 100:711-716, 1969.
3. Tomashefski JF: Benign endobronchial mesenchymal tumors: Their relationship to parenchymal pulmonary tumors. Am J Surg Pathol 6:531-540, 1982.
4. Fraser RS, Muller NL, Colman N, Pare PD: Diagnosis of Diseases of the Chest, 4th ed. Philadelphia, WB Saunders, 1999.
5. Carney JA: The triad of gastric epithelioid leiomyosarcoma, functioning extra-adrenal paraganglioma, and pulmonary chondroma. Cancer 43:374-382, 1979.
6. Schmutz GR, Fisch-Ponsot C, Sylvestre J: Carney syndrome: Radiologic features. J Can Assoc Radiol 45:148-150, 1994.
7. Dajee A, Dajee H, Hinrichs S, et al: Pulmonary chondroma, extra-adrenal paraganglioma, and gastric leiomyosarcoma: Carney's triad. J Thorac Cardiovasc Surg 84:377-381, 1982.

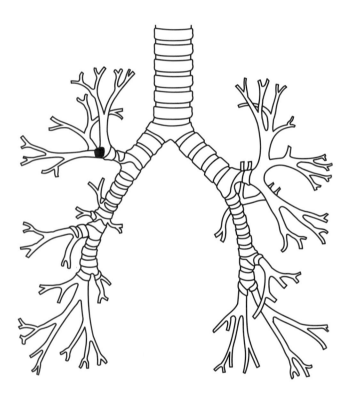

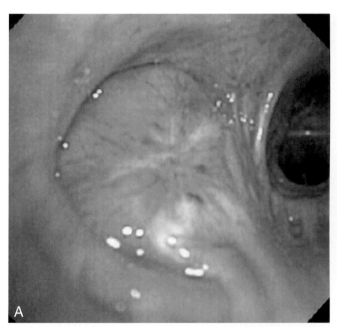

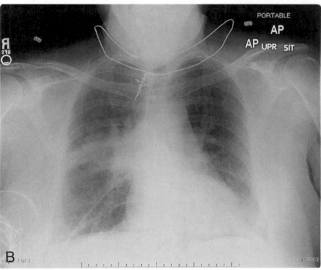

Figure 33-1. A, A smooth, pink, rubbery chondroma, which completely occludes the right upper lobe anterior segment. **B,** A chest radiograph showing an infiltrate and slight volume loss in the right upper lobe anterior segment. **C,** A CT scan demonstrating obstruction of the right upper lobe anterior segment with an impressive postobstructive pneumonia. The concave surface of the obstructing chondroma can be seen filling the bronchus. *Continued*

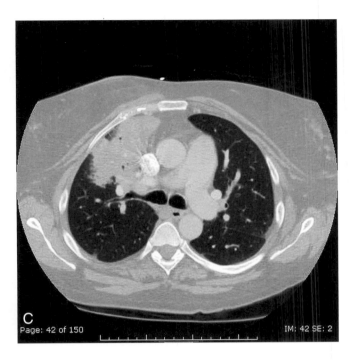

Figure 33-1, *cont'd.*

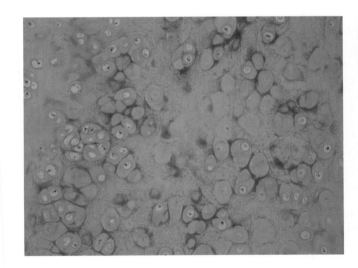

Figure 33-2. Bland chondrocytes surrounded by a blue chondroid matrix.

CHAPTER 34

Tracheal Stenosis

Jeffrey S. Prince
David R. Duhamel

Stenosis of the trachea can be due to multiple and varied etiologies but is most commonly associated with endotracheal intubation and tracheostomy tube placement. The incidence of postintubation stenosis is on the rise because the number of endotracheal intubations and emergency procedures has increased in general. Postintubation tracheal stenosis is believed to be due to the pressure exerted on the airway mucosa by the cuff of the endotracheal tube. A cuff pressure greater than 30 mm Hg exceeds the mucosal capillary perfusion pressure, which may lead to ulceration of the mucosa and chondritis of the tracheal cartilages.[1] The older style of endotracheal tubes with high-pressure, low-volume cuffs had a reported incidence of stenosis around 20%. The newer style of endotracheal tubes with high-volume, low-pressure cuffs is used much more commonly and has an incidence of stenosis that is lower than 1%. Mucosal injury can be further exacerbated by infection, mechanical irritation, steroid administration, and positive pressure ventilation. In the long term, this may lead to scarring and subsequent airway stenosis.[2]

In the past decade, the technique described by Ciaglia called *percutaneous dilational tracheostomy* has proved to be a safe and effective surgical method for performing tracheostomy. The technique in experienced hands has led to significantly lower rates of postoperative bleeding and stomal infection when compared with those in routine surgical tracheostomies.[3] More important, on follow-up CT scan after decannulation, evidence indicates that the incidence of tracheal stenosis with percutaneous tracheostomy is lower than that with surgical tracheostomy.[4] This is probably related to the greater tissue trauma and mucosal disruption associated with a surgical tracheostomy. It is also a common practice during the standard surgical procedure to remove a cartilaginous ring, which unfortunately contributes to the development of tracheomalacia as well as stenosis.

The presentation of airway stenosis varies from asymptomatic to life threatening, depending on the degree of stenosis and the cardiopulmonary reserve of the patient. In general, the tracheal lumen must be stenosed to 30% of its original size before a patient becomes symptomatic. A common presentation includes symptoms of dyspnea on exertion, stridor, and wheezing.[5] The wheeze heard in upper airway obstruction is classically described as monophonic, whereas the wheeze of asthma is described as polyphonic. Tracheal stenosis is frequently misdiagnosed as asthma for many months to even years before the actual diagnosis is made. Pulmonary function testing can sometimes be useful at suggesting the disease. The flow-volume loop exhibits a characteristic reduction in peak expiratory flow, with a plateau in the expiratory curve.[6] This classic pattern, however, is seen only in severe disease.

Bronchoscopic appearances can be varied, but the classic description is a dense, fibrotic, cicatricial ring. The lesion is typically circumferential but can be eccentric. The mucosa tends to be pale, smooth, and bland, consistent with fibrotic tissue. The lesion can be a focal, thin, weblike adhesion or a lengthy, complicated, and tortuous mass of fibrous tissue obstructing the lumen. The stenosis can occur at any one of four predictable locations in the trachea, as described by Montgomery[7]: (1) Stenosis in the high trachea due to trauma during intubation, "high" tracheotomy (above the first or second cartilaginous ring), or trauma to the anterior tracheal wall during tracheotomy; (2) narrowing at the level of the tracheotomy due to inflammatory changes caused by tissue disruption, infection, polyps, or granulation; (3) ulceration and necrosis of the tracheal mucosa and cartilage at the level of the endotracheal or tracheotomy tube cuff; and (4) recurrent trauma to the anterior tracheal wall distal to the tracheostomy tube, resulting in granulation tissue and loss of cartilaginous support.

Radiographic evidence of stenosis may be seen either on plain film, tomogram, or CT scan. Stenoses may occur at the site of the cuff, the subglottic region, or the stoma site in the case of tracheostomy.[8] The classic radiographic appearance of the stenosis is a short segmental focal stenosis with a symmetric hourglass shape. Eccentric stenosis is less common.[2] This narrowing is often seen on chest radiograph. Lateral and oblique views may also be helpful. Tomograms are felt to be useful in delineating the extent of the stenosis and its relationship to the glottis and the vocal cords.[8,9] CT with multiplanar reconstruction can give this same information and has essentially replaced standard tomography for detailed evaluation of these stenoses.[10]

The endoscopic approach to treating tracheal stenosis has undergone significant evolution in the past decade. Current endoscopic procedures are directed toward preserving the epithelium and minimizing thermal and mechanical mucosal injury. The standard approach is to mechanically dilate the stenosis with progressively larger bronchoscopes, balloons, or bougies. This can be somewhat disruptive to the mucosa and frequently leads to restenosis a short time later. In an attempt to prevent restenosis, a Silastic stent is sometimes necessary. Shapshay and co-workers are credited with the development of a technique to help minimize the mucosal disruption. Using a laser, they make small radial incisions in the stenosis at 3, 9, and 12 o'clock.[11] These incisions help to guide and control the tissue disruption that occurs with the subsequent mechanical dilation. Corticosteroids are frequently used intra- and postoperatively to minimize the acute inflammatory response and to inhibit further fibrosis during the healing phase. Intralesional corticosteroid injections have demonstrated little benefit. More recently, there has been very positive anecdotal experience using topical mitomycin C to help inhibit recurrent stenosis. It is important to realize that these lesions frequently require multiple successive procedures to obtain a satisfactory result. Aggressive endoscopic management does not preclude future open procedures if necessary. All conservative endoscopic techniques should be exhausted before committing a patient to the morbidity and mortality of an open surgical procedure. The surgical procedure typically requires resection of the diseased segment of trachea followed by anastomosis of the two ends.

REFERENCES

1. Knowlson GTG, Bassett HFM: The pressures exerted on the trachea by tracheal inflatable cuffs. Br J Anaesth 42:834-837, 1970.
2. Stark P: Imaging of tracheobronchial injuries. J Thoracic Imaging 10:206-219, 1995.
3. Cheng KT: Dilational versus surgical tracheostomy: A meta analysis. Ann Otol Rhinol Laryngol 109:803-807, 2000.
4. van Heurn LW, Goei I, de Ploeg I, et al: Late complications of percutaneous dilational tracheotomy. Chest 110:1572-1576,1996.
5. Grillo HC, Donahue DM: Postintubation tracheal stenosis. Chest Surg Clin North Am 6(4):725-731, 1996.
6. Spittle N, McCluskey A: Tracheal stenosis after intubation. BMJ 321:1000-1002, 2000.
7. Montgomery WW: Current modifications of the salivary by-pass tube and tracheal T-tube. Ann Otol Rhinol Laryngol 95:121-127, 1986.
8. Stauffer JL, Olson DE, Petty TL: Complications and consequences of endotracheal intubation and tracheotomy. Am J Med 70:65-75, 1981.
9. Kontos GJ, Hedges CP, Rost MC, et al: Postintubation tracheal stenosis: Diagnosis and management. S Dakota J Med 323-325, 1993.
10. Whyte RI, Quint LE, Kazerooni EA, et al: Helical computed tomography for the evaluation of tracheal stenosis. Ann Thorac Surg 60:27-30, 1995.
11. Shapshay SM, Beamis JF, Hybels RL, et al: Endoscopic treatment of subglottic and tracheal stenosis by radial laser incision and dilation. Ann Otol Rhinol Laryngol 96:661-667, 1987.

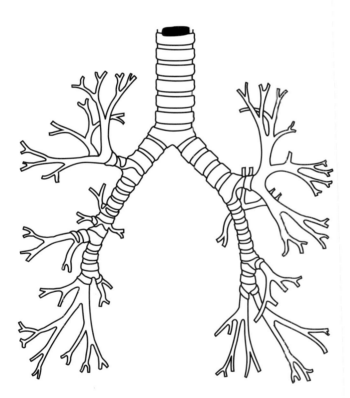

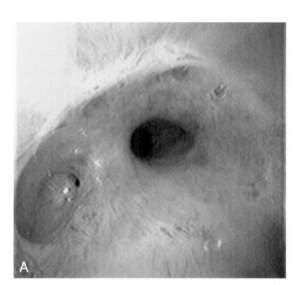

Figure 34-1. A, A stenotic proximal trachea that is bisected into two lumens by a thick fibrous band of scar tissue. The patient is a 34-year-old diabetic woman who was intubated for 12 hours during a bout of diabetic ketoacidosis.

Continued

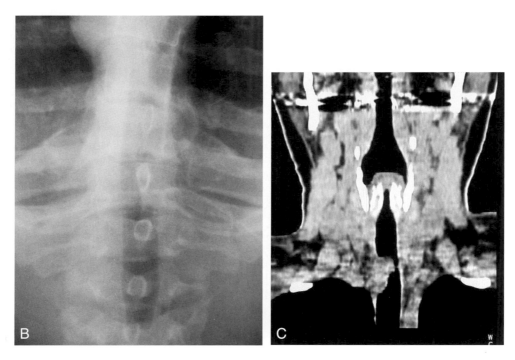

Figure 34-1, *cont'd.* **B,** Detail of the midtrachea obtained from a frontal radiograph demonstrates narrowing of the airway just distal to the thoracic inlet. A soft tissue density is present along the right lateral aspect of the trachea. **C,** Coronal reformation of the trachea from axial CT data again demonstrates a soft tissue mass arising from the right lateral tracheal wall with significant narrowing of the trachea.

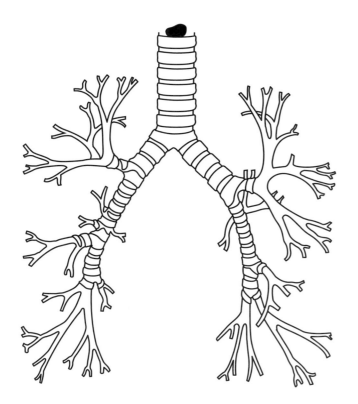

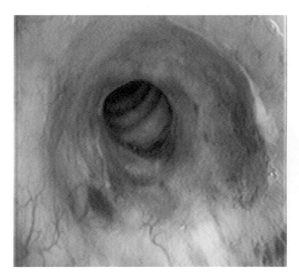

Figure 34-2. A circumferential band of inflammatory scar tissue in the proximal trachea.

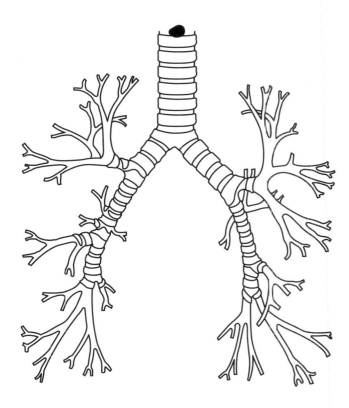

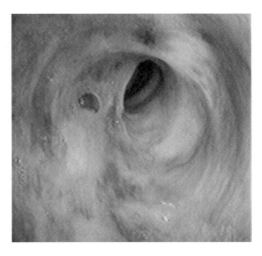

Figure 34-3. An eccentric web of bland scar tissue that has formed in the proximal trachea of a patient with multiple tracheal intubations.

CHAPTER 35

Idiopathic Subglottic Stenosis

Jeffrey S. Prince
David R. Duhamel

Stenosis in the area of the cricoid cartilage and first two or three cartilage rings of the trachea is considered subglottic stenosis. Subglottic stenosis can be the result of many different conditions. Most commonly, it is secondary to mucosal injury during intubation. Wegener's granulomatosis, postinfectious complications, collagen vascular diseases, blunt external trauma, congenital cartilaginous abnormalities, and surgery are other possible causes. A type of subglottic stenosis exists with which no etiology can be identified, called *idiopathic subglottic stenosis*. True idiopathic stenosis occurs in a small percentage of patients, most commonly women between the ages of 30 and 50.[1] Most of the other causes of subglottic stenosis are discussed in other sections of this atlas; therefore, the focus of this chapter is on idiopathic subglottic stenosis.

Patients may present with stridor, dyspnea, dysphonia, and life-threatening airway obstruction. Because these patients are otherwise healthy, they are often treated as asthmatics by their primary care physicians until they are referred for endoscopy or a tracheal imaging study. Grillo and colleagues found that symptoms lasted between 4 months and 15 years before evaluation, with most patients reporting symptoms from 1 to 3 years' duration.[2]

The cause of idiopathic subglottic stenosis remains unclear, but there are several theories. Gastroesophageal reflux disease is often described as a possible cause; however, conclusive evidence remains absent.[3] Either way, most experts agree that patients with idiopathic subglottic stenosis should be treated with a prolonged course of antireflux medications, especially in the perioperative period. Another theory blames a remote upper airway infection that causes circumferential mucosal injury and leads to cicatricial stenosis. Valdez and Shapshay have proposed that the stimulatory effect of estrogen on fibroblasts leads to excessive collagen deposition and stenosis in the setting of recent mucosal injury.

Histologically, dense collagenous tissue replaces the lamina propria of the trachea. There is no calcification or ossification. Fibroblasts are sparse. Histiocytes and lymphocytes are few in number and frequently are lacking. Mucous glands may be trapped by the fibrosis and become dilated. The epithelium often undergoes squamous metaplasia, and rarely granulation tissue is present. The cartilaginous rings remain intact without inflammation or erosion. Lacking is evidence of eosinophils, plasma cells, granulomas, vasculitis, or the changes that are characterisitic of relapsing polychondritis, Wegener's granulomatosis, amyloidosis, or other identifiable conditions.[3]

Viewed radiographically, this lesion appears as either a short- or long-segment circumferential narrowing of the upper trachea on chest or soft tissue neck radiographs.[4] CT has been shown to have good correlation with bronchoscopic methods of grading stenosis. These examinations must be performed with thin (1 mm) sections. It does not completely replace bronchoscopy in evaluation and management of this entity, but CT is a useful adjunct to bronchoscopy in evaluation of these lesions.[5]

Bronchoscopically, the lesion appears dense, bland, and fibrotic, although mucosal bleeding occurs easily on instrumentation. The length of the stenosis is usually between 2 and 3 cm with a range of 1.5 to 5 cm. The trachea distal to the lumen should be normal in appearance. Although the proximal end of the stricture sometimes begins gradually below the vocal cords, the distal end is often well defined.[3] Airway involvement is most often circumferential rather than eccentric. The lumen is typically narrowed to 5 to 7 mm but may be as narrow as 2 mm. The bronchoscopist should be extremely cautious when inspecting the stenotic area. Even the slightest trauma to the mucosal surface can cause rapid swelling or bleeding and convert a stable airway into an unstable one.

The endoscopic approach to treating tracheal and subglottic stenosis has undergone significant evolution in the past decade. Current endoscopic procedures are directed toward preserving the epithelium and minimizing thermal and mechanical mucosal injury. The standard approach is to mechanically dilate the stenosis with progressively larger bronchoscopes, balloons, or bougies. This can be somewhat disruptive to the mucosa and frequently leads to restenosis a short time later. In an attempt to prevent restenosis, a Silastic stent is sometimes necessary. Silastic stents are sometimes difficult to place in the high trachea or subglottic area owing to their tendency to migrate. The migration can usually be prevented by fixation of the stent using an external suture as described by Colt and colleagues.[6] In my opinion, metallic stents should be avoided in this situation because they cannot be removed and they tend to cause a severe granulation response. Shapshay is credited with the development of a technique to help minimize the mucosal disruption. Using a laser, he makes small radial incisions in the stenosis at 3, 9, and 12 o'clock.[7] These incisions

help to guide and control the tissue disruption that occurs with the subsequent mechanical dilation. Systemic corticosteroids are frequently used intra- and postoperatively to minimize the acute inflammatory response and to delay collagen synthesis during the healing phase. Intralesional corticosteroid injections have demonstrated little benefit. Empirical antireflux medications are given even if the patient is without symptoms. A short course of antibiotics is usually appropriate as prophylaxis against a mucosal superinfection at the site of dilation, which could exacerbate the scarring response. More recently, there has been very positive experience using topical mitomycin C to help inhibit recurrent stenosis.[8] Mitomycin is able to modulate the wound healing response by inhibiting the proliferation of fibroblasts. It is important to realize that these lesions frequently require multiple successive procedures to obtain a satisfactory result. Aggressive endoscopic management does not preclude future open procedures if necessary. All conservative endoscopic techniques should be exhausted before committing a patient to the morbidity and mortality of an open surgical procedure.

REFERENCES

1. Valdez TA, Shapshay SM: Idiopathic subglottic stenosis revisited. Ann Otol Rhinol Laryngol 11:690-695, 2002.
2. Grillo HC, Mark EJ, Mathisen DJ, et al: Idiopathic laryngotracheal stenosis and its management. Ann Thorac Surg 56:80-87, 1993.
3. Grillo HC: Management of idiopathic tracheal stenosis. Chest Surg Clin North Am 6:811-818, 1996.
4. Worrell JA: Radiology of the central airways. Otolaryngol Clin North Am 28:701-720, 1995.
5. Jewett BS, Cook RD, Johnson KL, et al: Subglottic stenosis: Correlation between computed tomography and bronchoscopy. Ann Otol Rhinol Laryngol 108:837-841, 1999.
6. Colt HG, Harrell JH, Neuman TR, et al: External fixation of subglottic tracheal stents. Chest 105:1653-1657, 1994.
7. Shapshay SM, Beamis JF, Hybels RL, et al: Endoscopic treatment of subglottic and tracheal stenosis by radial laser incision and dilation. Ann Otol Rhinol Laryngol 96:661-667, 1987.
8. Rhabar R, Valdez TA, Shapshay SM: Intraoperative application of mitomycin C in the treatment and prevention of glottic and subglottic stenosis. J Voice 14:282-286, 2000.

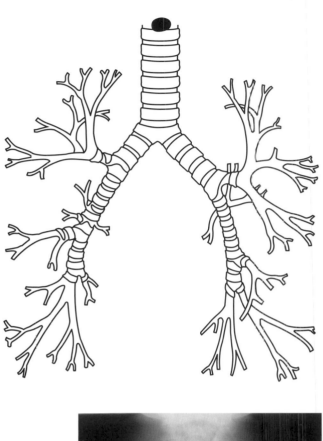

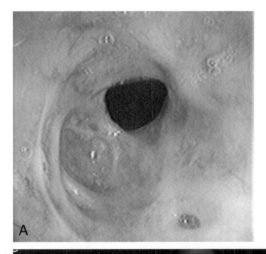

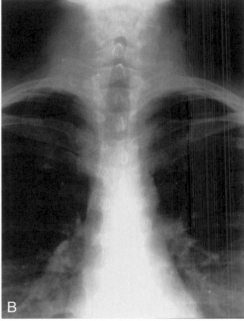

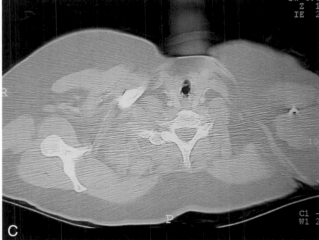

Figure 35-1. A, A thin eccentric web of bland stenotic tissue in the subglottic space. **B,** Detail of trachea from a frontal radiograph demonstrates subglottic narrowing. **C,** A CT image at the subglottic level identifies a thin soft tissue density anteriorly associated with slight narrowing.   *Continued*

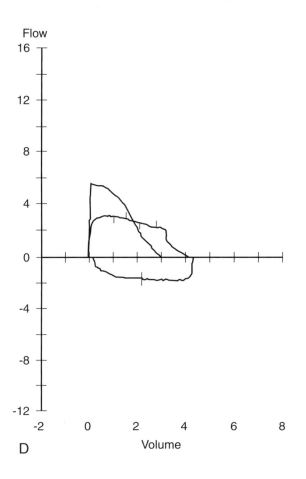

Figure 35-1, *cont'd.* **D,** A flow volume loop in the same patient demonstrates the classic pattern for a fixed tracheal obstruction. Note the flattening of both the inspiratory and expiratory flow patterns.

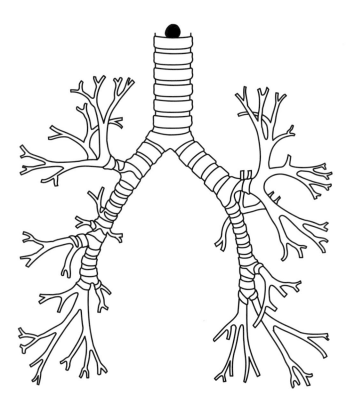

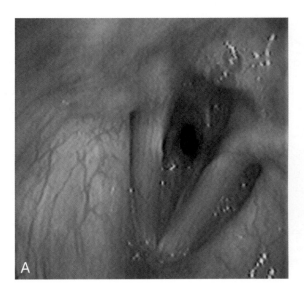

Figure 35-2. A, A view through the vocal cords of tight subglottic stenosis in an elderly patient who complained of only mild dyspnea. **B,** A frontal radiograph demonstrates an area of narrowing in the proximal trachea.

Continued

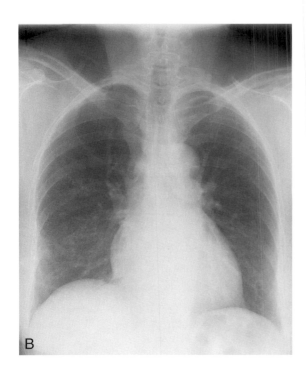

B

Figure 35-2, *cont'd.*

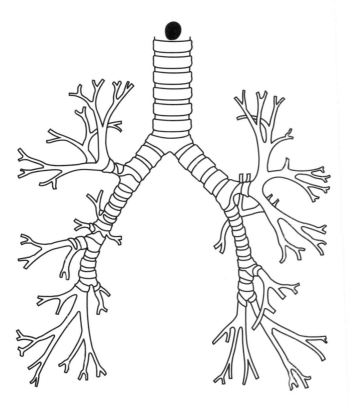

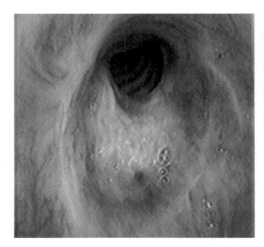

Figure 35-3. Extensive circumferential scarring in the subglottic space. The stenotic segment is approximately 1 cm long, with completely normal mucosa beyond the stenosis.

CHAPTER 36

Granulation Tissue

David R. Duhamel

A common complication of tracheostomy tube placement is the formation of granulation tissue. The tissue typically develops on the anterior tracheal surface, just superior to the tracheostomy tube or at the tip of the tube. The traditional explanation for this is local trauma due to excessive tube motion, suction catheters, or the fenestrations on a tracheostomy tube. Infection and localized perichondritis are also felt to play a role.[1] The exact incidence of tracheostomy-related granulation tissue in adults has not been studied, but in children it is between 1 in 294[2] and 50 in 319 (15.7%),[3] with one author anecdotally noting an incidence of about 50%.[4] Suprastomal granulation tissue should be considered if a patient has difficulty talking with a cuffless or deflated tracheostomy tube, or more typically if patients "fail" when the tracheostomy tube is capped. The granulation tissue may be a source of bleeding, present difficulties when the tracheostomy tube must be replaced, delay decannulation, or even cause airway obstruction. Multiple cases show granulation leading to complete airway obstruction and death.

Airway granulation tissue may also be seen at the site of tracheal or bronchial anastomosis after lung transplantation or bronchial sleeve resection. The suture material that remains at the anastomosis site is frequently an inciting cause of the granulation response. A granulation response is also commonly seen at the superior and inferior margins of a Silastic airway stent. The granulation tissue in this situation is frequently minimal and can sometimes be beneficial for securely anchoring the stent. On the other hand, the family of metallic airway stents is especially known for stimulating an excessive granulation response of the airway mucosa. The granulation tissue can be so intense that it results in occlusion of the airway.

Viewed bronchoscopically, the granulation tissue appears as a whitish endotracheal mass. It is usually soft and friable and typically arises from the proximal lip of the tracheostomy stoma or at the tip of the tracheostomy tube, where it abrades the mucosa. The ball of granulation tissue may be pedunculated and frequently obscures visualization of the tracheostomy tube when viewing through the subglottis. When the bronchoscope is passed through the lumen of the tracheostomy tube, "fingers" of granulation tissue may be noted growing through the fenestrations.

The occurrence of granulation tissue may be anticipated by the appropriate radiographs before bronchoscopy is performed. A high-kilovolt soft tissue lateral neck radiograph with the neck in hyperextension can often reveal the presence of abnormal tissue.[4]

The formation of granulation tissue is part of the normal wound healing process characterized by increased vascular permeability and angiogenesis. Vascular endothelial growth factor (VEGF) plays a crucial role in this process. There is some evidence that excessive production of VEGF induces continuous enhancement of vascular permeability and angiogenesis, resulting in aberrant growth of granulation tissue.[5] From a histologic standpoint, granulation tissue consists of immature stromal tissue and numerous small vessels. These vessels typically lack the well-developed tight junctions normally seen in capillaries. The lack of tight junctions makes the vessels "leaky" and results in localized tissue edema and extravasation of inflammatory cells into a background of granulation tissue.

The therapeutic options to treat suprastomal granulation tissue are multiple. The most widely accepted endoscopic technique remains ablation with the Nd:YAG laser. However, the surgeon must remember to exchange the plastic tracheostomy tube for a metal one, because there is a significant risk of airway fire. Others advocate "piecemeal" removal with cupped biopsy forceps. Reilly and Myers describe a surgical technique in which the mass of granulation is grasped and pulled up through the stoma and excised with scissors.[4] The latter two techniques have the potential risk of incomplete hemostasis. More recently Sato and colleagues have advocated the use of argon plasma coagulation (APC) to treat this process.[6] APC relies on high-frequency electrical current fed from a probe tip through ionized argon gas to superficially thermocoagulate the tissue. Sato and colleagues also used tranilast, an antiallergic agent used to treat keloids, to help prevent recurrence of the granulation tissue.[6] Mitomycin C applied topically has also been found to inhibit formation of granulation tissue. Its mechanism of action is believed to be fibroblast inhibition.[7]

REFERENCES

1. Maddwern B, Werkhaven J, Stool SE: Posttracheotomy granulation tissue managed by carbon dioxide laser excision. Ann Otol Rhinol Laryngol 98:828-830, 1989.
2. Oliver P, Richardson JR, Chubb RW, et al: Tracheostomy in children. N Engl J Med 267:631-637, 1962.
3. Crysdale WS, Feldman RI, Naito K: Tracheotomies: A 10-year experience in 319 children. Ann Otol Rhinol Laryngol 97:439-443, 1988.
4. Reilly JS, Myer CM III: Excision of suprastomal granulation tissue. Laryngoscope 95:1545-1546, 1985.
5. Pokharel RP, Maeda K, Yamamoto T, et al: Expression of vascular endothelial growth factor in exuberant tracheal granulation tissue in children. J Pathol 188:82-86, 1999.
6. Sato M, Terada Y, Nakagawa T, et al: Successful use of argon plasma coagulation and tranilast to treat granulation tissue obstructing the airway after tracheal anastomosis. Chest 118:1829-1831, 2000.
7. Rahbar R, Valdez TA, Shapshay SM: Preliminary results of intraoperative mitomycin C in the treatment and prevention of glottic and subglottic stenosis. J Voice 14:282-286, 2000.

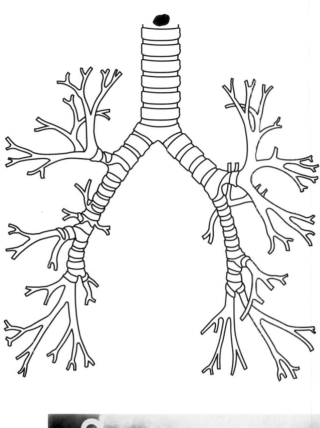

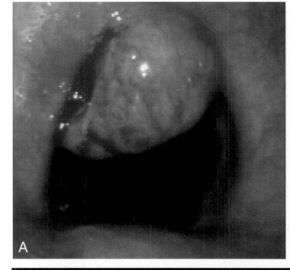

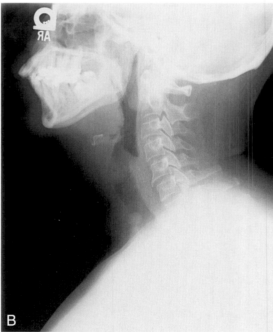

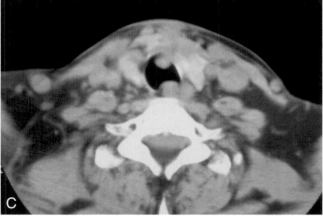

Figure 36-1. **A**, A large, reddish, friable deposit of granulation tissue on the anterior wall of the trachea. **B**, The lateral radiograph of the neck demonstrates a small soft tissue nodule associated with the anterior subglottic tracheal wall. **C**, The CT image demonstrates a noncalcified soft tissue nodule arising from the anterior tracheal wall.

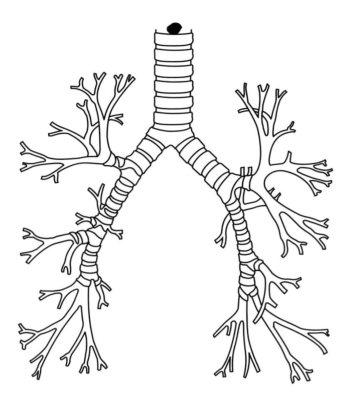

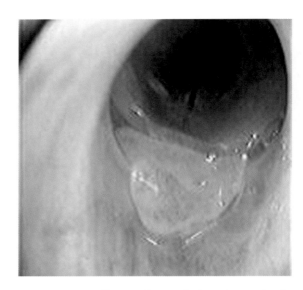

Figure 36-2. A small rim of granulation tissue that has formed at the proximal lip of a Silastic stent, which has been sutured into the trachea.

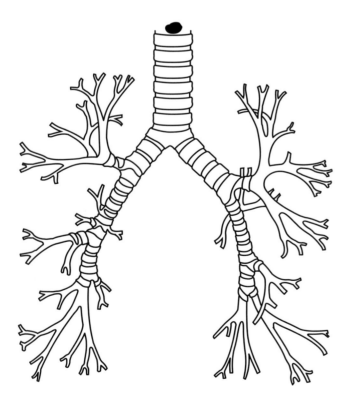

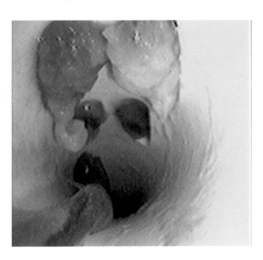

Figure 36-3. A view through the inner lumen of a fenestrated tracheostomy tube. Note the whitish-gray granulation tissue occluding and growing through the fenestrations.

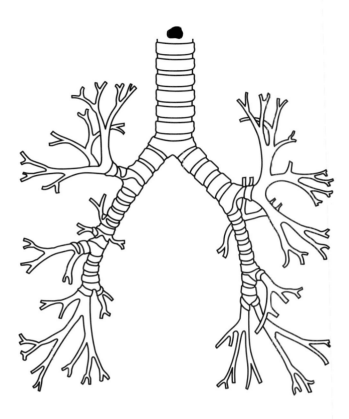

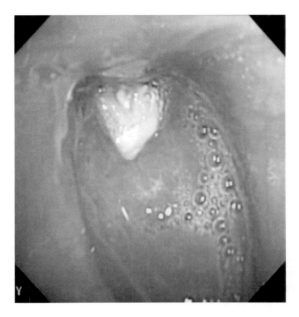

Figure 36-4. Extensive granulation tissue that has developed in the subglottic space just proximal to the tracheostomy tube. The airway obstruction was so extensive that the patient became immediately cyanotic when the tracheostomy tube was occluded. All that is seen of the tracheostomy tube in this picture is a small portion of white plastic.

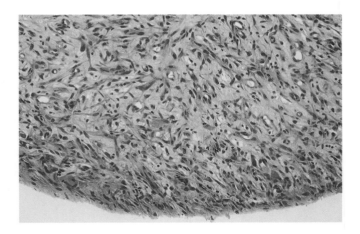

Figure 36-5. Granulation tissue formation is a common reaction to airway mucosal injury of any cause and is composed of fibroblastic/myofibroblastic stromal cells and newly formed vessels (H&E, ×200).

CHAPTER 37

Extrinsic Compression of the Trachea from the Thyroid

Gehan Devendra

Thyroid enlargement can be due to a benign or malignant primary goiter, thyroid involvement by a fibrosing or infectious process, or a thyrostimulatory goiter. The pathophysiology of tracheal obstruction due to the thyroid can be divided into two categories: extrinsic compression or actual tissue invasion. The focus of this summary is on extrinsic compression. The incidence of airway or esophageal compression due to a benign goiter has been reported as high as 33%.[1] However, this is subject to referral bias and worldwide the incidence is much less. Also the incidence of multinodular goiters is decreasing with increased use of iodine. However, in endemic areas it still represents a problem.

The thyroid gland usually enlarges anteriorly or laterally. Rarely, the enlargement extends inferiorly into the chest. Given the limited space of the thoracic inlet, symptoms tend to develop more rapidly with substernal goiters. The incidence of respiratory symptoms is up to 90% in cases of substernal goiters. Symptoms range from cough, hoarseness, and dyspnea, with about 70% of patients reporting a mass in their neck.[2] One third of patients with a substernal goiter have dysphagia.[2] Thyroid carcinoma can also cause airway obstruction, either laryngeal or tracheal, with actual compression or tracheal invasion.[3,4]

Pulmonary function testing may be helpful in diagnosing airway obstruction; however, the sensitivity is poor and a greater reduction in airway diameter is frequently necessary before a diagnosis can be made using this modality. Bronchoscopic findings for tracheal compression due to benign substernal goiters are that of airway narrowing without invasion of the mucosa. The lumen can be narrowed circumferentially, eccentrically, and in an anteroposterior or side-to-side direction. The mucosa typically remains intact without evidence of pathology.

Treatment for airway compression by the thyroid is surgical. In patients for whom surgery is not suitable, treatment can be accomplished by intervention or medical therapy. Medical therapy entails ^{131}I treatment, which may decrease the airflow obstruction in mild to moderate airway compression by the goiter.[5] Interventional therapy consists of stenting. Both metal and silicone stents have been implemented to relieve airway obstruction from substernal goiters.[6,7] The main caution with the use of metal stents is the inability to remove them, especially if the stent was placed as a bridge to surgery. It should be noted that the tracheal narrowing from a benign goiter tends to be elastic in nature, and can be easily dilated with a rigid bronchoscope before placement of a stent. If the patient were to undergo thyroidectomy, postoperative tracheomalacia at the site of compression is a well-documented complication. In severe cases, this complication manifests as acute stridor upon extubation. The tracheomalacia can be managed via surgical resection, stenting, endoprosthetic support, or tracheostomy.[8]

REFERENCES

1. Alfonso A, Christoudias G, Amaruddin Q, et al: Tracheal or esophageal compression due to benign thyroid disease. Am J Surg 142:350-354, 1981.
2. Newman E, Shaha A: Substernal goiter J Surg Onc 60:207-212, 1995.
3. Carter N, Milroy CM: Thyroid carcinoma causing fatal laryngeal occlusion. J Laryngol Otol 110:1176-1178, 1996.
4. Beasley NJ, Walfish PG, Witterick I, Freeman JL: Cause of death in patients with well-differentiated thyroid carcinoma. Laryngoscope 111:989-991, 2001.
5. Nygaard B, Søes-Petersen U, Høilund-Carlsen PF, et al: Improvement of upper airway obstruction after treatment of multinodular nontoxic goiter evaluated by flow volume loop curves. J Endocrinol Invest 19:71-75, 1996.
6. Nomori H, Kobayashi R, Kodera K, et al: Indications for an expandable metallic stent for tracheo-bronchial stenosis. Ann Thorac Surg 56:1324-1328, 1993.
7. Noppen M, Meysman M, Dhondr E, et al: Upper airway obstruction due to inoperable intrathoracic goiter treated by tracheal endoprosthesis. Thorax 49:1034-1036, 1994.
8. Geelhoed GW: Tracheomalacia from compressing goiter: Management after thyroidectomy. Surgery 104:1100-1108, 1988.

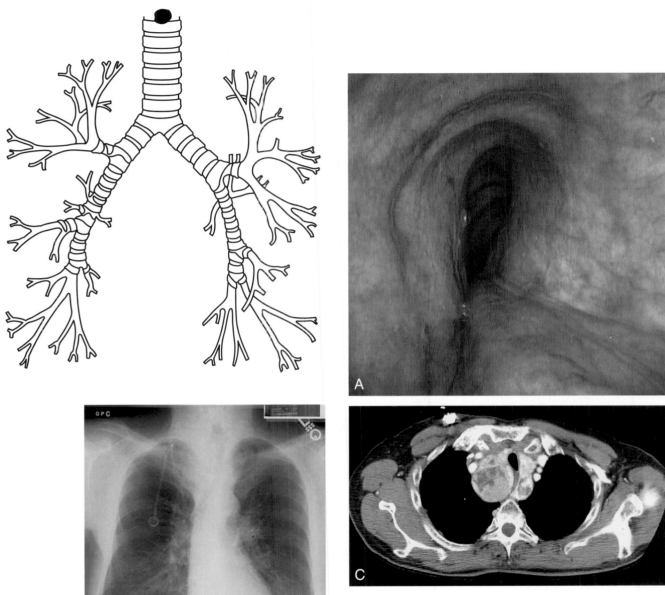

Figure 37-1. A, Extrinsic compression, narrowing, and deviation of the midtrachea by a massive substernal thyroid goiter. **B,** The frontal radiograph demonstrates displacement and narrowing of the trachea by a large mass arising within the right superior mediastinum. **C,** The contrast-enhanced CT image demonstrates a heterogeneously enhancing mass within both the right and the left superior mediastinum. The imaged features are typical of a thyroid goiter.

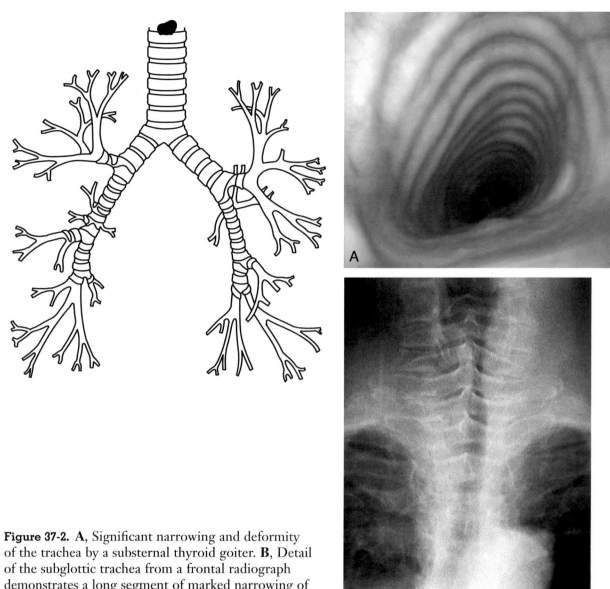

Figure 37-2. A, Significant narrowing and deformity of the trachea by a substernal thyroid goiter. **B,** Detail of the subglottic trachea from a frontal radiograph demonstrates a long segment of marked narrowing of the airway.

CHAPTER 38

Post-transplant Stricture

Jeffrey S. Prince

The first lung transplant was performed by Hardy in 1963. Since that time, lung transplantation has become a common procedure for the treatment of various pulmonary diseases, including chronic obstructive pulmonary disease, idiopathic pulmonary fibrosis, alpha$_1$-antitrypsin deficiency emphysema, primary pulmonary hypertension, and cystic fibrosis. Both single-lung transplant and bilateral single-lung transplant are performed.

In the past, airway complications were common in lung transplant. Early studies showed airway complications in 57% of patients.[1] This has been attributed to the fact that the arterial supply of the transplanted lung is not routinely anastomosed during surgery. The donor bronchus is completely dependent on low-pressure retrograde perfusion from pulmonary artery collaterals in the immediate post-operative period. Infection, rejection, and immuno-suppression may also contribute to the rate of complication in this area. Complications include formation of granulation tissue at the anastomosis and dehiscence of the surgical anastomosis. Stenosis at the anastomotic site is a late complication felt to be secondary to healing of early anastomotic complications or the result of chronic rejection. Changes in surgical technique have improved complication rates at the anastomosis. Wrapping of the anastomosis in an omental flap to increase vascularity was the first change in surgical technique. Telescoping of the bronchus and covering of the anastomosis with peribronchial tissue are current techniques used at the bronchial anastomosis that have been found to decrease the rate of anastomotic complication.[2] Current studies show the risk of complication at the anastomosis to range between 12% and 17% per anastomosis.[1] It has also been found that the modifications in the use of steroids and the increased use of cyclosporine have aided in decreasing airway complications.[3]

Clinical manifestations of anastomotic complications include failure of improvement of symptoms in the months after transplantation and decline in flow rates (FEV$_1$).

Bronchoscopy remains the gold standard of diagnosis. The bronchoscopic appearance is typically a dense bland fibrotic narrowing of the bronchus at the anastomosis site. It often affects the entire circumference of the bronchial lumen. The nonabsorbable suture material can frequently be seen within the fibrotic tissue. The suture material can on occasion stimulate a granulation tissue response, which also may lead to airway stenosis. Strictures may be treated with dilation by a rigid bronchoscope, olive-tipped bougies, balloon angioplasty, or laser therapy.[1] Once the lumen has been dilated properly, a stent is placed to maintain luminal patency. I prefer a Silastic stent in this situation because it can be removed easily to allow for further dilation and can be subsequently upsized. The metallic stents should be avoided because they are extremely difficult to remove and can greatly exacerbate the fibrotic and granulation response of the airway.

Radiographic manifestations of post-transplant stenosis are characterized by narrowing at the anastomotic site in the mainstem bronchus of the transplanted lung. Extra-luminal gas and mucosal ulcerations are signs of anastomotic dehiscence that may be seen in the postoperative period. Suggested radiographic methods include contiguous spiral HRCT with 2-mm collimation and planar reformats.[2] Multiplanar reformatting, three-dimensional reconstruction, and virtual bronchoscopy have all been suggested as methods for evaluation of the anastomotic area. Virtual bronchoscopy has been found to detect greater than 90% of stenoses found at fiberoptic bronchoscopy. Because of this, it has been suggested that virtual bronchoscopy may play a limited role in evaluation of the transplant anastomosis.[4]

REFERENCES

1. Shennib H, Massard G: Airway complications in lung transplantation. Ann Thorac Surg 57:506-511, 1994.
2. Alvarez A, Algar J, Santos F, et al: Airway complications after lung transplantation: A review of 51 anastomoses. Eur J Cardiothorac Surg 19:381-387, 2001.
3. Engeler CE: Heart and lung transplantation. Radiol Clin North Am 33:559-580, 1995.
4. McAdams HP, et al: Bronchial anastomotic complications in lung transplant recipients: Virtual bronchoscopy for noninvasive assessment. Radiology 209:689-695, 1998.

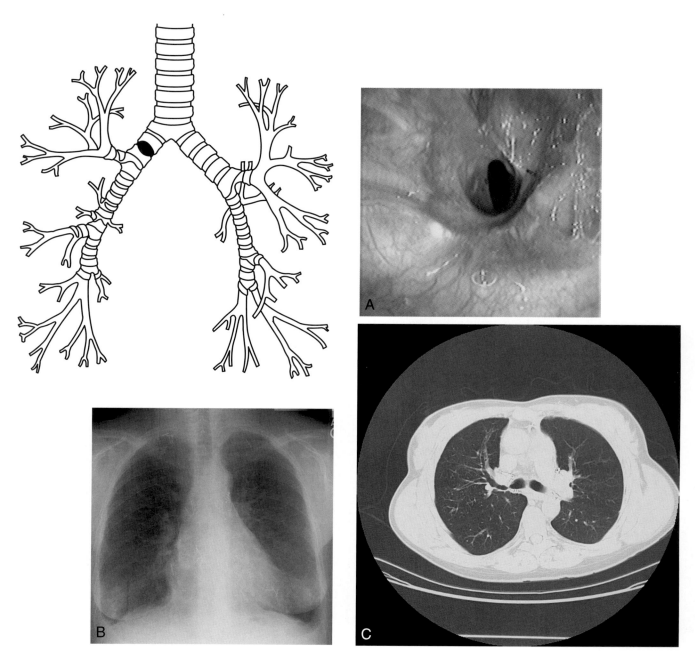

Figure 38-1. **A,** Tight stenosis of the right mainstem bronchus at the site of lung transplant anastomosis. Note the presence of the blue suture material within the scar tissue. **B,** The frontal radiograph demonstrates postsurgical changes from bilateral lung transplantation. No anastomotic narrowing is identified. **C,** The CT image demonstrates significant narrowing of the right anastomosis.

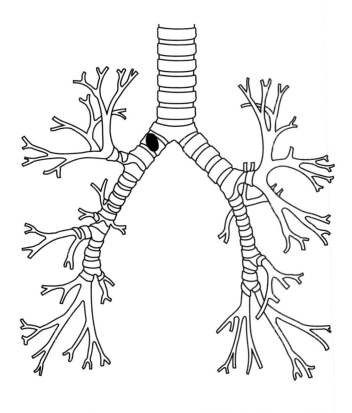

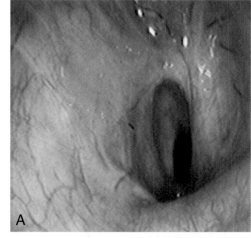

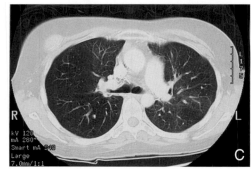

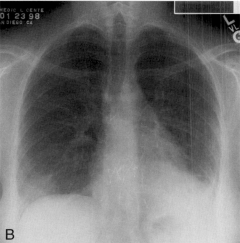

Figure 38-2. A, Dense stenosis and distortion of the right mainstem bronchus due to scar tissue formation at the transplant anastomosis. **B**, The frontal radiograph demonstrates postsurgical changes from bilateral lung transplantation. The airway is poorly visualized at the right anastomosis, but no definite narrowing is identified. **C**, The CT image demonstrates airway narrowing at the right anastomosis.

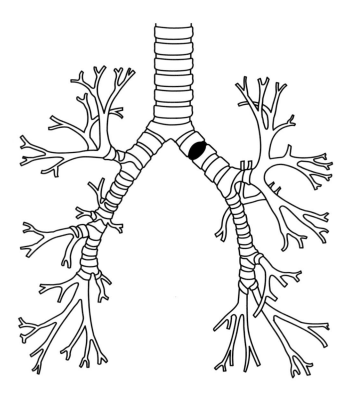

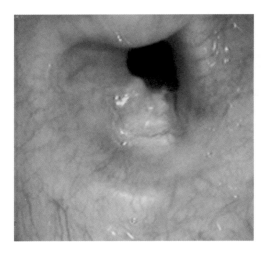

Figure 38-3. Granulation and scar tissue formation at the site of a transplant anastomosis. The sutures can sometimes cause irritation and stimulate a granuloma to form.

CHAPTER 39

Radiation Stenosis

David R. Duhamel

Radiation therapy is used to treat many pulmonary and endobronchial malignant lesions. Patients receive radiation therapy as part of their treatment for cure, palliation, or in combination with surgery, chemotherapy, or both. Most patients tolerate the therapy extremely well, with only subclinical manifestations of radiation-related changes. The two most common pulmonary complications of radiation therapy are pneumonitis and fibrosis. These processes predominantly affect the lung parenchyma and have a variable incidence and rate of clinical manifestation.[1] Endobronchial stenosis is a less common complication of radiation therapy but seems to have a rising incidence in recent years. This is mostly attributed to the increased use of endobronchial brachytherapy to treat malignant lesions of the airway.[2] Brachytherapy is a form of radiation therapy in which a very intense dose of radiation is given next to the lesion, thereby limiting the damage to surrounding healthy tissues.

This is accomplished in the lung by placing a hollow plastic catheter through a bronchoscope into the airway and adjacent to the lesion. Next, a very potent radioactive source is advanced through the catheter and positioned close to the lesion to deliver a very intense but localized dose of radiation.

After brachytherapy, the bronchoscopic incidence for any degree of bronchial stenosis is thought to be 9% to 12%.[2] The only identifiable risk factor for the development of stenosis appears to be length of survival. This may be explained by the fact that the longer a patient survives, the more radiation the patient is likely to receive and the greater the opportunity for clinically significant stenosis to develop. The use of endobronchial laser therapy, large cell carcinoma tissue type, and concurrent external beam radiation is felt to be a weak contributing factor.[2] The incidence of stenosis appears to be unaffected by other factors such as the technique used to deliver the radiation dose: high dose rate (HDR) versus medium dose rate (MDR) or single dose versus multiple fractionated doses.

A wide spectrum of clinical changes occurs in the tracheobronchial tree following radiation. Erythema and mucositis of the airway lumen are seen initially at the time of treatment. However, this is considered to be a normal reaction to radiation, and does not predispose to the development of stenosis.[2] Endobronchial stenosis is considered a late complication of radiation therapy and is typically identified on follow-up bronchoscopy. On average, patients are 40 weeks out from the date of their first radiation treatment before a fixed fibrotic bronchial stenosis is first diagnosed. The bronchoscopic findings range from a thin, whitish, circumferential membrane overlying the treated endo-bronchial mucosa to a more marked inflammatory exudate with a surrounding fibrotic reaction to the final stage of complete fibrosis with circumferential stenosis and narrowing of the airway.[2] In its final stage, the stenotic lesion is typically a hard, bland, fixed circumferential narrowing without evidence of active inflammation. These lesions are seen most commonly in the orifices of the lobar segments, less frequently in the mainstem bronchi, and rarely in the trachea. It is important to rule out recurrence of malignant disease as a cause of the narrowing.

The diagnosis of radiation stenosis can often be difficult to make based on radiography alone. The radiographic findings of radiation stenosis are very similar to those seen in radiation fibrosis, and both disease processes typically occur concurrently. They can both exhibit lobar volume loss, bronchial wall thickening, and atelectasis. In addition, radiation fibrosis manifests with linear stranding extending out from the hila, architectural distortion of interstitial markings, and pleural fibrosis.[3] A CT scan frequently under-estimates the degree of bronchial stenosis either as a result of slice selection or because of distorted anatomy in the setting of fibrosis. Therefore, a high index of suspicion for bronchial stenosis must be maintained in a lung cancer patient complaining of shortness of breath after radiation therapy

Most pathologic studies of the effect of radiation therapy focus on the lung parenchyma because it is much more radiosensitive than the tracheobronchial tree. In one autopsy study, external beam radiation was found to cause fibrosis of the bronchial wall and atrophy of the bronchial glands.[4] In another study, Jennins and Arden looked at the effect on the lung of a single large dose of radiation versus multiple fractionated doses. They found no significant difference between the treatment modalities, and both caused irregularity of the epithelial lining with loss of cilia after only 4 days.[5] In the early-stage bronchoscopic lesions described by Speiser and Spratling, the histopathologic changes consist of a mild mucosal inflammatory response characterized by amorphous fibrinous or eosinophilic debris containing varying amounts of entrapped white cells and necrotic tumor cells.[2] The late-stage stenotic lesions are characterized by a dense fibrotic stroma seen on biopsy. There is little evidence of active inflammation or necrosis at this point.

The treatment options for bronchial stenosis due to radiation therapy depend on the stage at which it is discovered. If the lesion is discovered early while an inflammatory exudate still exists, then systemic glucocorticoids may still be helpful in reversing the scarring process. The evidence to support this, however, is purely anecdotal. Once the stenosis has become fixed and fibrotic, there is little benefit to steroids, and interventional bronchoscopic techniques are required. The vast majority of lesions are best treated by bronchodilation with angioplasty balloons. These are the same balloons used to dilate stenotic lesions in the peripheral vascular system. They come in a wide range of balloon diameters and lengths and can be easily passed through a flexible or rigid bronchoscope. If a lesion is more proximal in the trachea or mainstem bronchi, the rigid bronchoscope can be used to mechanically dilate the lesions as well. Rarely are patients candidates for surgical resection of the stenotic segment of the airway mostly because of the confounding morbidities of their other medical illnesses.

REFERENCES

1. Movsas B, Raffin TA, Epstein AH, Link CJ: Pulmonary radiation injury. Chest 111:1061-1067, 1997.
2. Speiser BL, Spratling L: Radiation bronchitis and stenosis secondary to high dose endobronchial irradiation. Int J Radiat Oncol Biol Phys 25:589-597, 1993.
3. Libshitz HI: Radiation changes in the lung. Semin Roentgenol 28:303-325, 1993.
4. Boushy SF, Helgason AH, North LB: The effect of radiation on the lung and bronchial tree. Am J Roentgenol 108:284-292, 1970.
5. Jennins FL, Arden A: Development of experimental radiation pneumonitis. Arch Path 71:437-446, 1961.

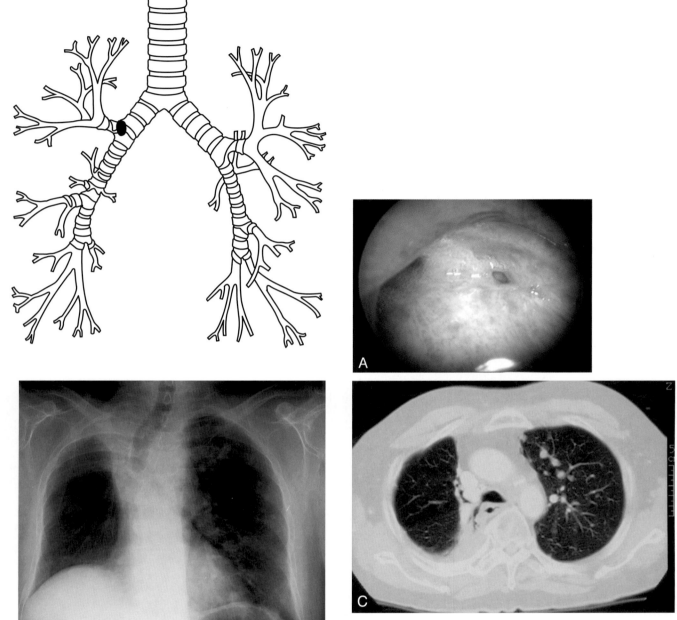

Figure 39-1. A, Tight stenosis of the right upper lobe orifice in a patient who received external beam radiation for lung cancer. **B,** The frontal radiograph demonstrates right-sided volume loss and post–radiation therapy changes. Multiple pulmonary metastases are present. **C,** The CT image demonstrates marked narrowing of the right upperlobe take-off.

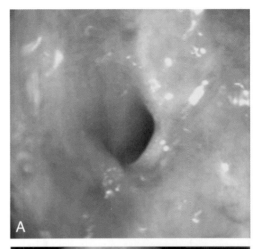

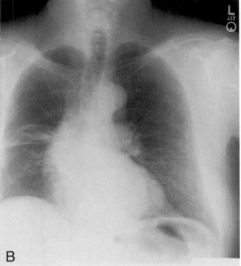

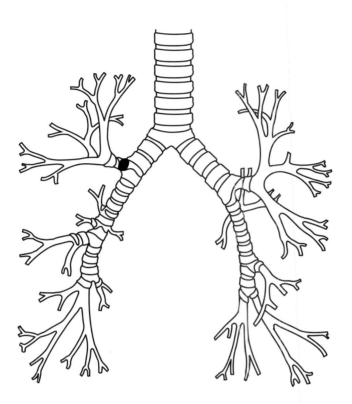

Figure 39-2. A, Extensive fibrosis and distortion of the right upper lobe bronchus after external beam radiation. **B**, The frontal radiograph demonstrates partial right upper lobe collapse. Post–radiation therapy changes are present with bilateral paramediastinal linear opacities.

CHAPTER 40

Coccidioidomycosis of the Airway

Gehan Devendra

Coccidioidomycosis is a disease caused by the dimorphic fungus *Coccidioides immitis*. It grows in alkaline soil in areas that are free from severe frost. It is found mainly in the Western Hemisphere, especially in California, Arizona, Texas, Utah, Nevada, New Mexico, and areas of Central and South America. *C. immitis* grows in the soil into a mycelium that produces several arthrospores. These arthrospores are

resistant to drying and are highly virulent. The arthrospores are inhaled by humans and develop into spherules that result in a bronchopneumonia typically labeled as *primary coccidioidomycosis*. If the infection lasts longer than 6 weeks, it is termed *persistent primary coccidioidomycosis* and is associated with progressive pneumonia, cavitation, nodules that can result in reactivation, or hematogenous dissemination. Chronic coccidioidomycosis is present in less than 1% of cases of pulmonary coccidioidomycosis.[1] Airway involvement of *Coccidioides* is a rare manifestation and is a chronic form of the disease, with fewer than 40 reported cases in the literature.[2]

Even the airway manifestations are varied, with bronchoscopic findings including mass lesions, extrinsic compression, granular lesions, irregularity of the trachea, endobronchial nodules, hyperemic patches, papillary lesions, and stenotic lesions.[2] Furthermore, airway stenosis has been described in only two patients.[3] Lesions are typically characterized as endobronchial nodules with yellow centers. Airway narrowing can be caused by extrinsic compression of the airway from lymph nodes. Hilar or mediastinal lymph nodes can also erode through the bronchus and cause obstruction.[4] Coccidiomas can also cause airway obstruction.[5]

The diagnosis is made by treating sputum, pus, or cutaneous lesions with a solution of 10% potassium hydroxide. Bronchoscopy is a proven method for obtaining samples. Results of cytologic examination are positive in less than 50%; however, culture positive for *C. immitis* was present in all cases. Transbronchial biopsy increased the yield on cytologic analysis.[6] Precaution has to be exercised when culturing *C. immitis*, given the virulence of the arthrospores.[7]

The mode of therapy depends on the endobronchial manifestation. Given the lack of cases, the best management for endobronchial disease is not known. However, my personal experience reveals that the treatment of stenotic lesions with balloon dilation with or without stent placement is optimal. Tracheal or laryngeal lesions can be treated with stenting, tracheotomy or surgical excision, and anastomosis. And unlike airway disease secondary to tuberculosis, which seems to respond to antituberculous therapy, the results with *Coccidioides* are much more variable. If a coccidioma is seen, initial treatment with amphotericin B with long-term treatment with an azole antifungal. Treatment is recommended for long term as in disseminated disease.[2]

REFERENCES

1. Bayer AS, Yoshikawa TT, Guze LB: Chronic progressive coccidioidal pneumonitis; report of six cases with clinical, roentgenographic, serologic, and therapeutic features. Arch Intern Med 139: 536, 1979.
2. Polesky A, Kirsch CM, Snyder LS, et al: Airway coccidioidomycosis—Report of cases and review. Clin Infect Dis 28: 1273-1280, 1999.
3. Winn WR, Harrell JHI, Warner GC: Endobronchial coccidioidomycosis. *In* Einstein HE, Pappagianis D, Catanzaro A (eds): Proceedings of the Centennial Conference on Coccidioidomycosis. Bethesda, MD, National Foundation for Infectious Diseases, 1997, pp 324-337.
4. Henley-Cohn J, Boles R, Weisberger E, Ballantyne J: Upper airway obstruction due to coccidioidomycosis. Laryngoscope 89:355-360, 1979.
5. Wallace JM, Catanzaro A, Moser KM, Harrell JHI: Flexible fiberoptic bronchoscopy for diagnosing pulmonary coccidioidomycosis. Am Rev Respir Dis 123:286-290, 1981.
6. DiTomasso JP, Ampel NM, Sobonya RE, Bloom JW: Bronchoscopic diagnosis of pulmonary coccidioidomycosis. Comparison of cytology, culture, and transbronchial biopsy. Diagn Microbiol Infect Dis 18:83-87, 1994.
7. Omieczynski DT: Safe isolation of *Coccidioides immitis* from clinical specimens. Health Lab Sci 7:227-232, 1970.

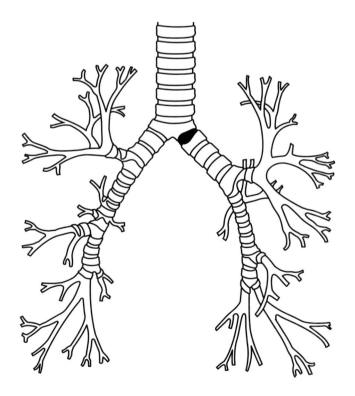

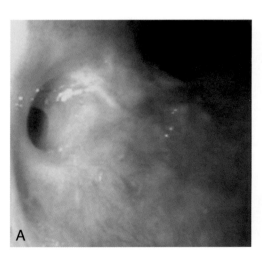

Figure 40-1. **A,** Fixed, tight stenosis of the proximal left mainstem bronchus at the level of the carina in a patient with coccidioidomycosis. **B,** Detail of the central airways from the frontal chest radiograph demonstrates narrowing of the left main bronchus. **C,** The CT image demonstrates marked narrowing of the left main bronchus. *Continued*

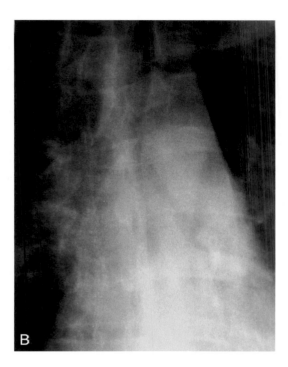

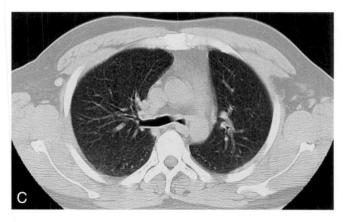

Figure 40-1, *cont'd.*

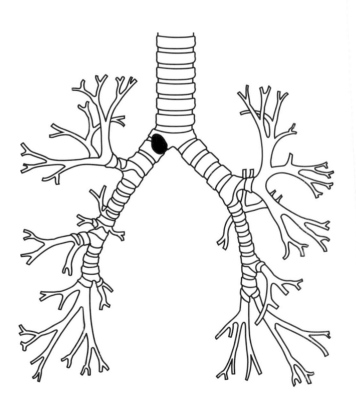

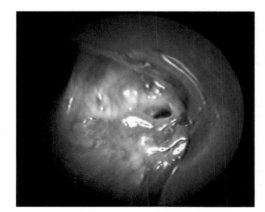

Figure 40-2. An enflamed fibrotic stenosis of the right mainstem bronchus that contained coccidioidomycosis on biopsy.

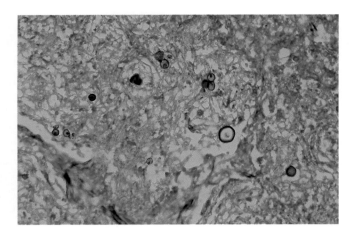

Figure 40-3. *Coccidioides* spherules highlighted by the special stain Gomori methenamine (×200).

CHAPTER 41

Tuberculous Stenosis

David R. Duhamel

Tuberculous stenosis is an endobronchial complication of pulmonary tuberculosis that can develop acutely at the time of infection or manifest 30 years later.[1] The greatest risk factor for developing this complication is endobronchial tuberculosis. Endobronchial tuberculosis has been reported in 10% to 37% of patients with pulmonary parenchymal tuberculosis who underwent bronchoscopy.[1-3] Some authors feel that as many as 90% of the patients with endobronchial tuberculosis will go on to develop some degree of tracheobronchial stenosis despite appropriate antituberculous therapy.[4] Tuberculous strictures are rarely encountered in developed countries; the incidence is much higher in Asia and Africa, where tuberculosis is common.[5] In the Asian literature, there is a four-times greater incidence of stenosis in women. This is believed to be due to the fact that the female bronchus is smaller and women expectorate less for social reasons, resulting in stasis of tuberculous sputum on bronchial walls.[6]

The strictures are characteristically cicatricial, extensive, and involve multiple levels of the tracheobronchial tree. The mucosa in between strictures may be completely normal. Active tuberculosis is not a requirement for the development of tracheobronchial stenosis. However, an alarmingly high number of patients are sputum negative despite having active disease.[7] The explanation for this may be the inability to expectorate the infected sputum past the stenotic area. The usual etiology of stenosis is believed to be necrosis and ulceration of the bronchial mucosa by active infection, subsequently causing granulation and fibrotic stenosis. It is important, however, that 20% of the stenoses are believed to be due to extrinsic compression of the bronchus by parabronchial lymph nodes.[1] On occasion, the caseating lymph node may even erode into the bronchus and manifest as an endobronchial mass.

Viewed bronchoscopically, the typical finding is localized endobronchial gelatinous granulation tissue. The mucosa may be red, nodular, and ulcerated and the diagnosis of bronchogenic cancer is suggested until microbiologic studies can be done. The radiographic findings in tuberculous stenosis may be nonspecific. The typical changes of post-tuberculous fibrocavitary parenchymal disease are frequently seen. Primary endobronchial tuberculosis leading to stenosis without parenchymal involvement is a very rare entity. Narrowing or obliteration of the tracheobronchial air column may be seen. A 30-degree left anterior oblique chest radiograph may better define the stenotic region. A CT scan shows inflammatory endobronchial narrowing frequently with associated lymphadenopathy. Calcification of the stenotic region is rarely seen.

The primary treatment for tuberculous stenosis due to active disease includes antituberculous chemotherapy sometimes combined with steroids. The role of steroids in this setting still has not been clearly defined because the majority of studies to evaluate it were too limited to be definitive.[1] In one double-blind study by Nemir and colleagues, it was found that steroids actually did not reduce the incidence of bronchostenosis.[8] However, once fibrotic stenosis is established, medical therapy alone is rarely useful; therefore, more aggressive interventions need to be done. Balloon dilation and mechanical dilation with the rigid bronchoscope are useful endoscopic techniques for the treatment of bronchial stenosis. There is a high rate of recurrence of the stenosis, and frequently multiple dilations are required. Once the stenosis is sufficiently dilated, a Silastic endobronchial stent can be deployed to help maintain patency. Surgery frequently is necessary for certain lesions that have failed endoscopic therapy. The surgical approach should be directed toward lung sparing and bronchoplastic procedures, especially if the parenchymal lung is not involved. The ideal surgical procedure is a sleeve resection in which the stenotic segment of bronchus is resected and the two healthy ends are reanastomosed.

REFERENCES

1. Kim YH, Kim HT, Lee KS, et al: Serial fiberoptic bronchoscopic observations of endobronchial tuberculosis before and early after antituberculosis chemotherapy. Chest 103:673-677, 1993.
2. So SY, Lam WK, Yu DYC: Rapid diagnosis of suspected pulmonary tuberculosis by fiberoptic bronchoscopy. Tubercle 63:195-200, 1982.
3. McIndoe RB, Steele JD, Samsom PC, et al: Routine bronchoscopy in patients with active pulmonary tuberculosis. Am Rev Tuberc 39:617-628, 1939.
4. Han JK, Im JG, Park JH, et al: Bronchial stenosis due to endobronchial tuberculosis: Successful treatment with self-expanding metallic stent. Am J Roentgenol 159:971-972, 1992.
5. Tong MCF, van Hasselt CA: Tuberculous tracheobronchial strictures: Clinicopathological features and management with the bronchoscopic carbon dioxide laser. Eur Arch Otorhinolaryngol 250:110-114, 1993.
6. Ozawa K. Wada S, Hirose Y, et al: Bronchial tuberculosis: A clinical study on 26 cases. Jpn J Chest Dis 40:42-48, 1982.
7. Ip MSM, So SY, Lam WK, Mok CK: Endobronchial tuberculosis revisited. Chest 89:727-730, 1986.
8. Nemir RL, Cardona J, Lacoius A, David M: Prednisone therapy as an adjunct in the treatment of lymph node bronchial tuberculosis in children. Am Rev Tuberc 74:189-198, 1963.

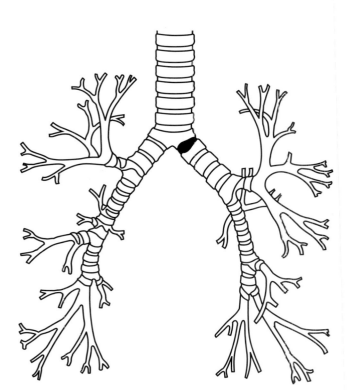

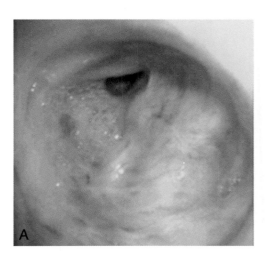

Figure 41-1. A, Bland fibrotic stenosis of the left mainstem bronchus in a patient with inactive tuberculosis. *Continued*

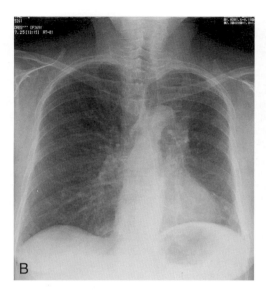

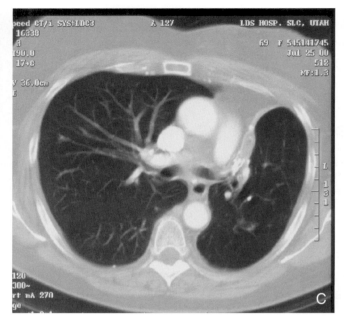

Figure 41-1, *cont'd.* **B**, The frontal radiograph demonstrates partial left upper lobe collapse. The left upper lobe bronchus is not identified. **C**, The CT image demonstrates calcified left hilar lymph nodes and narrowing of the upper left lobe bronchus.

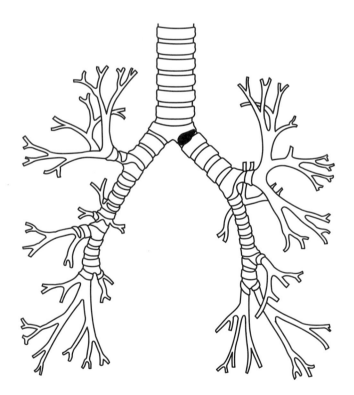

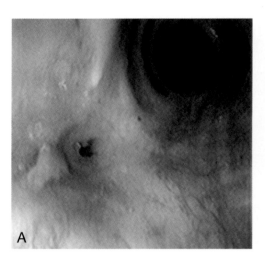

Figure 41-2. A, Near complete obstruction of the left mainstem bronchus at the level of the carina in a patient with active tuberculosis. **B**, The frontal radiograph demonstrates left lower lobe air-space opacity. The left main bronchus is not well identified. **C**, The CT image demonstrates marked narrowing of the left main bronchus.

Continued

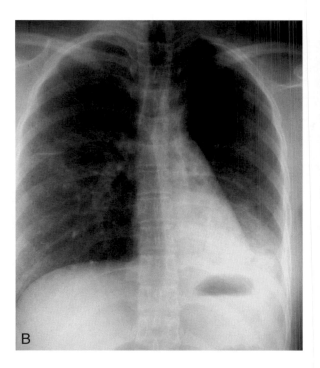

B

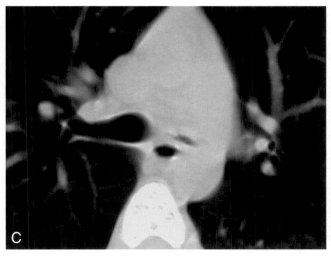

C

Figure 41-2, *cont'd.*

Figure 41-3. Caseating granuloma associated with tuberculosis (H&E, ×200).

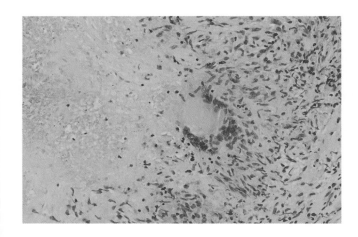

CHAPTER 42

Sarcoidosis

Jeffrey S. Prince

Sarcoidosis is a multisystem granulomatous disorder of unknown etiology. It is characterized by the formation of noncaseating granulomas in the affected tissue. Because other diseases such as tuberculosis, fungal infections, allergic alveolitis, or lymphoma can simulate the histologic and radiologic features of the disease, it is frequently a diagnosis of exclusion. The disease is found worldwide, but the epidemiology varies based on geographic location. In the United States it is most common in young adult African-American women. Worldwide it has an equal sex distribution and is most common in adults younger than the age of 40.

Hilar and mediastinal lymph nodes as well as the interstitium of the lung are the most common areas of involvement. This leads to the common radiographic presentation of symmetrical hilar adenopathy with or without pulmonary nodules. Common presenting symptoms are dry cough and shortness of breath. Systemic symptoms such as weight loss, fatigue, and malaise may also be present. However, up to 50% of patients may be asymptomatic, and the sarcoidosis is picked up incidentally on chest radiographs performed for other indications. Granulomas may also be found in the eyes, heart, liver, brain, kidneys, salivary glands, and skin.[1]

Sarcoidosis primarily affects the hila and the lung parenchyma; however, 1% to 3% of patients exhibit involvement of the airway mucosa. This most often affects the upper trachea but may extend to the distal trachea and mainstem bronchi. Patients with symptomatic tracheal involvement present with symptoms common to large airway disease, namely, stridor and wheezing. Narrowing of the trachea may be secondary to extrinsic compression from mediastinal lymph nodes or may be the result of granuloma formation in the tracheal mucosa and submucosa. This results in a thickening of the tracheal mucosa on radiographic examination.[2,3]

Airways obstruction in sarcoidosis is a complex topic. It is well documented that sarcoidosis patients may exhibit physiologic signs of airway obstruction characterized by reduced volume and flow rate on spirometry. The nature of this change is controversial and is most likely attributable to a combination of factors. Small airway compression secondary to peribronchiolar granulomas, submucosal granulomas in the central airways, extrinsic compression from enlarged lymph nodes, and late-stage interstitial changes in the lung all seem to contribute to these changes. Patients without extensive interstitial involvement on high-resolution CT of the chest seem to benefit from steroid therapy, but even this remains controversial.[4-7]

Bronchoscopic findings include endobronchial plaques and areas of narrowing and stenosis of the trachea and bronchi. A diffuse nodular or plaquelike appearance of the airway is frequently seen, which represents granulomatous involvement of the bronchial mucosa. It is sometimes referred to as "cobblestoning" and carries a very high yield on biopsy for noncaseating granulomas. The other airway manifestation of sarcoidosis is fibrotic stenosis of the tracheal and bronchial lumen. This is frequently a late finding and may only be discovered after a period of quiescent disease. The stenotic area is bland and fibrotic without evidence of active inflammation. Biopsy of the stenotic area is often void of granulomas, especially if the lesion is chronic and fibrotic. It is important to note that bronchoscopy often underestimates the extent and severity of the bronchial stenosis. The presence of bronchiectasis is also difficult to detect at bronchoscopy.[8]

The pathologic hallmark of sarcoidosis is the granuloma, a more or less well-circumscribed collection of epithelioid histiocytes sometimes associated with multinucleated giant cells. The vast majority of sarcoid granulomas are described as noncaseating, or without evidence of necrosis. Some granulomas resolve over time, with many undergoing progressive fibrosis.[9] It is this tendency toward lamellar fibrosis that undoubtedly leads to the end-stage airway findings of cicatricial stenosis. The finding of non-necrotizing granulomas does not constitute absolute evidence of sarcoidosis because such lesions are in no way specific. In many cases, ancillary testing such as culture, histochemical staining, immunohistochemical reactions, polymerase chain reactions, or polarization microscopy may be necessary to elucidate the etiology of the granulomatous process.

REFERENCES

1. Fraser RS, Paré JAP, Fraser RG, Paré PD: Synopsis of Diseases of the Chest, 2nd ed. Philadelphia, WB Saunders, 1994.
2. Kwong JS, Mueller NL, Miller RR: Diseases of the trachea and main-stem bronchi: Correlation of CT with pathologic findings. Radiographics 12:645-657, 1992.
3. Stark P: Radiology of the Trachea. Stuttgart, Georg Thieme Verlag, 1991.
4. Cieslichk J, Zych D, Zielinski J: Airways obstruction in patients with sarcoidosis. Sarcoidosis 8:42-44, 1991.
5. Gleeson FV, Traill ZC, Hansell DM: Evidence on expiratory CT scans of small-airway obstruction in sarcoidosis. Am J Roentgenol 166:1052-1054, 1996.
6. Hansell DM, Milne DG, Wilsher ML, Wells AU: Pulmonary sarcoidosis: Morphologic association of airflow obstruction at thin-section CT. Radiology 209:697-704, 1998.
7. Lavergne F, Clerici C, Sadoun D, et al: Airway obstruction in bronchial sarcoidosis. Chest 116:1194-1199, 1999.
8. Udwadia ZF, Pilling JR, Jenkins PF, Harrison BD: Bronchoscopic and bronchographic findings in 12 patients with sarcoidosis and severe or progressive airways obstruction. Thorax 45:272-275, 1990.
9. Mitchell DN, Scadding JG, Heard BE, et al: Sarcoidosis: Histopathological definition and clinical diagnosis. J Clin Pathol 30:395-401, 1977.

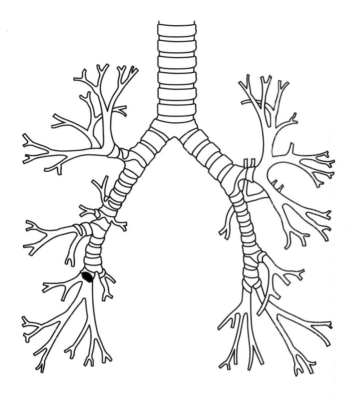

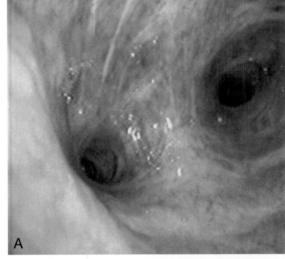

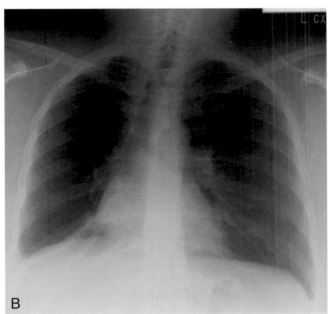

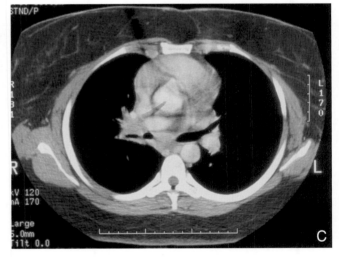

Figure 42-1. A, Erythema and dense fibrotic stenosis of the right lower lobe superior segment and basilar segment orifices in a patient with sarcoidosis. Note the grainy texture of the mucosal surface, which frequently demonstrates granulomas on biopsy. **B,** The frontal radiograph demonstrates narrowing of the right lower lobe bronchus with right lower lobe volume loss. **C,** The CT image demonstrates abnormal soft tissue within the right hilum, with slight narrowing of the right lower lobe bronchus.

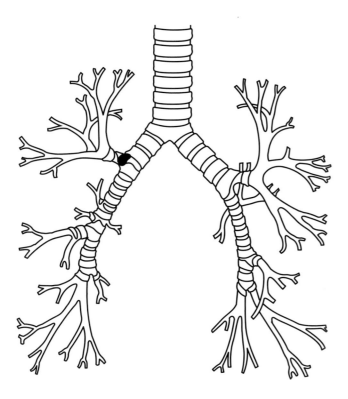

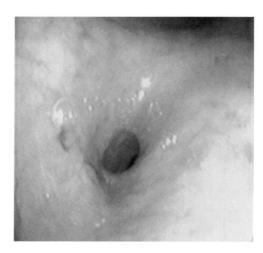

Figure 42-2. Bland stenosis and scarring of the right upper lobe bronchial orifice in a patient with chronic sarcoidosis.

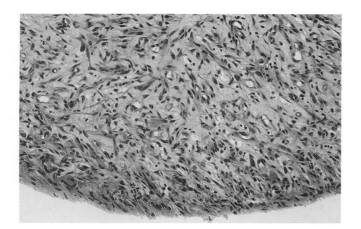

Figure 42-3. Noncaseating granulomas with no detectable infectious organisms are consistent with sarcoidosis. Sarcoid granulomas often involve small airway mucosa as well as alveolar interstitium (H&E, ×20).

CHAPTER 43

Inflammatory Bowel Disease of the Airway

Jeffrey S. Prince

Crohn's disease is classically described as a chronic inflammatory disease of the terminal ileum. However, it is widely accepted that the disease may affect all segments of the gastrointestinal tract. Other less common manifestations of Crohn's disease and ulcerative colitis that affect the respiratory tract have been described. Clinically apparent respiratory involvement in these disorders is rare; in one study, only three cases were identified in a series of more than 1400 patients followed for more than 40 years.[1]

The earliest reported cases of Crohn's disease of the airway come from Kelly and associates.[2] Both presented with stridor. These cases showed involvement of the hypopharynx and the subglottic trachea. Airway involvement is attributed to either direct obstruction from submucosal edema from chronic inflammation or obstruction secondary to inflammation of the cricoarytenoid joint.[2] Chronic bronchitis and bronchiectasis have also been seen in a number of inflammatory bowel disease patients who had no history of smoking. Subglottic stenosis has been described in both ulcerative colitis and Crohn's disease patients.[3]

Several other cases have since been reported in the literature. In the majority of these cases, the initial manifestation of the patient's Crohn's disease has been gastrointestinal in nature, with the respiratory symptoms following remotely. Kuzniar and colleagues reviewed all the cases in the literature and showed seven of nine to have tracheobronchitis. Five of nine presented with airway obstruction. All showed improvement with oral corticosteroid therapy.[4] Inhaled corticosteroids have been found to be beneficial in airway involvement, especially in those patients with chronic bronchitis and bronchiectasis. Interestingly, pulmonary disease has a tendency to flare up after bowel resection.

Presenting symptoms included stridor, dyspnea, dysphagia, productive cough, and hoarseness. Bronchoscopic findings are described as epiglottic and arytenoid edema,[1,3] inflammation of the tracheal and bronchial mucosa, as well as stricture and stenosis of the airway.[2] The edematous airway has a bland nonvascular appearance, and the airway is occluded with swollen, boggy, patulous tissue. The mucosa at this stage is soft and pliable; however, in late-stage obstruction and stenosis the tissue is fixed and fibrotic. Bronchial biopsy in general reveals acute and chronic inflammation of the mucosa and submucosa with associated peribronchial fibrosis.[5]

Radiologic manifestations in the reported cases have included edema of the epiglottis, aryepiglottic folds, and arytenoids,[1] tracheal deformity and thickening with mucoid impaction on CT,[2] and diffuse soft tissue swelling involving the hypopharynx and larynx.[6]

REFERENCES

1. Kraft SC, Earle RH, Roesler M, et al: Unexplained bronchopulmonary disease with inflammatory bowel disease. Arch Intern Med 136:454-460, 1976.
2. Kelly JH, Montgomery WW, Goodman ML, Mulvaney TJ: Upper airway obstruction associated with regional enteritis. Ann Otolaryngol 88:95-99, 1979.
3. Wilcox P, Miller R, Miller G, et al: Airway involvement in ulcerative colitis. Chest 92:18-23, 1987.
4. Kuzniar, T, Sleiman, C, Brugiere, O, et al: Severe tracheobronchial stenosis in a patient with Crohn's disease. Eur Respir J 15:209-212, 2000.
5. Garg K, Lynch DA, Newell JD: Inflammatory airways disease in ulcerative colitis: CT and high-resolution CT features. J Thorac Imaging 8:159-170, 1993.
6. Ulrich R, Goldberg R, Line WS: Crohn's disease: A rare cause of upper airway obstruction. J Emerg Med 19:331-332, 2000.

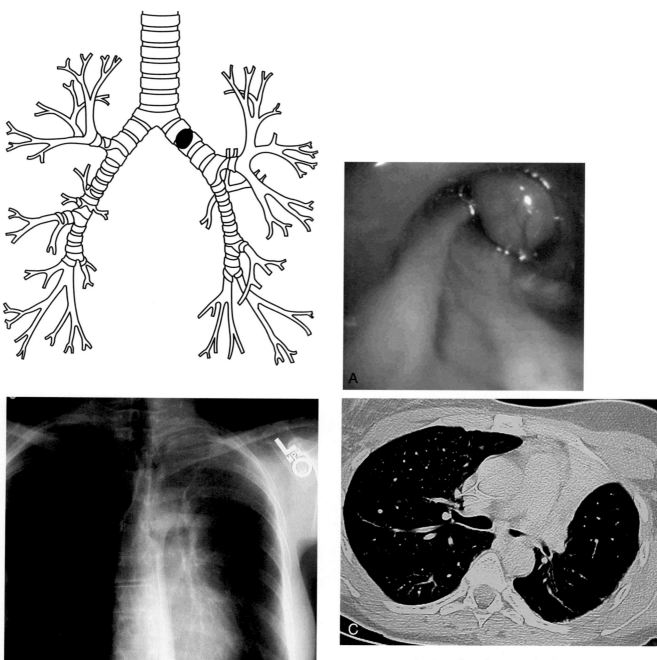

Figure 43-1. A, A pink soft mass of edematous tissue, which completely obstructs the left mainstem bronchus in a patient with Crohn's disease. **B,** The frontal radiograph demonstrates left upper lobe collapse. The left main bronchus is markedly narrowed at its origin. **C,** The CT image demonstrates marked narrowing of the left main bronchus and left upper lobe collapse.

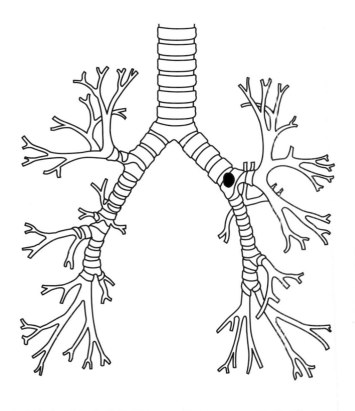

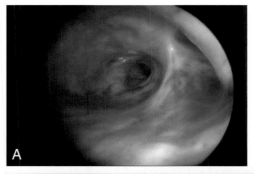

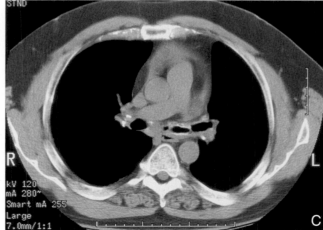

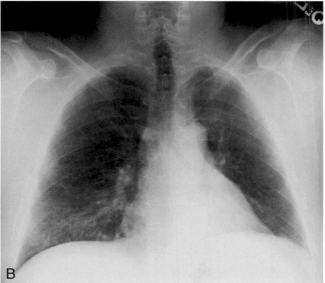

Figure 43-2. A, Erythematous and enflamed mucosa in the left mainstem bronchus at the bifurcation between left upper and lower lobes. The patient has severe Crohn's disease and chronic respiratory complaints. **B,** The frontal radiograph demonstrates subtle narrowing of the mid and distal left main bronchus. **C,** The CT image identifies partially calcified soft tissue density within the left main bronchus.

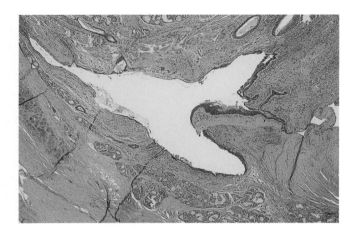

Figure 43-3. Severe chronic bronchitis and fibrosis with luminal stenosis in a large airway of a patient who has a history of Crohn's disease (H&E, ×100).

CHAPTER 44

Behçet's Disease of the Airway

Gehan Devendra

In 1937, a Turkish dermatologist, Hulusi Behçet, first described the triad of orogenital ulcers, uveitis, and arthritis that now bears his name. In addition, a wide variety of other structures and organ systems may be affected, including the kidneys, joints, central nervous system, gastrointestinal tract, and pericardium. Men are affected more often than women, and the age of onset is usually between 20 and 30 years. The incidence is highest in the Middle East and Japan. The mechanism of the disease is a nonspecific vasculitis with perivascular infiltration, possibly due to immune complex deposition. Although the cause is unknown, there has been some speculation that it may be a virus.[1] An increased frequency of HLA B5 has been reported, suggesting a genetic component in pathogenesis.[2]

Lung involvement is a rare phenomenon, occurring in about 5% of cases.[3] Clinical manifestations include dyspnea, hemoptysis, cough, pleuritic chest pain, and fever. Results on chest radiography are abnormal in about 90% of patients with pulmonary involvement and can show either unilateral or bilateral parenchymal infiltrate. Prominent hilar vessels can also be seen and were indicative of pulmonary hypertension secondary to pulmonary arterial involvement. Pleural effusions have also been described. Aneurismal dilation of both major and minor vessels can also be seen.[4] Pulmonary function test results in patients with Behçet's disease can be anywhere from normal to obstructive.[5,6]

Endobronchial manifestations of the disease vary. Ulcerative lesions similar to those seen in the gastrointestinal tract have also been reported in the trachea and bronchi. The associated mucosal edema of the airway may result in irregular narrowing of the tracheal lumen. This may on occasion be seen on chest radiograph.[7] The other airway manifestation of Behçet's disease is dense fibrotic stenosis of the bronchial lumen. The cicatricial bronchial stenosis seen in this disease is probably the end-stage fibroinflammatory healing response to an airway ulceration. Therapy is with corticosteroids for the aphthous ulceration. Stenosis can be treated with Nd:YAG laser therapy or balloon dilatation in addition to immunosuppression.[7]

REFERENCES

1. Slavin RE, de Groot WJ: Pathology of lung in Behçet's disease: Case report and review of the literature. Am J Surg Pathol 5:779-783, 1981.
2. Yang CW, Park IS, Kim Sy, et al: Antineutrophil cytoplasmic autoantibody associated vasculitis and renal failure in Behçet's disease. Nephrol Dial Transplant 8:871-876, 1993.
3. Raz I, Okon E, Chajek-Shaul T: Pulmonary manifestations in Behçet's syndrome. Chest 1989: 95:585-589.
4. Rosenbeger A, Adler OB, Haim S: Radiological aspects of Behçet's disease. Radiology 144:261-264, 1982.
5. Tatsis G, Vaiopoulos G, Tassiopoulos T, et al: Lung function in Adamantiades-Behçet's disease. Rheumatology 38:1018-1019, 1999.
6. Evans WV, Jenkins RM: Pulmonary function in Behçet's syndrome. Scand J Resp Dis 60:314-316, 1979.
7. Witt C, John M, Martin H, et al: Behçet's syndrome with pulmonary involvement—Combined therapy for endobronchial stenosis using neodymium-YAG laser, balloon dilatation and immunosuppression. Respiration 63:195-198, 1996.

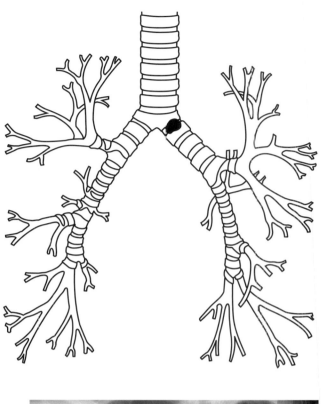

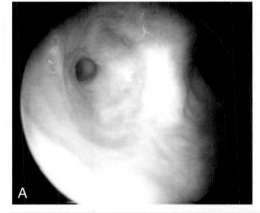

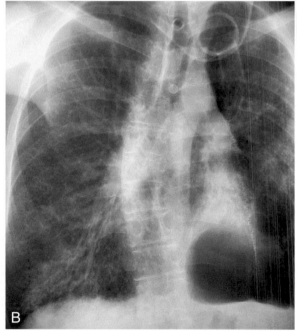

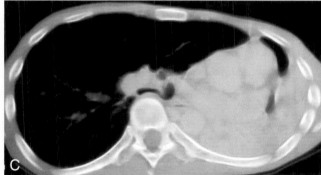

Figure 44-1. A, Extensive bland stenosis of the left mainstem bronchus, which extends the length of the bronchus in a patient with Behçet's disease.
B, The frontal radiograph demonstrates a long segment of marked narowing of the left main bronchus. **C,** The CT image demonstrates near complete collapse of the left lung, with marked shift of the mediastinum.

CHAPTER 45

Bronchopleural Fistulas

David R. Duhamel

A bronchopleural fistula is a process, not a specific disease, in which there is direct communication between the pleural cavity and the bronchial tree. Large airway or central bronchopleural fistulas usually occur after blunt or penetrating trauma and at the suture line after surgical resection of lung parenchyma. Small airway or peripheral bronchopleural fistulas usually occur in the setting of major parenchymal lung infection or empyema. Other potential causes include necrotizing malignancy, penetrating chest wall trauma from stab and gunshot wounds, complications of chest tube placement or thoracentesis, and mechanical ventilation with positive end-expiratory pressure. Bronchopleural fistula after lung resection is the most feared complication of thoracic surgery. In general, it is the only type of fistula amenable to bronchoscopic evaluation; therefore, this is the focus of my discussion.

The incidence of bronchopleural fistula after surgical resection is reported to be between 2% and 13%.[1] The early symptoms of a postoperative fistula are dramatic, with the sudden onset of breathlessness as the patient aspirates fluid from the thoracic space through the fistula. Another early sign is the development of explosive coughing on changing position in bed.[2] Frequently, the patient expectorates "muddy" watery sputum with old blood from the pleural space, and at least one patient is reported to have coughed up the staples used to close his bronchial stump.

Bronchoscopy can be extremely useful in the diagnosis of a fistula. The findings range from a small separation of the two opposed layers at the suture line to a widely patent aperture in the bronchial stump. The passage of fluid from the thoracic space into the bronchial lumen can sometimes be observed, especially with gentle coughing. Bronchoscopists have even used methylene blue injected into the pleural space to help confirm the diagnosis. The finding of blue secretions is strong evidence of a bronchopleural connection.

CT scanning is the imaging technique of choice for visualizing and characterizing bronchopleural fistulas.[3] Helical CT techniques are especially useful for imaging the entire course of a peripheral bronchopleural fistula.[4] Chest radiographs are also useful for suggesting the possibility that a fistula may exist. The classic radiographic finding is an intrapleural air-fluid collection, or hydropneumothorax. The air-fluid level typically extends to the chest wall, and this helps to distinguish it from an intraparenchymal fluid collection.[3] In patients who have undergone a pneumonectomy, a hydropneumothorax is to be expected postoperatively. However, in the setting of bronchial stump dehiscence, new or increased intrathoracic air with displacement of the mediastinum away from the resected side may be seen.[5]

The pathologic cause of postsurgical bronchopleural fistula is necrosis of the bronchial stump with subsequent wound dehiscence as the sutures or staples tear through the friable granulating tissue. The blood supply to the cartilage and posterior membrane is fragile and very susceptible to damage during intraoperative manipulation. Other risk factors for the development of a postoperative fistula include a malnourished state, steroid use, diabetes, prior radiation therapy, residual carcinomatosis at the suture line, preoperative pleuropulmonary infection, postoperative mechanical ventilation, intraoperative lymph node dissection, right-sided lung resection, the length of the bronchial stump, and the intraoperative buttressing of the stump with muscle, fat, or pericardium.[6,7]

The mortality rate for bronchopleural fistula from all causes ranges from 16.4% to 66.6%. If the fistula develops after surgical resection for malignancy, the mortality appears to be consistently worse, 50% to 71%.[6] Aspiration pneumonia is the major cause of mortality in bronchopleural fistula, especially when it develops in the early postoperative period.[1] The situation is made worse when the diagnosis is delayed by unsuspecting clinicians. The treatment for bronchopleural fistula begins with immediate drainage of the thoracic cavity to prevent recurrent aspiration. If an empyema exists, many investigators advocate the early creation of an open thoracostomy by the Eloesser flap procedure. Surgical repair of the fistula should be attempted only after the infection has been controlled. The repair consists of resection of any necrotic tissue, reclosure of the bronchial stump, and reinforcement of the suture line with vascularized tissue. The endoscopic closure of a bronchopleural fistula has been shown to be increasingly useful, especially if it avoids a repeat thoracotomy. The procedure entails the bronchoscopic administration of various fibrin "glue" compounds to the bronchial stump to create a plug for the fistula. Becker has reported successful closure in 35 of 45 patients, with increased success in smaller fistulas.[8]

REFERENCES

1. Hollaus PH, Lax F, El-Nashef BB, et al: Natural history of bronchopleural fistula after pneumonectomy: A review of 96 cases. Ann Thorac Surg 63:1391-1397, 1997.
2. Williams NS, Lewis CT: Bronchopleural fistula: A review of 86 cases. Br J Surg 63:520-522, 1976.
3. Stern EJ, Sun H, Haramati LB: Peripheral bronchopleural fistulas: CT imaging features. Am J Roentgenol 167:117-120, 1996.
4. Vogel N, Wolcke B, Kauczor HU, et al: Detection of a bronchopleural fistula with spiral CT and 3D reconstruction. Aktuelle Radiol 5:176-178, 1995.
5. Lauckner ME, Beggs I, Armstrong RF: The radiologic characteristics of bronchopleural fistula following pneumonectomy. Anaesthesia 38:452-456, 1983.
6. Asamura H, Naruke T, Tsuchiya R, et al: Bronchopleural fistulas associated with lung cancer operations. Univariate and multivariate analysis of risk factors, management, and outcome. J Thorac Cardiovasc Surg 104:1456-1464, 1992.

7. Wright CD, Wain JC, Mathisen DJ, et al: Post-pneumonectomy bronchopleural fistula after sutured bronchial closure: Incidence, risk factors, and management. J Thorac Cardiovasc Surg 112:1367-1371, 1996.

8. Becker HD: Treatment of postoperative bronchial fistulas by endoscopic fibrin application. *In* Schlag G, Wolner E, Eckersberger F (eds): Fibrin Sealing in Surgical and Nonsurgical Fields: Cardiovascular Surgery, Thoracic Surgery. New York, Springer, 1995, pp 187-193.

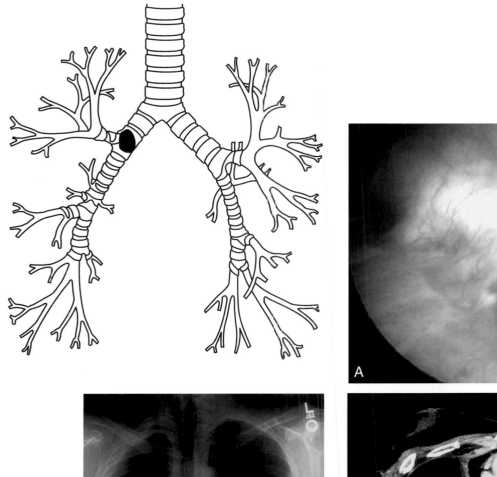

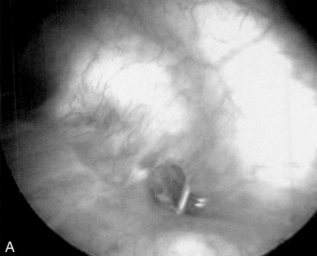

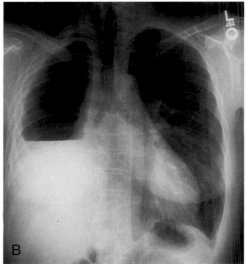

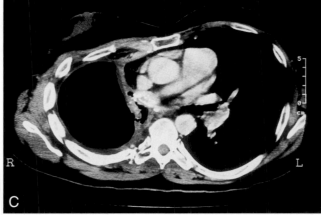

Figure 45-1. A, A view of a right mainstem bronchial stump after pneumonectomy for non–small cell lung cancer, which shows evidence of breakdown and dehiscence and subsequently formed a bronchopleural fistula. **B,** The frontal radiograph demonstrates a large right hydropneumothorax. The right bronchus intermedius terminates abruptly. **C,** The CT image demonstrates a patent fistula extending into the right pleural space.

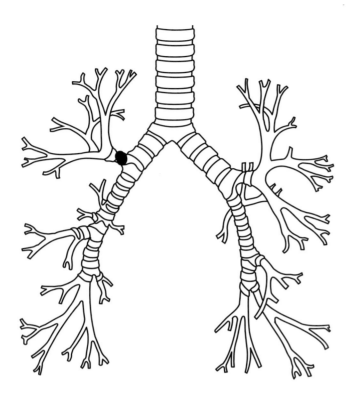

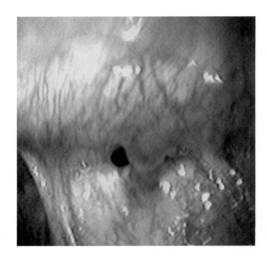

Figure 45-2. A view of a right upper lobe bronchial stump after a lobectomy for non–small cell lung cancer. Note the small area of recurrent tumor with early dehiscence and breakdown at the suture line.

CHAPTER 46

Tracheoesophageal Fistulas

David R. Duhamel

Tracheoesophageal fistulas in adults are either congenital or acquired. Congenital tracheoesophageal fistula is rarely encountered beyond infancy, but there are case reports of it being discovered in adolescents and adults. The H-type fistula is the only type found in adults because the others are not consistent with prolonged life.[1] The most common cause of acquired fistula is esophageal carcinoma.[2] It may be apparent at initial presentation, or, more typically, it develops after radiation therapy to the area.[3] The tumor initially invades both the trachea and the esophagus; next necrosis of the lesion occurs either spontaneously or following radiation therapy, allowing the fistula to develop. It is a known complication in 5% to 13% of patients with carcinoma of the esophagus.[4] Other causes of acquired tracheoesophageal fistula include pressure necrosis from the endotracheal tube cuff, especially as it exerts pressure against a rigid nasogastric tube, surgical injuries, blunt trauma, endoscopic laser therapy, and foreign bodies.[5] The

classic presentation includes violent bouts of coughing following ingestion of food or liquid and is called Ono's sign. Other symptoms of congenital fistulas include frothy stools in infants and excessive flatus in adolescents resulting from the involuntary aerophagia.

The radiographic findings on barium swallow include the passage of radiopaque material into the tracheobronchial tree. It is important to confirm that the contrast in the airway has not resulted from aspiration in the setting of an obstructed esophagus. Couraud and colleagues[6] found that barium swallow revealed only 70% of fistulas; therefore, if the clinical suspicion remains high, other diagnostic studies should be pursued. The finding of a thickened retrotracheal stripe on the lateral chest radiograph has been shown to be a useful diagnostic indicator of fistula formation.[7] CT has also been used to diagnose tracheoesophageal fistulas, especially in intubated patients who are unable to swallow barium.[8]

The diagnosis can frequently be made by bronchoscopy. Most fistulas affect the trachea, but the mainstem, lobar, and segmental bronchus may also be involved. Bronchoscopy in general is superior to esophagoscopy for making the diagnosis because esophagoscopy may not discover a small fistula hidden behind a mucosal fold.[6] The bronchoscopic appearance can be highly variable. A fungating tumor mass protruding through the membranous portion of the trachea has been described, as well as the more subtle bulging posterior membrane or extrinsically compressed bronchus.[2] In nonmalignant fistulas, the perforation may be very difficult to detect. The bubbling of secretions over the site can be the only helpful finding. Methylene blue dye has been used to assist in confirming the diagnosis. The patient swallows the dye before bronchoscopy, and the subsequent presence of blue secretions in the airway strongly suggests a communication.

From a histologic standpoint, the vast majority of malignant tracheoesophageal fistulas are due to squamous cell carcinoma of the esophagus. Bronchogenic carcinoma, also of the squamous cell type, is known to cause a fistula occasionally. The second most common cause of acquired fistula is probably a complication of prolonged endotracheal tube insertion. The pathologic findings in this situation include circumferential tracheal necrosis most likely due to ischemia from an overinflated cuff. In a congenital fistula, a definite muscularis mucosae is present microscopically, and the tract is lined by either columnar or squamous epithelium.[9]

The fatal consequences of this complication of esophageal cancer are reflected by the fact that 100% of untreated patients die within 6 weeks of making the diagnosis.[2] The vast majority of these patients succumb to overwhelming mediastinal and pulmonary infections rather than complications of metastatic disease. Treatment options are limited and geared toward palliation, because cure is not a realistic goal. One option includes surgical esophageal bypass using a section of colon or stomach to bypass the ligated esophagus above and below the tumor. Esophageal intubation is a second option that includes the endoscopic insertion of a tubular device into the esophageal lumen, which occludes the fistula and helps to prevent aspiration of food and saliva into the airway. Stenting of the airway with a Silastic stent has been performed with some success and helps to lessen symptoms of recurrent aspiration as well. It is important to stent the airway before esophageal intubation because a fully stented esophagus can worsen extrinsic compression of the trachea and potentially occlude it. Early surgical repair is the usual treatment for acquired nonmalignant fistulas. These patients typically have a very good prognosis and recover without significant sequelae if the fistula can be detected early and the infection controlled.

REFERENCES

1. Grant DM, Thompson GE: Diagnosis of congenital tracheoesophageal fistula in the adolescent and adult. Anesthesiology 49:139-140, 1978.
2. Little AG, Ferguson MK, DeMeester TR, et al: Esophageal carcinoma with respiratory tract fistula. Cancer 53:1322-1328, 1984.
3. Symbas PN, McKeown PP, Hatcher CR, et al: Tracheoesophageal fistula from carcinoma of the esophagus. Ann Thorac Surg 38:382-386, 1984.
4. Fitzgerald RH, Bartles DM, Parker EF: Tracheoesophageal fistulas secondary to carcinoma of the esophagus. J Thorac Cardiovasc Surg 82:194-197, 1981.
5. Hilgenberg AD, Grillo HC: Acquired nonmalignant tracheoesophageal fistula. J Thorac Cardiovasc Surg 85:492-498, 1983.
6. Couraud L, Ballester MJ, Delaisement C: Acquired tracheoesophageal fistula and its management. Semin Thorac Cardiovasc Surg 8:392-399, 1996.
7. Daffner RH, Postlethwait RW, Putnam CE: Retrotracheal abnormalities in esophageal carcinoma: Prognostic implications. Am J Roentgenol 130:719-723, 1978.
8. Leeds WM, Morley TF, Zappasodi SJ, et al: Computed tomography for diagnosis of tracheoesophageal fistula. Crit Care Med 14:591-592, 1986.
9. Kim JH, Park KH, Sung SW, et al: Congenital bronchoesophageal fistulas in adult patients. Ann Thorac Surg 60:151-155, 1995.

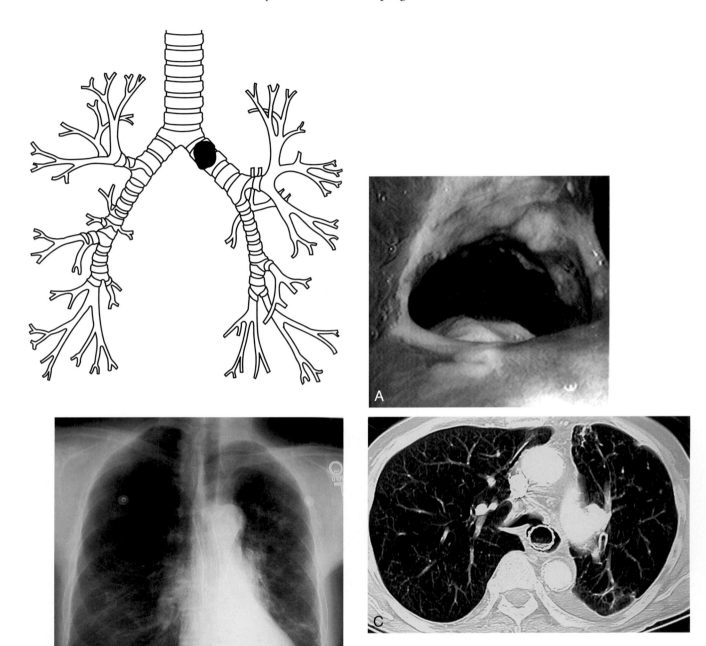

Figure 46-1. A, Complete absence of the posterior membrane of the left mainstem bronchus in a patient who has received radiation for esophageal cancer. The external surface of the mesh-covered esophageal stent can be seen easily through the tracheoesophageal fistula. **B,** The frontal radiograph demonstrates a mesh esophageal stent. Left lower lobe air-space opacity is present. **C,** The CT image demonstrates a connection between the posterior wall of the left main bronchus and the esophagus.

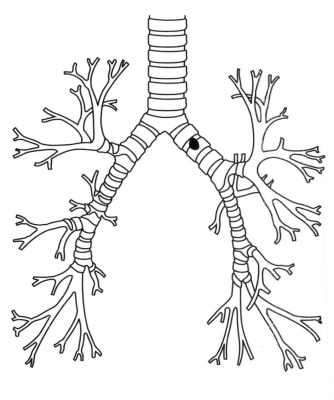

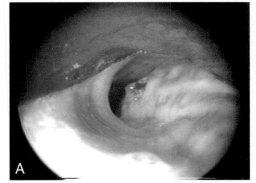

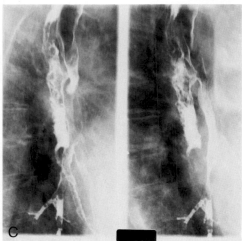

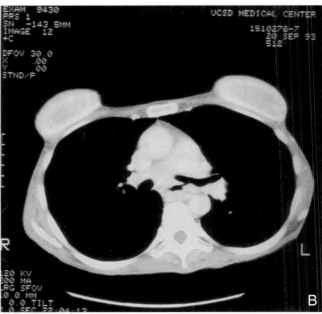

Figure 46-2. A, A small raised mound of friable tumor tissue on the posterior membrane of the left mainstem bronchus that connects to the esophagus through a fistulous tract. **B,** The CT image demonstrates a fistula tract between the left main bronchus and the esophagus. **C,** A single image from an esophagram demonstrates a fistulous connection with the left main bronchus.

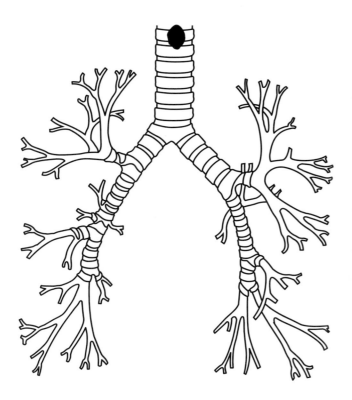

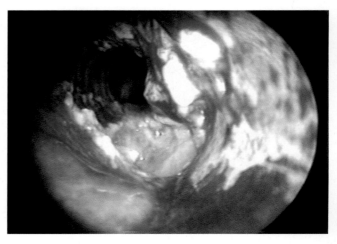

Figure 46-3. A large perforation in the posterior membrane of the trachea connecting to the esophagus in a patient who suffered neck trauma from a motor vehicle accident and difficult intubation.

CHAPTER 47

Foreign Body Aspiration

David R. Duhamel

Suffocation caused by an ingested object accounted for 3200 (1.2 per 100,000) deaths in the United States in 1998.[1] Death from suffocation demonstrates a bimodal pattern, with peaks at ages less than 1 year (1.9 per 100,000) and greater than 75 years (10.7 per 100,000).[1] Nonasphyxiating aspirated foreign bodies, however, are much more common in children than in adults. Approximately 85% of all foreign body aspirations occur in children younger than 15 years, and its occurrence is due to children's propensity to put objects in their mouths.[2] Adults tend to aspirate from failure of their airway protective mechanisms. Factors contributing to this failure include alcohol intoxication, sedative drug use, poor dentition, senility, primary neurologic disorders, trauma with loss of consciousness, seizure, and general anesthesia.[2]

The clinical presentation of an aspirated foreign body can be highly variable and depends greatly on the location of the object. If the object is lodged in the trachea or subglottic space, inspiratory stridor and paroxysms of coughing may be noted. An object located in the bronchus may be surprisingly asymptomatic, with localized wheezing being the only finding. Because of the paucity of symptoms with aspirated objects in adults, the diagnosis is often delayed for months to years and even as late as 25 years after aspiration.[3] Limper and Prakash reported on 60 adults who presented with foreign body aspiration. In this series, cough was the most frequent presenting symptom, occurring in 94% of patients.[3] Metrangelo and associates reported that the presence of a choking crisis is one of the most accurate indicators of a foreign body aspiration, with a sensitivity of 96% and a specificity of 76%.[4] Interestingly, 40% to 70% of objects come to rest in the right bronchus and 30% to 40% end up in the left bronchus. This is due to the fact that the right bronchus is larger and more vertically continuous with the trachea. The remaining 10% to 20% are found in the laryngotracheal region.[5,6]

Radiographic evaluation is helpful in diagnosing foreign bodies, but flexible bronchoscopy remains the gold standard in the identification and localization of the aspirated object. The chest radiograph is not always helpful because only a small percentage of aspirated objects are radiopaque. Other more subtle radiographic signs may be helpful when present, including air trapping, atelectasis, pulmonary infiltrates, and mediastinal shift.[2] Limper and Prakash found the chest radiograph to be useful in 41 of 57 cases (72%).[3] Silva and associates studied the usefulness of conventional roentgenograms in the diagnosis and management of children who have suspected foreign bodies. In their series, the sensitivity and specificity of the imaging studies in identifying the presence of a foreign body was 73% and 45%, respectively. They conclude that radiography may be helpful in cases without a suspicious history of aspiration, but if the clinical suspicion is high, then the routine use of radiography is less efficient and cost effective.[7]

The types of aspirated foreign bodies are highly variable but in general can be classified as either organic or inorganic substances. Peanuts are the most common aspirated foreign body in children, with 38% reported in one series and 34% in another. In adults, dental and medical appliances tend to occur more frequently than food particles.[8] Organic materials such as nuts, seeds, meat, and bones elicit a more severe mucosal reaction, with rapid development of granulation tissue.[2] The inorganic materials such as dental appliances, tacks, and coins are usually inert and may be tolerated for many years without symptoms.

In 1897 Gustav Killian was the first to use a rigid bronchoscope to remove a foreign body in a patient who aspirated a chicken neck bone.[9] Because of the efforts of Chevalier Jackson, the rigid bronchoscope soon became firmly established as the vital instrument in foreign body removal. It was not until the 1970s with the invention of the flexible bronchoscope by Shigeto Ikeda that alternative methods of foreign body removal became available. At present, the vast array of endobronchial instruments available to the bronchoscopist, including grasping forceps, snares, baskets, and Fogarty balloons, has made foreign body removal with a flexible bronchoscope much easier and highly successful. Review of the large series of foreign body removals indicates a success rate of 86% in more than 400 procedures with a flexible bronchoscope.[2]

Inflatable angioplasty balloon catheters are extremely useful in removing foreign bodies, especially when the object is impacted in a distal orifice. The catheter can be inserted beyond the object and the balloon inflated; with gentle pressure, most objects can be dislodged and subsequently grasped and removed.[2] Glucocorticoids are sometimes used to decrease local mucosal inflammation surrounding an impacted endobronchial foreign body before attempting removal. Cryotherapy is a relatively new bronchoscopic technology that is ideally suited for foreign body removal.

A cryogen or coolant such as nitrogen is delivered to a cryoprobe catheter tip that has been passed through the working channel of a flexible bronchoscope. The catheter tip is supercooled by the nitrogen to the point where it freezes to the foreign body. The foreign body, cryoprobe, and bronchoscope are then removed as one contiguous unit. This technique is particularly useful in the removal of blood clots, mucous plugs, necrotic organic material, and small inorganic objects.[2] The ideal instrument for foreign body removal remains to be determined. It is extremely difficult to create a single instrument that is suitable for the removal of every different type and texture of foreign body. One thing is clear: when dealing with foreign bodies it is best to be prepared. This may mean having both rigid and flexible bronchoscopes available along with a full array of endoscopic instruments in order to safely handle any foreign body that comes along.

REFERENCES

1. The National Safety Council: Injury Facts (formerly Accident Facts). Itasca, Ill, 1999, pp 9-12, 43.
2. Rafanen AL, Mehta AC: Adult airway foreign body removal. Clin Chest Med 22:319-330, 2001.
3. Limper AH, Prakash UB: Tracheobronchial foreign bodies in adults. Ann Intern Med 112:604-609, 1990.
4. Metrangelo S, Monetti C, Meneghini L: Eight-years' experience with foreign body aspiration in children. What is really important for a timely diagnosis? J Pediatr Surg 34:1229-1231, 1999.
5. Abdulmajid OA, Ebeid AM, Motaweh MM, et al: Aspirated foreign bodies in the tracheobronchial tree: Report of 250 cases. Thorax 31:635-640, 1976.
6. McGuirt W, Holmes K, Feehs R, et al: Tracheobronchial foreign bodies. Laryngoscope 98:614-618, 1988.
7. Silva AB, Muntz HR, Clary R: Utility of conventional radiography in the diagnosis and management of pediatric airway foreign bodies. Ann Otol Rhinol Laryngol 107:834-838, 1998.
8. Swanson KL, Edell ES: Tracheobronchial foreign bodies. Chest Surg Clin North Am 11:861-872, 2001.
9. Killian G: Meeting of the Society of Physicians of Freiburg, Dec. 17, 1897. Munchen Med Wschr 45:378-384, 1898.

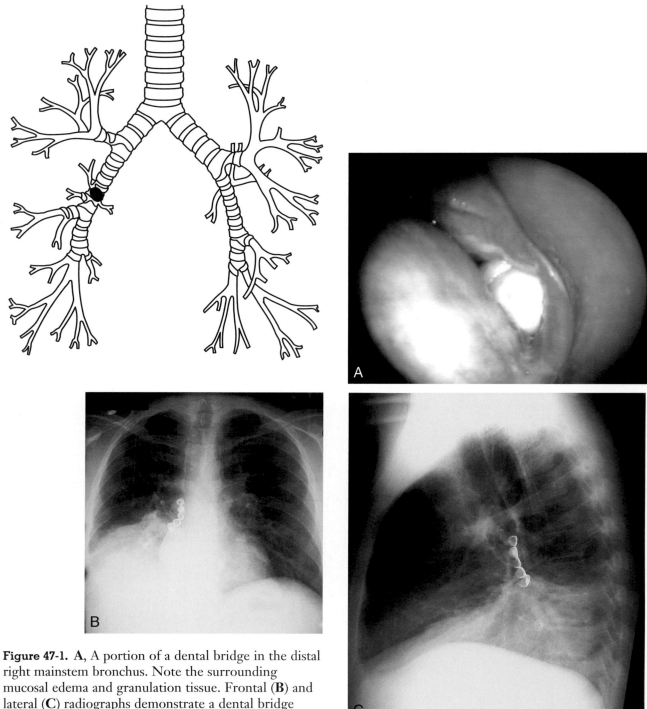

Figure 47-1. A, A portion of a dental bridge in the distal right mainstem bronchus. Note the surrounding mucosal edema and granulation tissue. Frontal (**B**) and lateral (**C**) radiographs demonstrate a dental bridge lodged within the right main bronchus and bronchus intermedius. The right lower lobe is consolidated with slight volume loss.

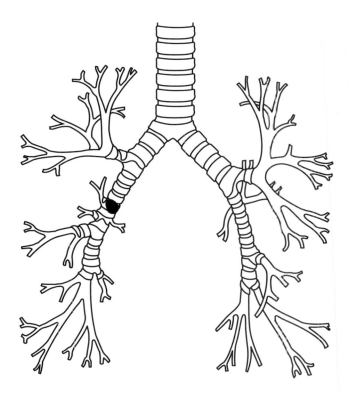

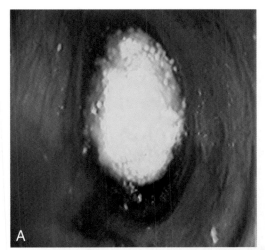

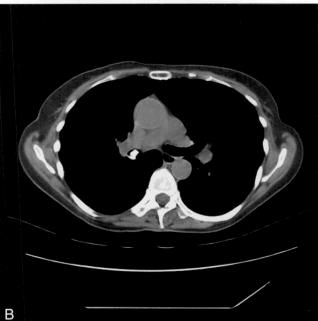

Figure 47-2. **A**, A partially dissolved calcium pill in the distal bronchus intermedius. **B**, A single image from a noncontrast CT scan demonstrates a radiodense foreign body within the bronchus intermedius corrresponding with the aspirated calcium pill.

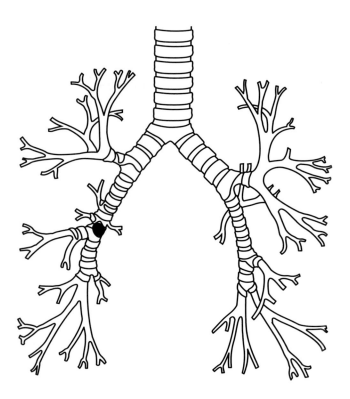

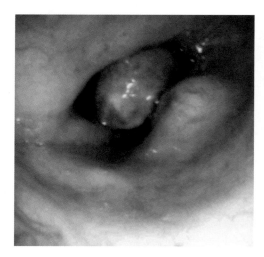

Figure 47-3. An olive pit in the bronchus intermedius that was probably aspirated 2 years before bronchoscopy. Upon initial evaluation, the lesion appeared to be an endobronchial tumor.

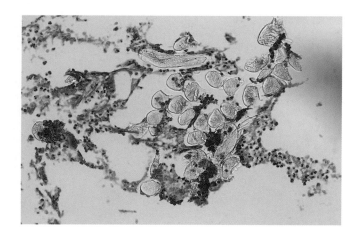

Figure 47-4. Aspirated foreign material consistent with plant or vegetable matter (H&E, ×200).

CHAPTER 48

Inhalation Injury

David R. Duhamel

Pulmonary pathology, primarily as a result of inhalation injury, accounts for 20% to 84% of burn mortality.[1] Some researchers feel that the presence or absence of inhalation injury may be a better determinant of mortality than the size of the burn injury.[1] Clinical indicators of potential inhalation injury include the presence of facial burns, singed eyebrows or nasal vibrissae, voice changes, bronchorrhea, wheezes on auscultation, carbonaceous sputum, and a history of closed-space smoke exposure or loss of consciousness. Laboratory findings of hypoxemia and elevated carbon monoxide may also be present. When bronchoscopy and xenon 133 (^{133}Xe) scanning along with clinical criteria are used to screen for inhalation injury, the reported incidence is as high as 33% of all major burn cases.[2] The clinical course of patients with inhalation injury has been well described by Stone and Martin.[3] The first stage is acute pulmonary insufficiency, the second is pulmonary edema, and the last is bronchopneumonia.

Fiberoptic bronchoscopy is now the standard technique for diagnosis of inhalation injury, and is performed routinely on admission to most burn centers. Bronchoscopic findings include airway edema and inflammation, mucosal ulceration and necrosis, and the presence of soot in the airway.[4] The absence of the cough reflex is a diagnostic sign of severe inhalation injury similar to the absence of pain in a full-thickness burn of the skin.[5] The areas of bifurcation such as the carina and lower lobe divisions are typically most severely involved. This is because the products of combustion are deposited most heavily there. When compared with the use of indirect clinical criteria to determine the presence of inhalation injury, bronchoscopy identified approximately twice as many true cases. Some investigators recommend endobronchial brush or biopsy to help make the diagnosis if the bronchoscopic findings are nonspecific.[5] The late bronchoscopic findings 48 to 72 hours after the initial injury include massive sloughing of airway epithelium. Large casts of denuded tissue and carbonaceous deposits accumulate and can occlude the airway, necessitating copious bronchoscopic lavage. After 72 hours, when the healing process has begun, characteristic patches of white granulation tissue can be seen on the airway bifurcations.

Standard chest radiographs have been found to be a very insensitive measure of inhalation injury. Putnam and co-workers reported that 13 of 21 patients with inhalation injury eventually produced abnormal chest radiographic results consisting of focal infiltrates, diffuse patchy infiltrates, and pulmonary edema. The more important point, however, is that the admission film results were normal, and many remained so up to 7 days after the injury.[6] ^{133}Xe scanning is another radiologic study used to screen for inhalation injury. It is useful to identify areas of air trapping caused by small-airway obstruction. It involves intravenous injection of radioactive xenon gas followed by serial chest scintiphotograms. Areas of decreased alveolar washout or air trapping will be identified. The decreased clearance is typically due to airway edema, mucosal sloughing, or bronchial casts causing small airway obstruction.

The mechanism of action in inhalation injury is complex. Upper airway edema occurs as a result of direct thermal injury, but because of efficient heat exchange in the oropharynx, the lower airways are typically spared. Thermal insult, however, is not the only contributing factor in inhalation injury. Smoke is composed of gas and suspended particulate materials. Gases such as hydrogen chloride, which are released by the combustion polyvinyl chloride materials, cause severe burns of the airway mucosa. Other products of combustion such as oxides of sulfur and nitrogen combine with water in the lung to yield corrosive acids and alkali. These and other chemicals contribute significantly to the lung injury caused by smoke inhalation.

Inhalation injury has a fairly dismal mortality, with reported incidences between 45% and 78% despite major advances in burn resuscitation.[1] In patients who have survived inhalation injury, the long-term pulmonary sequelae are few. Bronchiectasis developed in two patients in one series of inhalation injury survivors. Subglottic stenosis occurred in 2 of 38 survivors who underwent endotracheal intubation at the time of injury.[7] The most critically injured patients, however, die during the acute phase of injury.

REFERENCES

1. Herndon DN, Thompson PB, Traber DL: Pulmonary injury in burned patients. Crit Care Clin 1:79-96, 1985.
2. Moylan JA, Alexander G: Diagnosis and treatment of inhalation injury. World J Surg 2:185-191, 1978.
3. Stone HH, Martin JD: Pulmonary injury associated with thermal burns. Surg Gynecol Obstet 129:1242-1246, 1969.
4. Moylan JA, Adib K, Birnbaum M: Fiberoptic bronchoscopy following thermal injury. Surg Gynecol Obstet 140:541-543, 1975.
5. Masanes MJ, Legendre C, Lioret N, et al: Using bronchoscopy and biopsy to diagnose early inhalation injury, macroscopic and histologic findings. Chest 107:1365-1369, 1995.
6. Putnam CE, Loke J, Matthay RA, et al: Radiographic manifestations of acute smoke inhalation. Am J Roentgenol 129:865-870, 1977.
7. Herndon DN, Langner F, Thompson P, et al: Pulmonary injury in burned patients. Surg Clin North Am 67:31-46, 1987.

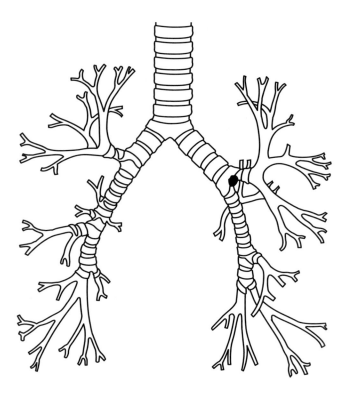

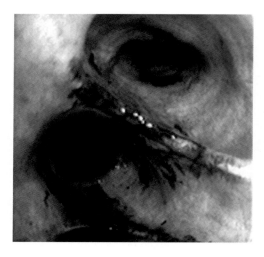

Figure 48-1. Intense deposition of soot on the bifurcation between left upper and lower lobes in a young man who was found unconscious in a burning bedroom. Note the adjacent mucosal erythema and irritation caused by the inhalation of noxious chemicals and products of combustion. It is unusual to have thermal injury in the distal airways.

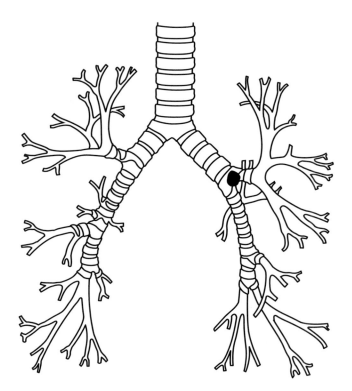

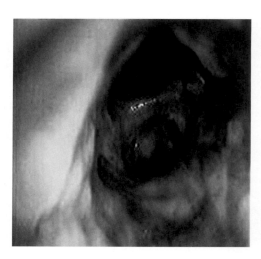

Figure 48-2. In the left mainstem bronchus, carbonaceous sputum and sloughing necrotic airway mucosa can be seen. These findings typically develop 2 to 10 days after the inhalation injury.

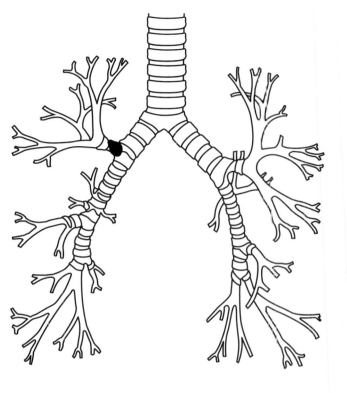

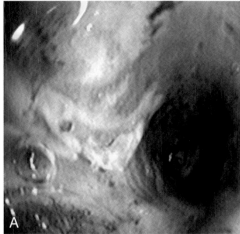

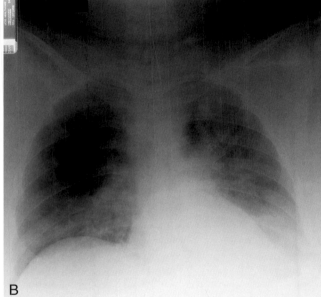

Figure 48-3. A, At the opening to the right upper lobe, more carbonaceous sputum and sloughing mucosa can be seen. **B,** Bedside radiograph demonstrates diffuse air-space opacity that is most consolidative within the left lower lobe.

CHAPTER 49

Wegener's Granulomatosis

David R. Duhamel

Wegener's granulomatosis is a disease of unknown etiology characterized by a necrotizing granulomatous vasculitis capable of affecting all organs but having a predilection for the upper and lower respiratory tracts.[1] Wegener's granulomatosis may affect persons of all ages but is most common in middle-aged patients. The disease is more prevalent in males. Sinusitis is the most common presenting symptom, followed by fever, arthralgias, cough, rhinitis, hemoptysis, otitis, and ocular inflammation.[2] Liebow described an entity called "limited Wegener's granulomatosis," which has the typical clinical and histopathologic features of the disease, without renal involvement. Cases of isolated involvement of the subglottic space or tracheobronchial tree have been reported but are rare.[3,4] Laryngeal and endobronchial involvement occurs more commonly as a late complication of fully developed or previously treated Wegener's granulomatosis.[5]

The bronchoscopic findings in Wegener's granulomatosis are highly variable. Cordier and co-workers reported that 55% of their series of patients who had Wegener's that affected the lung had bronchoscopic abnormalities. Subglottic stenosis can be found in anywhere from 8.5% to 16% of cases. Cicatricial tracheal or bronchial stenosis is seen much less frequently.[1] A cobblestone appearance of the mucosa is sometimes seen as well.[3] Inflammatory ulcers are the most prevalent finding and can be particularly impressive.[6] It is important to watch for these on the turbinates and nasopharynx as well. These ulcers can be erythematous, hemorrhagic, or black and necrotic appearing. Occasionally, a yellow-green plaque is found endobronchially, and this correlates with active disease and an increased diagnostic biopsy rate. Obstructing endobronchial pseudotumors of inflammatory granulomatous tissue have been reported. Other bronchoscopic findings include isolated lobar hemorrhage or purulent secretions.

The predominant radiographic features noted on review of chest radiographs and CT scans in a large case series were diverse.[1] They included unilateral and bilateral nodular opacities in 70% of cases. These nodules typically cavitate and often increase in quantity, especially if the disease is untreated. Infiltrates, both unilateral and bilateral, were seen in 53% of cases. Pleural opacities or effusions were seen in 12% of patients. Lobar or segmental atelectasis was seen in only 4% of cases, and is believed due to bronchial wall thickening with subsequent airway narrowing. These bronchial wall abnormalities are seldom seen on radiograph but are easily visualized on CT scan. The tracheal rings may be abnormally thickened and calcified, and, rarely, a tracheobronchial fistula may be seen. Subglottic stenosis is the most commonly reported airway manifestation and can be very difficult to see on radiograph.

The diagnosis of Wegener's granulomatosis is sometimes very difficult to make. Biopsies from the upper respiratory tract have a notoriously low yield when the strict pathologic criteria of vasculitis are required.[6] Many clinicians feel that the finding of vasculitis is not necessary to confirm the diagnosis when a patient has other classic clinical manifestations. A positive biopsy typically reveals parenchymal necrosis; granulomatous inflammation accompanied by an infiltrate consisting of a mixture of neutrophils, lymphocytes, plasma cells, eosinophils, and histiocytes; and vasculitis with blood vessel obstruction and bland infarct.[3] The c-ANCA is a fairly specific test for Wegener's granulomatosis; however, in Daum and colleagues' series of patients with endobronchial involvement, it was found not to be very predictive of disease presence or activity.[5] Although isolated Wegener's of the larynx and tracheobronchial tree is unusual, the literature suggests that early treatment with corticosteroids and cyclophosphamide is warranted.[7] The invasive management options for treating the subglottic and laryngotracheal manifestations of Wegener's granulomatosis include laryngoplastic surgery, mechanical and balloon dilation with a rigid bronchoscope and subsequent Silastic stent placement, intralesional glucocorticoid injections, and Nd:YAG or CO_2 laser resection.

REFERENCES

1. Cordier JF, Valeyre D, Guillevin L, et al: Pulmonary Wegener's granulomatosis a clinical and imaging study of 77 cases. Chest 97:906-912, 1990.
2. Fauci AS, Haynes BF, Katz P, et al: Wegener's granulomatosis: Prospective clinical and therapeutic experience with patients for 21 years. Ann Intern Med 98:76-85, 1983.
3. Scully RE, Mark EJ, McNeely WF, et al. Case records of the Massachusetts General Hospital, weekly clinicopathologic exercises. Case#50-1985. N Engl J Med 313:1530-1537, 1985.
4. Morris CJ, Byrd RP, Roy TM: Wegener's granulomatosis presenting as subglottic stenosis. J Ky Med Assoc 88:547-550, 1990.
5. Stein MG, Gamsu G, Webb WR, Stulbarg MS: Computed tomography of diffuse tracheal stenosis in Wegener's granulomatosis. J Comput Assist Tomogr 8:327-329, 1984.
6. Daum TE, Specks U, Colby TV, et al: Tracheobronchial involvement in Wegener's granulomatosis. Am J Respir Crit Care Med 151:552-526, 1995.
7. Hellman D, Laing T, Petri M, et al: Wegener's granulomatosis: Isolated involvement of the trachea and larynx. Ann Rheum Dis 46:628-63, 1987.

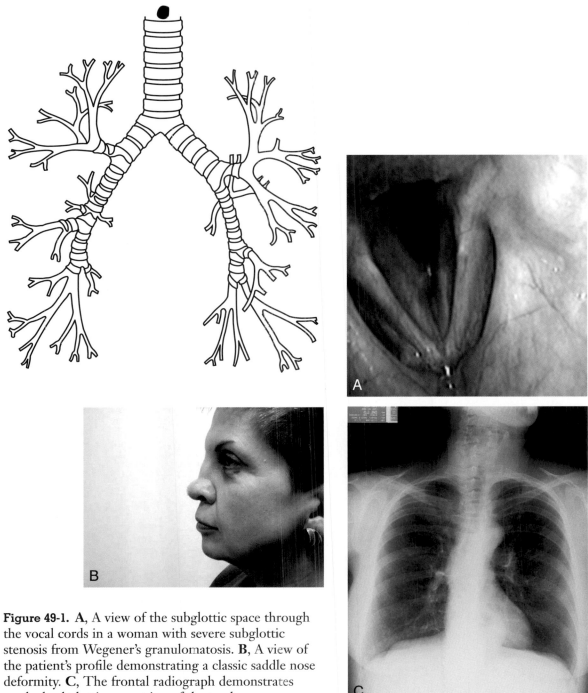

Figure 49-1. A, A view of the subglottic space through the vocal cords in a woman with severe subglottic stenosis from Wegener's granulomatosis. **B,** A view of the patient's profile demonstrating a classic saddle nose deformity. **C,** The frontal radiograph demonstrates marked subglottic narrowing of the trachea.

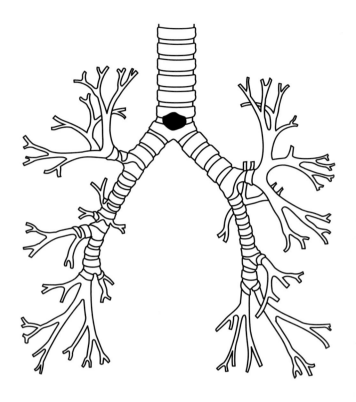

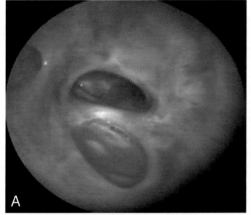

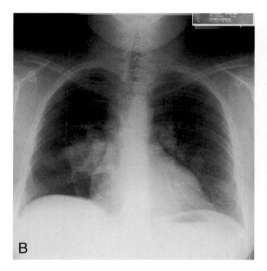

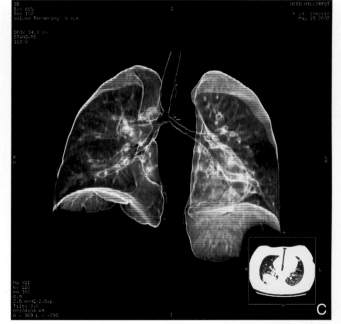

Figure 49-2. **A,** A view of the carina from the distal trachea. The airway is so distorted from chronic inflammation and scarring that only the right mainstem bronchus is identifiable. A blind ending pouch is seen just inferiorly to the orifice of the right mainstem bronchus. **B,** The frontal radiograph demonstrates multiple parenchymal air-space opacities. The distal trachea is markedly narrowed and distorted. **C,** A three-dimensional reconstruction of CT image data demonstrates marked irregularity of the distal trachea and proximal main bronchi.

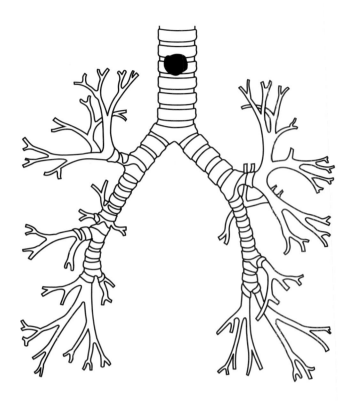

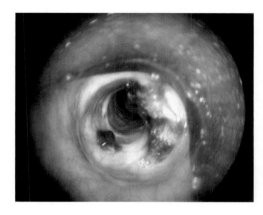

Figure 49-3. Black necrotic exudates of inflammatory tissue overlying areas of mucosal ulceration are seen in the midtrachea of a young woman with active Wegener's granulomatosis. On biopsy, these lesions are highly consistent with Wegener's granulomatosis.

Figure 49-4. Microabscesses, scattered hyperchromatic multinucleated giant cells, and heavy inflammatory background in the airways are consistent with Wegener's granulomatosis in patients with other clinical and laboratory findings (H&E, ×200, original magnification).

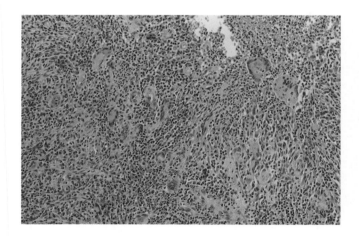

CHAPTER 50

Tracheobronchial Amyloidosis

David R. Duhamel

Amyloidosis refers to a process manifested by abnormal deposition of extracellular protein fibrils either systemically, involving multiple organs, or locally, confined to one system. Tracheobronchial amyloidosis is among the localized variants of amyloidosis. This disease can be idiopathic in etiology or associated with various inflammatory, hereditary, or neoplastic conditions. Amyloid protein takes up Congo red stain and exhibits apple-green birefringence under polarized microscopy. Pulmonary amyloidosis may be part of a widespread process involving many organs or may be localized to the airways and lung parenchyma. Primary pulmonary amyloidosis refers to amyloidosis that is confined to the pulmonary system; patients who have systemic amyloidosis are not included here.[1] It occurs in three forms: diffuse interstitial deposits, single or multiple pulmonary nodules, and, most commonly, tracheobronchial deposits.[2]

Primary pulmonary amyloidosis is relatively uncommon. Thompson and Citron reviewed the world literature and found 126 cases, of which 67 were tracheobronchial and the rest were either interstitial or parenchymal nodular.[3] The mean age at diagnosis appears to be the mid-50s.[1] The male-to-female ratio was 1:1. Patients with tracheobronchial amyloid may be asymptomatic or may have dyspnea, hemoptysis, cough, and hoarseness. Atelectasis and post-obstructive pneumonia have been reported as well. These findings usually indicate amyloid deposition involving the lobar or segmental bronchi. The localized form of pulmonary amyloidosis typically manifests with no evidence of disease outside the tracheobronchial system. In a review of 17 cases of tracheobronchial amyloidosis at the Mayo Clinic, only 1 was associated with a systemic illness—multiple myeloma.[4] Typically, parenchymal and tracheobronchial amyloid do not occur together.

The bronchoscopic findings may include multifocal flat plaques of grayish-white amyloid material distributed throughout the trachea and bronchial lumens. The entire endobronchial lumen may be involved, and there is no sparing of the posterior membrane as seen in tracheopathia osteoplastica. Less commonly seen is a raised endobronchial tumor-like mass of amyloid material that is easily mistaken for neoplasm.[1] Other bronchoscopic findings have included nodular and polypoid lesions. Although bronchoscopic biopsy is the mainstay of diagnosis, there is concern for an increased bleeding risk. The amyloid deposition in the vascular wall is thought to inhibit appropriate hemostatic mechanisms.

The radiographic findings were normal in one quarter of the cases of tracheobronchial disease.[5] The typical radiographic appearance is that of multiple nodules protruding from the wall of the trachea. Occasionally, the disease manifests with unifocal, multifocal, or diffuse narrowing of the tracheobronchial lumen. An amyloid tumor-like mass may cause endobronchial obstruction with collapse, air trapping, and pneumonia.[6] On CT scan, the tracheal or bronchial walls are much thicker in the affected areas. In certain cases of diffuse involvement, there is a significant component of calcification and ossification of the lesions, which leads to a second diagnosis of tracheopathia osteoplastica. This has led some researchers to suggest that tracheopathia osteoplastica may represent end-stage pulmonary amyloidosis.[5]

Amyloid deposits have characteristic tinctorial properties, which greatly facilitiates making a histologic diagnosis. Most notably is the apple-green birefringence seen with polarized light on Congo red–stained tissue. Currently it is felt that amyloid material is made up of segments of light chain immunoglobulin, usually of the lambda type.

Although it may exhibit a relatively stable course, tracheobronchial amyloidosis also can cause severe morbidity with its potential for extensive airway involvement. In an article by Hui and associates, three of seven patients with tracheobronchial disease died of respiratory failure or recurrent pneumonia due to endobronchial obstruction.[7] Some investigators believe that the mortality rate with tracheobronchial amyloidosis is as high as 20%.[5] Management options are fairly limited. Endobronchial resection of obstructing lesions using Nd:YAG laser has had some success, and there are reports of surgical treatments including pneumonectomy.[8,9] One option that appears promising is the placement of an endobronchial silicone stent to help maintain airway patency. Others have advocated the use of radiation therapy for diffuse or multifocal tracheobronchial involvement.[5]

REFERENCES

1. Utz JP, Swenswn SJ, Gertz MA: Pulmonary amyloidosis the Mayo Clinic experience from 1980 to 1993. Ann Int Med 124:407-413, 1996.
2. Rubinow A, Celli BR, Cohen AS, et al: Localized amyloidosis of the lower respiratory tract. Am Rev Respir Dis 118:603-611, 1978.
3. Thompson PJ, Citron KM: Amyloid and the lower respiratory tract. Thorax 38:84-87, 1983.
4. Capizzi SA, Betancourt E, Prakash UBS: Tracheobronchial amyloidosis. Mayo Clin Proc 75:1148-1152, 2000.
5. Chen KTK: Amyloidosis presenting in the respiratory tract. Pathol Ann 24(Part 1):253-273, 1989.
6. Gross BH, Felson B, Birnberg FA: The respiratory tract in amyloidosis and the plasma cell dyscrasias. Semin Roentgenol 21:113-127, 1986.
7. Hui AN, Koss MN, Hochholzer L, Wehunt WD: Amyloidosis presenting in the lower respiratory tract. Arch Pathol Lab Med 110:212-218, 1986.
8. Flemming AF, Fairfax AJ, Arnold AG, Lane DJ: Treatment of endobronchial amyloidosis by intermittent bronchoscopic resection. Br J Dis Chest 74:183-188, 1980.
9. Weismann RE, Clagett OT, McDonald JR: Amyloid disease of the lung treated by pneumonectomy. J Thorac Cardiovasc Surg 16: 269-281, 1947.

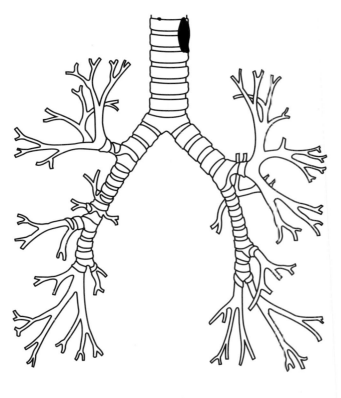

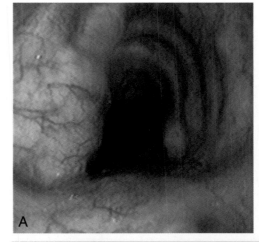

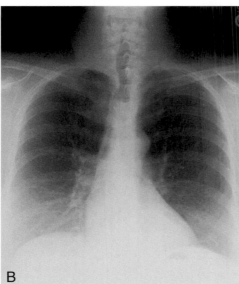

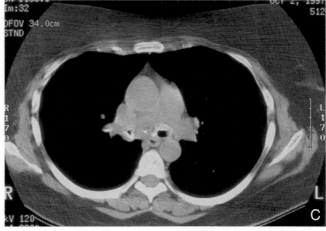

Figure 50-1. A, Yellowish waxy plaques and deposits of amyloid material in the left lateral tracheal wall. **B,** The frontal radiograph demonstrates multiple regions of airway narrowing involving the trachea and proximal bronchi. **C,** The CT image through proximal bronchi demonstrates marked thickening of the airway walls. Scattered calcifications are present.

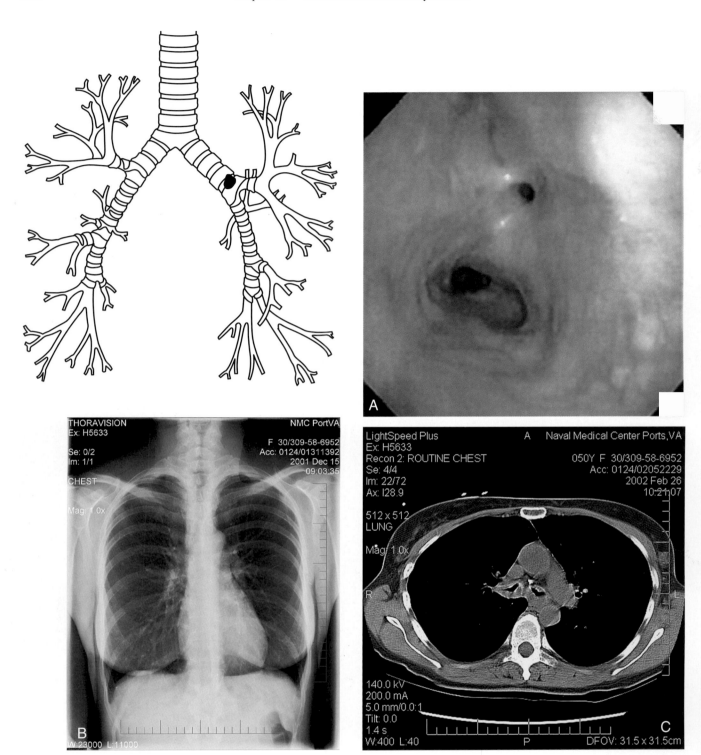

Figure 50-2. A, Extensive yellow-gray deposits of amyloid material in the left upper lobe bronchus that infiltrate the bronchial mucosa and narrow the airway lumen. **B,** The frontal radiograph demonstrates marked irregularity of the airways, primarily affecting the trachea. **C,** The CT image through proximal bronchi demonstrates thickening of the airways.

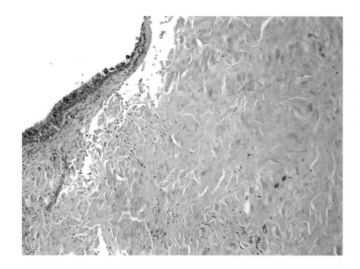

Figure 50-3. Amorphous homogeneous eosinophilic material consistent with tracheobronchial amyloid (H&E, ×100).

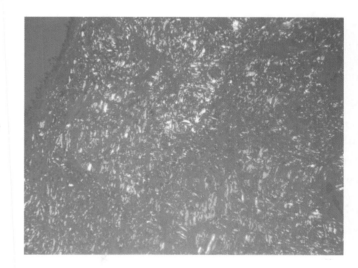

Figure 50-4. Apple-green birefringence demonstrated by polarized light.

CHAPTER 51

Tracheopathia Osteoplastica

David R. Duhamel

Tracheopathia osteoplastica (TPO) is a rare, benign disease of the trachea and major bronchi in which multiple submucosal osteocartilaginous nodules project into the airway lumen. These nodules can be focal or diffuse throughout the entire tracheobronchial tree, but classically they affect the lower two thirds of the trachea and proximal portion of the main bronchi.[1] It may on occasion affect the larynx and subglottic space. There is a 3:1 male predilection, and the disease typically manifests in patients in their mid-50s. The incidence of TPO found during routine bronchoscopy for pulmonary complaints ranges from 0.02%[2] to 0.7%.[3] However, many experienced bronchoscopists feel it occurs much more commonly than is reported and is not recognized due to its indolent course.[4] The characteristic symptoms include cough, dyspnea on exertion, recurrent infection, wheeze, and, on occasion, hemoptysis. The last-mentioned symptom is seen when two opposing nodules rub against each other, causing erosion of the mucosa and subsequent bleeding. Quite frequently the patient is asymptomatic, and the condition is discovered by chance after a difficult intubation or during a bronchoscopy or CT scan for nonrelated events.[5] Pathologically, the nodules are composed of submucosal islands of hyaline cartilage with areas of lamellar bone and occasional marrow elements. The mucosal surface is typically intact, and a connection to the perichondrium of a tracheal ring is frequently seen.[6]

The etiology of this disease remains unclear, but many theories exist. There is some evidence for a congenital process or inherited trait that predisposes an individual. The most compelling evidence is the high number of reported cases of TPO in Finland and Sweden.[5] One case report, however, appears to contradict the theory of congenital disease. A 55-year-old woman underwent bronchoscopy for unrelated reasons and reportedly had a normal trachea. She underwent bronchoscopy again at age 70 and was found to have severe TPO. Local metabolic or inflammatory factors and infections or chemical irritation have all been suggested as etiologic factors.[5] *Klebsiella ozaenae*, a bacterium that causes a chronic tracheal infection, is believed to be associated with TPO.[5] At least three early reports of TPO found an association with tracheal amyloidosis, causing some investigators to suggest that TPO represents the end stage of amyloidosis.[4] There is little other evidence to support this theory, and in a review of 245 cases of TPO by Martin no association with amyloid was found.[7]

The typical bronchoscopic appearance is that of multiple, smooth, raised, white, bony-appearing nodules protruding into the airway lumen. Some experts have described the airway as having a beaded appearance.[4] These nodules are typically distributed over the anterolateral walls in association with the cartilaginous rings but classically spare the posterior membrane. The lack of involvement of the posterior membrane is an important diagnostic point and helps to rule out other diseases of the tracheobronchial tree.[1-3] These lesions are typically very hard, and the bronchoscopist will find it extremely difficult, if not impossible, to perform a biopsy with a flexible bronchoscope. A rigid bronchoscope is frequently required for adequate biopsy specimens, but the diagnosis is often made with visual inspection. In certain cases, the trachea may be narrowed or distorted so severely that it prevents the passage of the rigid bronchoscope or endotracheal tube.

On CT scan the classic description is thickened tracheal cartilage with irregular calcification. There are multiple nodules with or without calcification that project into the airway lumen from the anterior and lateral walls.[6] Once again it is pathognomonic for TPO that the nodules spare the posterior membrane. In mild disease the radiograph results are usually normal.[8] In moderate to severe disease the radiograph may reveal tracheal scalloping, calcified nodules, or irregular asymmetric stenosis.[1]

Currently there is no treatment to remove the abnormal tissue growth or to prevent new nodules from growing. Most patients are without symptoms and need no treatment, but on occasion the disease process is so severe that it threatens to completely occlude the airway. These situations call for more invasive therapy. Attempted treatments have included Nd:YAG laser ablation, cryotherapy, and external beam radiation, none of which provided significant benefit.[4,5] The literature does include a description of a surgical procedure in which the trachea is split and the nodules are scraped out. The trachea is then closed over a silicone stent or Silastic T tube.[1] This treatment is rather extreme but fortunately very rarely needed.

REFERENCES

1. Case 32-1999. Tracheopathia osteoplastica. Case records of the Massachusetts General Hospital. N Engl J Med 341:1292-1299, 1999.
2. van Nierop MAMF, Wagenaar SS, van den Bosch JMM, et al: Tracheopathia osteochondroplastica. Report of four cases. Eur J Respir Dis 64:129-133, 1983.
3. Primer G: Tracheopathia osteochondroplastica. Prax Pneumol 33:1060-1063, 1979.
4. Prakash UBS, McCullough AE, Edell ES, Nienhuis DM: Tracheopathia osteoplastica. Familial occurrence. Mayo Clin Proc 64:1091-1096, 1989.
5. Vilkman S, Keistinen T: Tracheopathia osteoplastica. Report of a young man with severe disease and retrospective review of 18 cases. Respiration 62:151-154, 1995.
6. Kwong JS, Muller NS, Miller RR: Diseases of the trachea and main-stem bronchi: Correlation of CT with pathologic findings. Radiographics 12:645-657, 1992.
7. Martin CJ: Tracheobronchopathia osteochondroplastica. Arch Otolaryngol 100:290-293, 1974.
8. Meyer CA, White CS: Cartilaginous disorders of the chest. Sci Exhibit 18:1109-1123, 1998.

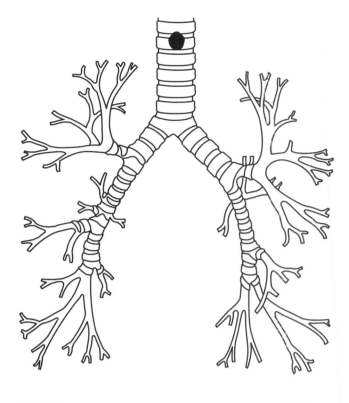

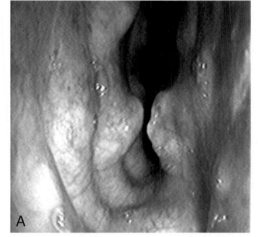

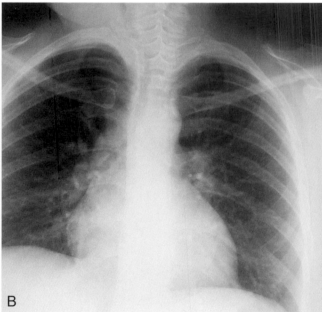

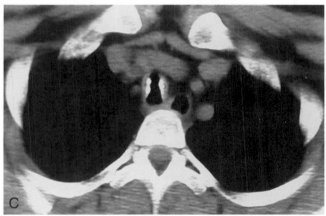

Figure 51-1. A, Multiple, white, bony protuberances arising from the cartilaginous rings of the trachea and occluding the airway lumen. **B,** The frontal radiograph demonstrates marked irregularity and narrowing of the trachea. **C,** A single image from a CT study demonstrates dense calcification and nodularity of the cartilaginous portions of the trachea. The posterior membrane is normal. The overall dimension of the airway is reduced.

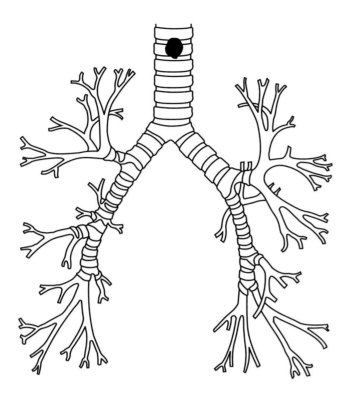

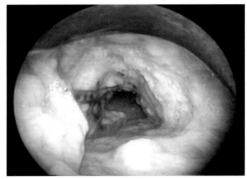

Figure 51-2. Extensive, diffuse, growth of yellowish-white bony material throughout the entire trachea. Note the sparing of the posterior membrane, which is characteristic of tracheopathia osteoplastica.

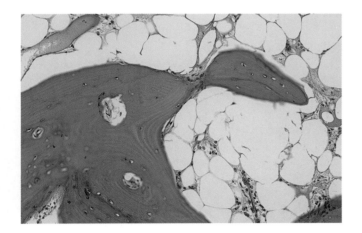

Figure 51-3. Submucosal nodules of benign metaplastic bone protrude into the bronchial lumen (H&E, ×20).

CHAPTER 52

Relapsing Polychondritis

David R. Duhamel

Relapsing polychondritis is a rare syndrome characterized by recurrent episodes of painful inflammation that affect cartilaginous structures, with subsequent degeneration and fibrosis. Cartilaginous destruction of the ear, nose, peripheral joints, larynx, and tracheobronchial tree may develop as a result of this process.[1] Laryngotracheobronchial involvement is a presenting manifestation in 10% of cases, but 50% of all polychondritis patients eventually develop it.[2,3] Involvement of the respiratory tract carries a worse overall prognosis, with 50% of all deaths being due to some aspect of airway disease.[2] The classic manifestations of airway involvement include hoarseness, aphonia, tenderness over the laryngeal and thyroid cartilages, stridor, dyspnea, cough, and recurrent infection.

The disease affects males and females equally, but airway involvement is seen more commonly in females. The peak incidence occurs between 40 and 60 years of age. It predominantly affects whites but has been reported rarely in other races and ethnic origins. It is considered an autoimmune process, and autoantibodies have been found directed against cartilage and type II collagen. The diagnosis can be made on clinical grounds when three or more of the following features are present: bilateral auricular chondritis, nonerosive seronegative inflammatory polyarthritis, nasal chondritis, ocular inflammation, respiratory tract chondritis, and audiovestibular damage.[2]

The bronchoscopic findings early in the disease course may include diffuse narrowing of lumen primarily from inflammatory mucosal erythema and edema. Later, tracheobronchomalacia may be seen with floppy collapsible airways due to softening and destruction of the cartilaginous rings. The lumen opens easily on passage of the bronchoscope but collapses back down with removal. Finally, fixed narrowing and stenosis may develop from granulation tissue and peribronchial fibrosis.[4]

Radiographically diffuse or localized airway involvement may be seen. It most commonly involves the larynx and upper trachea, but it may even involve the bronchus out to the subsegments.[1,5] Mediastinal lymphadenopathy has not been reported in relapsing polychondritis, and this finding on CT scan should raise questions about the diagnosis.[1]

The pathologic characteristics of the lesion are loss of basophilic staining and metachromasia of the cartilage matrix, which appears to be the result of loss of the acid mucopolysaccharides. In early phases of the disease, a loss of lacunae and occasionally a neutrophilic infiltrate of the cartilage matrix have been observed.[3]

The approaches to treatment are varied. If the disease is limited to the larynx and upper trachea, a tracheostomy can be performed, but it is of no value when there is bronchial obstruction. Other invasive techniques include placement of endobronchial Silastic stents to help maintain airway patency. Surgical resection is of limited value in treating inflammatory lesions, but may have a role in isolated fixed stenosis.[5] Some investigators advocate the surgical technique of external airway splinting with pericardium or dura mater for cases of extensive tracheobronchial involvement.[5] It should be reinforced that early and decisive intervention is vital in managing these patients' airways because they can develop rapid and complete occlusion. Sudden death due to tracheal collapse has been reported with bronchoscopy, intubation, and tracheostomy.[2,6] The mainstay of treatment remains medical management with corticosteroids. Most patients require chronic low doses of steroids with intermittent boluses during episodes of acute inflammation. Patients with milder disease have been managed with nonsteroidal anti-inflammatory drugs and dapsone. Success has also been reported with immunosuppressive drugs such as azathioprine and cyclosporin A.[5]

REFERENCES

1. Davis SD, Berkmen YM, King T: Peripheral bronchial involvement in relapsing polychondritis: Demonstration by thin-section CT. Am J Roentgenol 153:953-954, 1989.
2. McAdam LP, O'Hanlan MA, Bluestone R, Pearson CM: Relapsing polychondritis: Prospective study of 23 patients and a review of the literature. Medicine 55:193-215, 1976.
3. Scully RE, Mark EJ, McNeely BU: Case records of the Massachusetts General Hospital, weekly clinico-pathological exercises. Case #50-1985. N Engl J Med 313:1530-1537, 1985.
4. Dolan Dl, Lemmon GD, Teitelbaum SL: Relapsing polychondritis. Am J Med 41:285-299, 1966.
5. Eng J, Sabanathan S: Airway complications in relapsing polychondritis. Ann Thorac Surg 51:686-692, 1991.
6. Purcelli FM, Nahum M, Monell C: Relapsing polychondritis with tracheal collapse. Ann Otol Rhinol Laryngol 71:1120-1129, 1962.

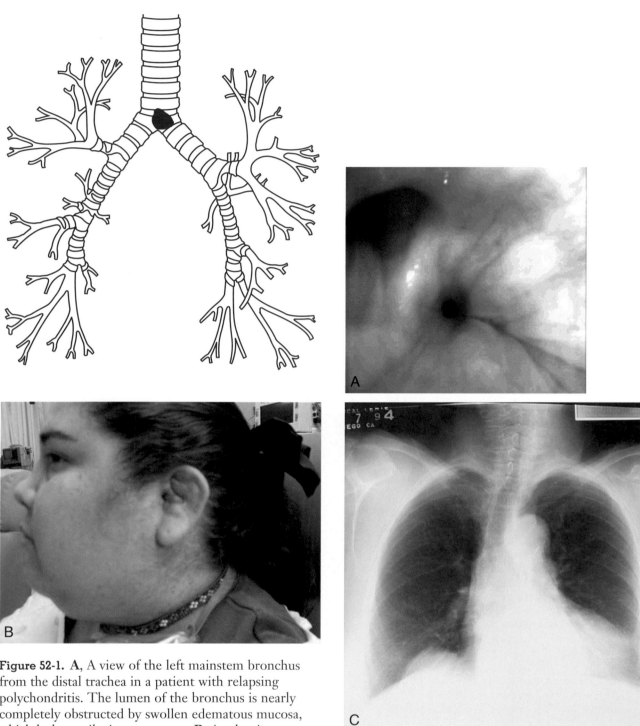

Figure 52-1. A, A view of the left mainstem bronchus from the distal trachea in a patient with relapsing polychondritis. The lumen of the bronchus is nearly completely obstructed by swollen edematous mucosa, which lacks cartilaginous support. **B,** A relapsing polychondritis patient with what is described as a "cauliflower ear." The distortion and edema of the ear are caused by the inflammatory destruction of the cartilaginous structures. **C,** The frontal chest radiograph demonstrates a long segment of marked tracheal narrowing proximal to the thoracic inlet. The intrathoracic trachea is relatively normal.

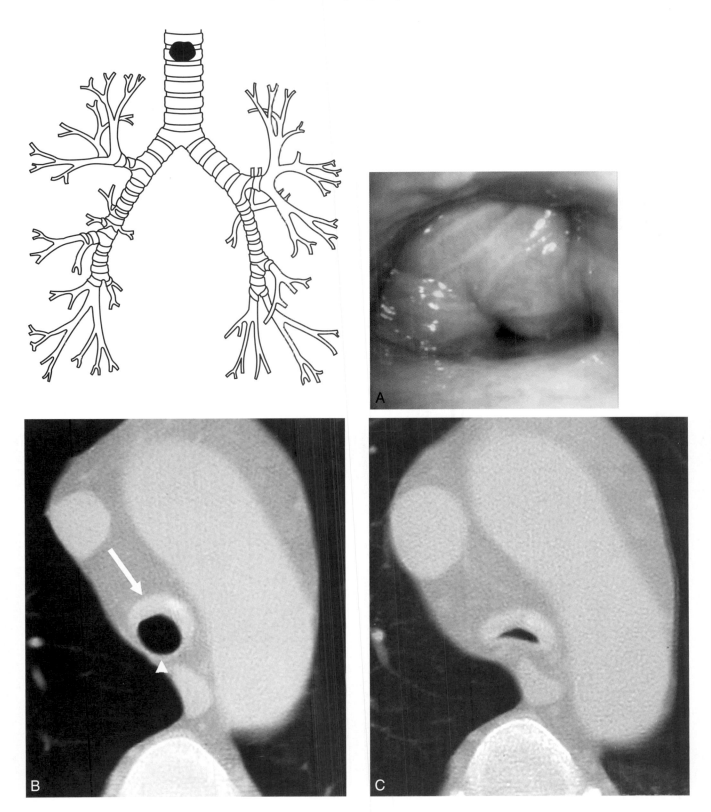

Figure 52-2. A, A view of the midtrachea in a patient with relapsing polychondritis, demonstrating the boggy edema and inflammation of the airway mucosa, as well as the loss of structural support and dynamic collapse of the lumen. Images from a dynamic CT scan obtained during inspiration (**B**) and expiration (**C**) demonstrate anterior motion of the posterior membrane with expiration. This results in dynamic collapse. The cartilagenous portion of the trachea is thickened and abnormally calcified.

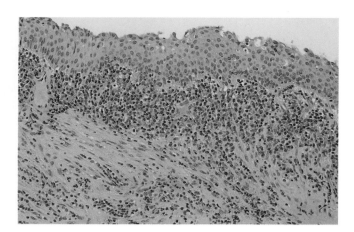

Figure 52-3. Recurrent destructive inflammation in the bronchial cartilage may result in a complete loss of cartilaginous plates of the bronchi with severe inflammatory reactions (H&E, ×20).

CHAPTER 53

Rhinoscleroma

David R. Duhamel

Rhinoscleroma is a chronic, progressive, granulomatous infection that affects the respiratory tract from the nose to the bronchi.[1] The etiologic agent, a gram-negative diplobacillus named *Klebsiella rhinoscleromatis*, was discovered by Von Frisch in 1882.[2] The disease is endemic in several places, including Central America, Central Europe, Africa, and Asia, but remains fairly rare in the United States. The increase in sporadic cases in recent years is apparently due to immigration to the United States from endemic regions. Untreated rhinoscleroma tends to progress slowly over many years, characterized by periods of remission and relapse. The disease manifests as four overlapping stages: the catarrhal stage, characterized by prolonged purulent rhinorrhea; the atrophic stage, with mucosal changes and crust formation; the granulomatous stage, characterized by granulomatous nodules in the nose, with or without involvement of other parts of the respiratory tract; and the sclerotic stage, with dense cicatricial fibrosis of the affected tissue.[3]

Rhinoscleroma originates in the nose but may progress and involve any part of the airway. Symptoms in the early stages are nonspecific and simulate simple rhinitis or sinusitis. Late-stage symptoms that indicate laryngotracheal involvement include dysphonia, dyspnea, stridor, and productive cough. Laryngeal involvement is seen in 15% to 80% of cases, but tracheobronchial disease is far less common.[4] Rhinoscleroma is not highly contagious. Poor hygiene, prolonged close contact, and malnutrition increase the potential for infection and transmission.[5] Mortality from rhinoscleroma is extremely rare and classically occurs in patients with newly diagnosed or undiagnosed disease.[6]

A positive culture of *K. rhinoscleromatis* is diagnostic of the disease but occurs in less than 60% of cases.[2] Immunocytochemistry using antibodies to the O2K3 capsular antigen on *K. rhinoscleromatis* can be used to make a definitive diagnosis. The histologic findings include numerous proliferating small blood vessels. A lymphocytic infiltrate is typically seen with a predominance of highly vacuolated foamy macrophages called Mikulicz cells. These cells frequently contain the intracellular gram-negative diplobacillus. Large degenerated plasma cells called Russell bodies are also seen.

The bronchoscopic findings are variable. During the earlier stages of disease, adherent whitish-green plaques may be seen in the airway. Culture of this material shows a high yield of the organism. In the late stages of the disease, bland densely fibrotic areas of scarring and stenosis may be seen focally or diffusely throughout the entire tracheobronchial tree. There may even be fibrosis and scarring at the orifice to the lobar segments. The radiographic findings are fairly nonspecific. Focal or diffuse areas of tracheobronchial narrowing are seen. The stenotic areas are of soft tissue density and are noncalcified. Concurrent nasal and sinus disease is almost always seen and represents an important diagnostic clue.

Antimicrobial therapy remains the cornerstone of therapy. Tetracycline or quinolones for a prolonged period of 6 months or until nasal biopsy results are negative are recommended. Significant fibrotic stenosis of the trachea and bronchus can sometimes be treated by balloon dilation or mechanical dilation with the rigid bronchoscope. A tracheostomy is occasionally required for severe involvement of the larynx or subglottic space.

REFERENCES

1. Yigla M, Ben-Izhak O, Oren I, Hashman N, Lejbkowicz F: Laryngotracheobronchial involvement in a patient with nonendemic rhinoscleroma. Chest 117:1795-1798, 2000.
2. Omeroglu A, Weisenberg E, Baim HM, Rhone DP: Pathologic quiz case: Supraglottic granulomas in a young Central American man. Arch Pathol Lab Med 125:157-158, 2001.
3. Amoils CP, Shindo ML: Laryngotracheal manifestations of rhinoscleroma. Ann Otol Rhinol Laryngol 105:336-340, 1996.
4. Soni NK: Scleroma of the respiratory tract: A bronchoscopic study. J Laryngol Otol 108:484-485, 1994.
5. Batsakis JG, El-Naggar AK: Rhinoscleroma and rhinosporidiosis: Pathology consultation. Ann Otol Rhinol Laryngol 101:879-882, 1992.
6. Miller RH, Shulman JB, Canlais RF, et al: *Klebsiella rhinoscleromatis:* A clinical and pathogenic enigma. Otolaryngol Head Neck Surg 87:212-221, 1979.

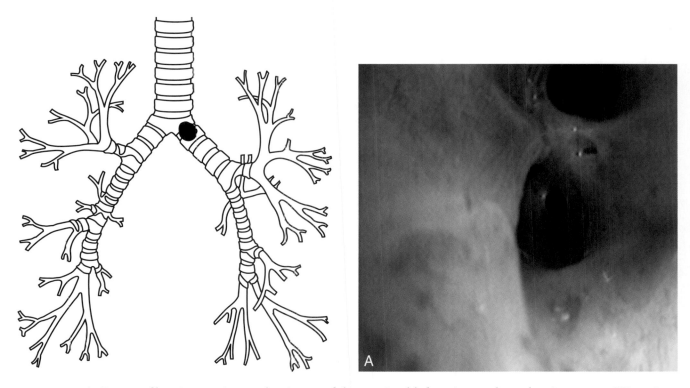

Figure 53-1. A, Intense fibrosis, scarring, and stricture of the proximal left mainstem bronchus in a young Hispanic woman with cicatricial *Klebsiella* rhinoscleroma. The lumen of the bronchus is transected by bands and webs of fibrotic tissue.

Continued

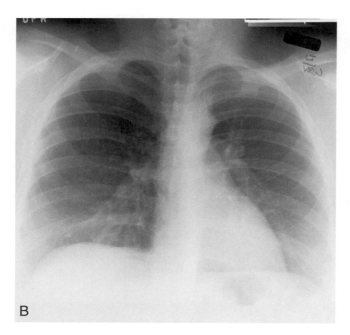

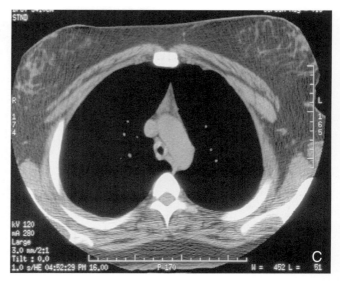

Figure 53-1, *cont'd.* **B,** The frontal radiograph demonstrates marked narrowing over a long segment of the trachea. **C,** A single image from a CT study at the level of the carina demonstrates marked circumferential thickening of the airways.

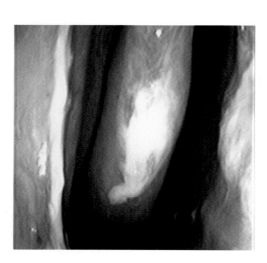

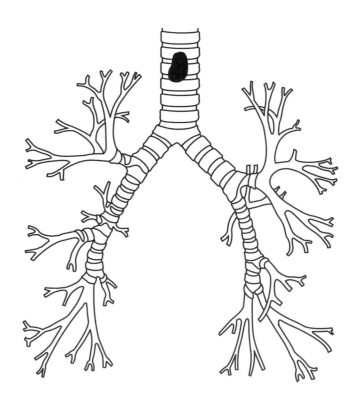

Figure 53-2. Adherent yellow-green plaques of mucoid material on the inferior turbinate of a patient with *Klebsiella* rhinoscleroma.

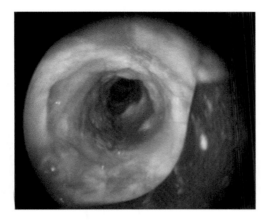

Figure 53-3. Yellow-green deposits of mucoid material along with mucosal inflammation and scarring of the midtrachea. Culture of the yellow material grew *Klebsiella rhinoscleromatis.*

Figure 53-4. Rhinoscleroma occurs primarily in the sinonasal mucosa and shows a diffuse submucosal infiltrate composed of numerous macrophages with clear to foamy cytoplasm in a mixed, nonspecific inflammatory background (H&E, ×200).

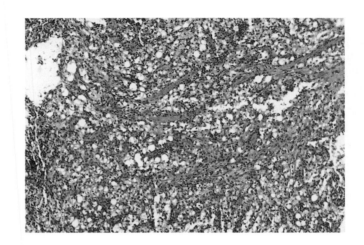

CHAPTER 54

Pseudomembranous Disease of the Airway

Gehan Devendra

Pseudomembranes are a coagulum of inflammatory material and fibrin with points of attachment at mucosal erosion. These pseudomembranes can be found at many sites throughout the body. This chapter focuses on the etiologic agents of pseudomembrane formation in the airways. The major cause for pseudomembrane production is usually the result of an infectious organism. Many agents have been associated with airway pseudomembrane formation (Table 54-1).

Diphtheria is the classic etiologic cause of pseudomembranes in the airway. It is transmitted by direct contact or by sneezing or coughing. Tracheobronchial diphtheria is uncommon. Symptoms include hoarseness, dyspnea, cough, and stridor. Edema and pseudomembrane formation of the tracheobronchial tree can cause respiratory failure from obstruction of the main airways. Initially the membrane is white but then becomes gray. Patches of green or black, or both, can occur later in the infection. The membrane may or may not be attached firmly. Underneath the membrane is hyperemic tissue, and bleeding can occur when the membrane is torn off. The infection can spread around the trachea and then down to the level of the bronchioles and alveoli, causing pneumonia. Viewed histologically, the pseudomembrane contains heavy amounts of pleomorphic

TABLE 54–1

Causative Agents of Pseudomembrane Formation

Infectious	Noninfectious
Corynebacterium diphtheriae[5]	Tracheal intubation[6]
Corynebacterium pseudodiphtheriticum[7]	Stevens-Johnson syndrome[8]
Staphylococcus aureus[9]	Paraquat ingestion[10]
Bacillus cereus[11]	Ligneous conjunctivitis[12]
Aspergillus species[13]	Smoke inhalation[15]
Haemophilus influenzae b[14]	

gram-positive bacilli with clubbed ends. Lesions have vascular congestion, edema, neutrophils, and fibrin exudation.[1] Treatment of diphtheria is with either penicillin or erythromycin.[2]

Corynebacterium pseudodiphtheriticum is a gram-positive bacillus with a clubbed end. It is a normal airway colonizer but can produce disease in immunocompromised patients. Unlike *Corynebacterium diphtheriae*, *C. pseudodiphtheriticum* does not have an endotoxin. Clinical presentation is like that of *C. diphtheriae*. The treatment depends on sensitivity testing. Care must be taken not to confuse this organism with *C. diphtheriae* so as to prevent unnecessary outbreak control measures.[3]

Aspergillus can also cause tracheobronchial pseudomembranes. Patients who acquire this form are immunosuppressed from either human immunodeficiency virus (HIV) or transplantation. Patients complain of dyspnea or wheezing that can rapidly progression to respiratory failure.[1-4] Treatment is with amphotericin B; however, success with itraconazole has been documented.[1]

REFERENCES

1. Kramer MR, Denning DW, Marshall SE, et al: Ulcerative tracheobronchitis after lung transplantation. A new form of invasive aspergillosis. Am Rev Respir Dis 144:552-556, 1991.
2. MacGregor RR: *Corynebacterium diphtheriae*. *In* Mandell GL, Bennett JE, Dolin R (eds): Principles and Practice of Infectious Disease, 4th ed. New York, Churchill Livingstone, 1995.
3. Izurieta HS, Strebel PM, Youngblood T, et al: Exudative pharyngitis possibly due to *Corynebacterium pseudodiphtheriticum*, a new challenge in the differential diagnosis of diphtheria. Emerg Infect Dis 3:65-68, 1997.
4. Pervez NK, Kleinerman J, Kattan M, et al: Pseudomembranous necrotizing bronchial aspergillosis. A variant of invasive aspergillosis in a patient with hemophilia and acquired immune deficiency syndrome. Am Rev Respir Dis 131:961-963, 1985.
5. Hadfield TL, McEvoy P, Polotsky Y, et al: The pathology of diphtheria. J Infect Dis 181(Suppl 1):S116-S120, 2000.
6. Deslee G, Brichet A, Lebuffe G, et al: Obstructive fibrinous tracheal pseudomembrane. A potentially fatal complication of tracheal intubation. Am J Respir Crit Care Med 162:1169-1171, 2000.
7. Colt HG, Morris JF, Marston BJ, Sewell DL: Necrotizing tracheitis caused by *Corynebacterium pseudodiphtheriticum*: Unique case and review. Rev Infect Dis 13:73-76, 1991.
8. Koch WM, McDonald GA: Stevens-Johnson syndrome with supraglottic laryngeal obstruction. Arch Otolaryngol Head Neck Surg 115:1381-1383, 1989.
9. Yamazaki Y, Hirai K, Honda T: Pseudomembranous tracheobronchitis caused by methicillin-resistant *Staphylococcus aureus*. Scand J Infect Dis 34:211-213, 2002.
10. Stephens DS, Walker DH, Schaffner W, et al: Pseudodiphtheria: Prominent pharyngeal membrane associated with fatal paraquat ingestion. Ann Intern Med 94:202-904, 1981.
11. Strauss R, Mueller A, Wehler M, et al: Pseudomembranous tracheobronchitis due to *Bacillus cereus*. Clin Infect Dis 33:E39-E41, 2001.
12. Ozcelik U, Akcoren Z, Anadol D, et al: Pulmonary involvement in a child with ligneous conjunctivitis and homozygous type I plasminogen deficiency. Pediatr Pulmonol 32:179-183, 2001.
13. Machida U, Kami M, Kanda Y, et al: Aspergillus tracheobronchitis after allogeneic bone marrow transplantation. Bone Marrow Transplant 24:1145-1149, 1999.
14. Oymar K: Bacterial tracheitis in children. Tidsskr Nor Laegeforen 120:1417-1419, 2000.
15. Hubbard GB, Langlinais PC, Shimazu T, et al: The morphology of smoke inhalation in sheep. J Trauma 31:1477-1486, 1991.

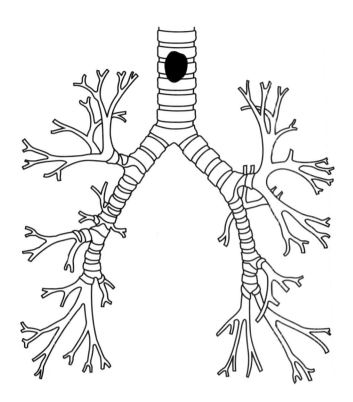

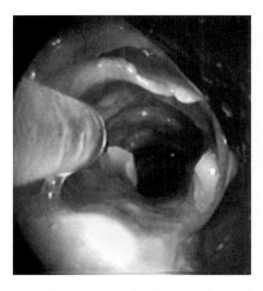

Figure 54-1. Classic gray and yellow pseudomembranes in the trachea of a patient infected with *Corynebacterium diphtheriae*. Note the erythematous and hyperemic mucosa below the sloughing membranes.

CHAPTER 55

Herpes Tracheobronchitis

David R. Duhamel

Herpes simplex virus (HSV) is a well-known and frequently encountered cause of mucocutaneous lesions, but only in recent years has it been recognized as a cause of respiratory tract infections. The herpesviruses are double-stranded deoxyribonucleic acid (DNA) viruses capable of lying dormant within a cell without causing clinical disease. Although it can be isolated from the oral secretions of 1% to 5% of asymptomatic normal individuals, immunologically competent patients rarely develop tracheobronchitis.[1] In the general population the incidence is thought to be around 1%, based on an autopsy study of 1000 patients.[2] However, in certain circumstances such as when a patient is immunocompromised from acquired immunodeficiency syndrome (AIDS), cancer, severe burns, or steroids, reactivation occurs with much higher frequency and the patient goes on to develop clinically apparent herpes tracheobronchitis. Evidence for this comes from a classic autopsy study by Nash and Foley of burn patients, which reported a 10% incidence of herpes tracheobronchitis.[3] Tracheobronchitis has also been reported occasionally in immunocompetent patients with recent myocardial infarcts or chronic obstructive pulmonary disease (COPD)[4] and in elderly but otherwise healthy individuals.[5] The clinical manifestations of tracheobronchitis include fever, productive cough, and in some patients bronchospasm and hemoptysis.

There are more than 70 subtypes in the family of herpesviruses, with only a few of them known to cause pulmonary disease. Herpes simplex virus type 1 is the most commonly recognized cause of tracheobronchitis, although varicella zoster virus and cytomegalovirus have been reported as well. The process by which these herpesviruses cause tracheobronchitis is unclear, but many theories exist. Some clinicians feel this develops from hematogenous spread in the setting of disseminated disease. Others feel that tracheobronchitis represents reactivation of the virus in the adjacent cervical and vagal nerve ganglions.[6] However, most investigators agree that some combination of contiguous spread and aspirated infected secretions is responsible.[3] It is also believed that instrumentation and mechanical trauma of the airway may predispose to herpetic infection because herpesvirus preferentially infects squamous epithelium, and factors that promote squamous metaplasia are associated with an increased risk for HSV infection. These factors include trauma, thermal injury, chemotherapy, radiation therapy, and smoking.[4]

The characteristic bronchoscopic appearance of an HSV infection is a necrotizing inflammation of the bronchi. The bronchial mucosa may be diffusely erythematous and edematous, and copious thin secretions are typical. The infection is also manifested by ulceration of the mucosa, accompanied by a gray to pearly white fibrinopurulent exudate that overlies the denuded surface.[5] These pearly white exudates are often referred to as pseudomembranes and have been reported to cause partial airway obstruction and difficulty with ventilation. Bronchoscopic brushings or biopsy of these areas is generally high yield for making the diagnosis. In most patients the herpetic infection affects the trachea and large bronchi. Herpetic mouth sores and oropharyngeal lesions have been reported to occur in association with tracheobronchitis but are not always present.[5] Bacterial or fungal superinfection of the mucosal ulcerations is not an uncommon occurrence, especially for immunocompromised patients.

The radiographic manifestations of herpetic tracheobronchitis tend to be underwhelming. In the setting of disseminated herpes, the interstitial parenchymal infiltrates of herpetic pneumonia may be apparent, but in general the airway manifestations are minimal. If the exudative pseudomembranes are large enough to cause airway obstruction, lobar collapse or atelectasis may be appreciated. Interestingly, there is a strong association between HSV infection and acute respiratory distress syndrome (ARDS). In one study, 13 of 16 (81%) patients with ARDS were recognized to have herpetic tracheobronchitis.[7]

The diagnosis of HSV infection can be made by cytologic examination of the lower respiratory tract secretions, which may demonstrate the characteristic viral cellular changes and nuclear inclusions. These changes include "ground glass" nuclei filled with basophilic inclusion material, multinucleated giant cells, and eosinophilic Cowdry type A intranuclear inclusions. These Cowdry type A inclusions refer to the characteristic nuclear molding and perinuclear halo effect seen on the nuclei of infected cells.[8] Other diagnostic techniques include immunoperoxidase staining for the presence of viral proteins or in situ hybridization to demonstrate the presence of viral ribonucleic acid (RNA) or DNA. Cell culture is also used to confirm the presence of virus in infected secretions by demonstrating the characteristic viral cytopathic effect on a line of cultured cells. Rapid detection of viral infection is crucial because symptomatic clinical illness is usually late in the course of infection and often coincides with the peak of viral replication. Once the infection has been identified, appropriate therapy with antiviral medications such as acyclovir can be initiated. Clinically acyclovir appears to shorten the severity and length of viral infection, although no randomized study has been done to confirm this in tracheobronchitis.

REFERENCES

1. Chakraborty A, Forker A, Reese H, et al: Tracheobronchitis and pneumonia due to herpes simplex virus infection. Nebr Med J 73:347-350, 1988.
2. Nash G: Necrotizing tracheobronchitis and bronchopneumonia consistent with herpetic infection. Human Pathol 3:283-291, 1972.
3. Nash G, Foley FD: Herpetic infection of the middle and lower respiratory tract. Am J Clin Pathol 54:857-863, 1970.
4. Schuller D, Spessert C, Fraser VJ, et al: Herpes simplex virus from respiratory tract secretions: Epidemiology, clinical characteristics, and outcome in immunocompromised and nonimmunocompromised hosts. Am J Med 94:29-33, 1993.
5. Sherry MK, Klainer AS, Wolff M, et al: Herpetic tracheobronchitis, Ann Int Med 109:229-233, 1988.
6. Remy DP, Kuzmowych TV, Rohatgi P, et al: Herpetic tracheobronchitis with a broncho-oesophageal fistula Thorax 50:906-907, 1995.
7. Byers RJ, Hasleton PS, Quigley A, et al: Pulmonary herpes simplex in burn patients. Eur Respir J 9:2313-2317, 1996.
8. Vernon SE: Herpetic tracheobronchitis: Immunohistologic demonstration of herpes simplex virus antigen. Human Pathol 13:683-686, 1982.

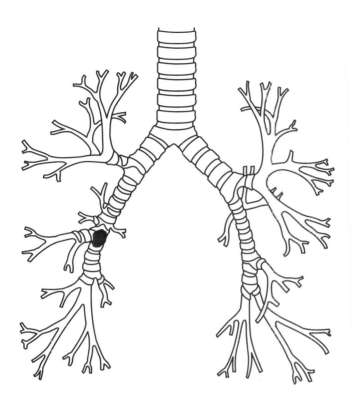

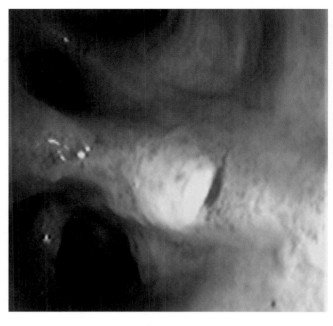

Figure 55-1. A gray and white fibropurulent exudate overlying a mucosal ulceration at the bifurcation between the superior segment and basilar segments of the right lower lobe. Note the surrounding mucosa is edematous and friable. On culture the herpesvirus was isolated.

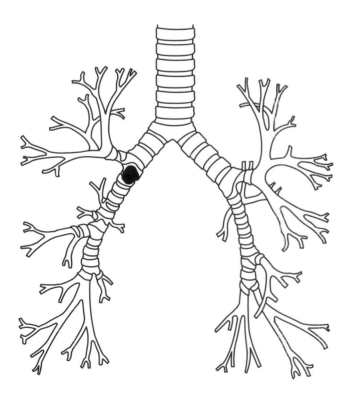

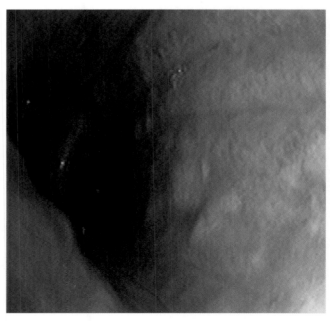

Figure 55-2. Additional whitish exudates along with mucosal erythema and edema on the posterior membrane of the right mainstem bronchus in the same patient.

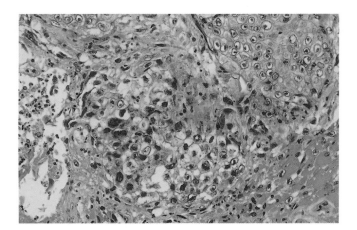

Figure 55-3. Nuclear changes associated with herpesvirus infection include multinucleation, nuclear molding, and glassy or marginated nuclear chromatin (H&E, ×400).

CHAPTER 56

Candidal Tracheobronchitis

Gehan Devendra

Candida is a common human saprophitic fungus. The yeast forms are roughly 2 to 4 μm in size with walls that are weakly gram positive and stain with periodic acid–Schiff (PAS) and Grocott's methenamine silver. *Candida albicans* is commonly found in the gastrointestinal tract and on most mucocutaneous surfaces. Most adults develop defense mechanisms to control the growth of such yeast. The overgrowth of *Candida* is kept under control by saprophytic bacteria that normally colonize the body. Overgrowth of *Candida* is often accompanied by a decrease in the bacterial load typically due to the use of antibiotics. Also inhaled corticosteroids can cause oral candidiasis.

Colonization of *Candida* is common in patients with indwelling catheters, diabetes, and prolonged hospital stays. Pulmonary candidiasis is less common. This seems to occur in about 5% of pulmonary infections in immunocompromised hosts and is rarely seen in immunocompetent individuals.[1] Conditions that are risk factors for the development of visceral candidiasis include chemotherapy, lymphoma/leukemia, extensive burns, major abdominal surgery, total parenteral nutrition (TPN) use, diabetes, organ and bone marrow transplantation, intravenous drug abuse, and acquired immunodeficiency syndrome (AIDS), to name a few.

Symptoms include dyspnea, cough, purulent secretions, stridor, and hemoptysis. Pathologically, washings show hyphae, pseudohyphae, and round or oval yeast buds. The major difficulty in diagnosis is to distinguish actual infection from colonization. Biopsy showing tissue invasion is required for accurate diagnosis.

Radiologic manifestations of *Candida* infection range from a normal chest radiograph result to bilateral parenchymal infiltrates to overt tracheal narrowing. Lateral neck radiographs may also be useful depending on the clinical scenario.

Bronchoscopic manifestations include mass lesions, mucosal plaques,[2] or bronchial striping. In my experience, the tracheobronchial striping is one of the most common manifestations of airway infection. The typical appearance is that of a raised whitish stripe of candidal overgrowth that develops on top of the bands of fibroelastic connective tissue that line the posterior membrane. Upper airway obstruction due to involvement of the vocal cords with *Candida* and resulting in stridor has also been described. Vegetating masses of *Candida* causing a tracheoesophageal fistula have been reported.[3] *Candida* can also cause a condition similar to allergic bronchopulmonary aspergillosis.[4] Treatment is with fluconazole; however, large mass lesions are treated with amphotericin B.[5]

REFERENCES

1. Logan PM, Primack SL, Staples C, et al: Acute lung disease in the immunocompromised host: Diagnostic accuracy of the chest radiograph. Chest 108:1283-1287, 1995.
2. Spear RK, Walker PD, Lampton LM: Tracheal obstruction associated with a fungus ball: A case of primary tracheal candidiasis. Chest 70:662-663, 1976.
3. Rusconi S, Meroni L, Galli M: Tracheoesophageal fistula in an HIV-1–positive man due to dual infect with *Candida albicans* and cytomegalovirus. Chest 106:284-285, 1994.
4. Lee TM, Greenberger PA, Oh S, et al: Allergic bronchopulmonary candidiasis: Case report and suggested diagnostic criteria. J Allergy Clin Immunol 80: 816-820, 1987.
5. Ganesan S, Harar RPS, Dawkins RS, Prior AJ: Invasive laryngeal candidiasis: A cause of stridor in the previously irradiated patient. J Laryngol Otol 112:575-578, 1998.

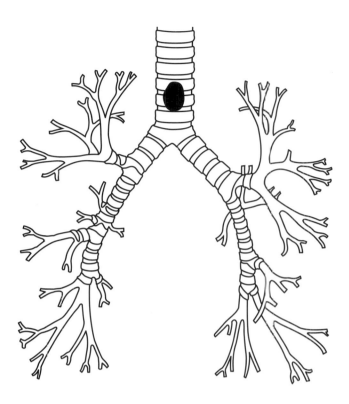

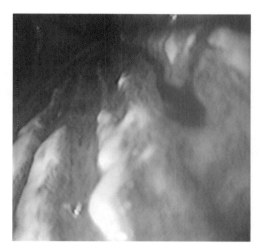

Figure 56-1. Characteristic whitish plaques and exudates that collect along the fibroelastic stripes of connective tissue on the posterior membrane of the airway. *Candida* was cultured from brushings of this whitish material.

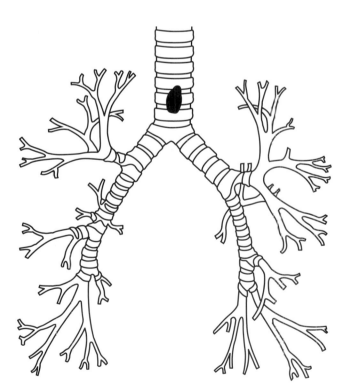

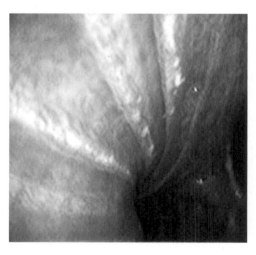

Figure 56-2. Significant improvement in the extensive plaquing of the posterior tracheal membrane after 48 hours of antifungal therapy.

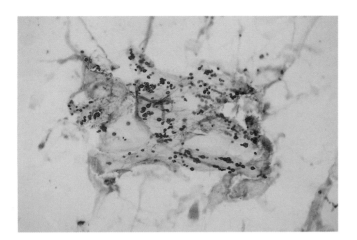

Figure 56-3. Pulmonary candidiasis with budding yeasts in bronchial washing cytology specimen; a possibility of oral contamination should be excluded (Papanicolaou stain, ×200).

CHAPTER 57

Radiation Necrosis of the Airway

David R. Duhamel

Radiation therapy produces dramatic effects in the lung. Most studies dealing with the effects of radiation on the lung focus on the lung parenchyma, which is considerably more radiosensitive than the tracheobronchial tree. The effects of radiation on the airway can develop early or late and be highly varied. These side effects include inflammation, fibrosis, stenosis, and the dreaded complication of necrosis. Radiation necrosis occurs as a late complication due to ischemia from a progressive obliterative endarteritis. The necrotizing process is sometimes exacerbated by other factors, including trauma, infection, or the compromised circulation of the elderly.[1] In the past two decades, with the development of a new technique to deliver radiation therapy, called *brachytherapy*, the incidence of airway necrosis has been increasing. Brachytherapy is a form of radiation therapy that utilizes a hollow plastic catheter inserted bronchoscopically into the airway adjacent to the neoplastic lesion to deliver a very potent radioactive source. The end result is an intense localized dose of radiation, delivered in the airway lumen.

Very little literature exists on this dreaded complication; however, Speiser and Spratling devised a gradation system to describe this entity, which they refer to as *radiation bronchitis*.[2] They accurately describe the raised, whitish, waxy, exudative membrane and plaques that cover the bronchial mucosa. These membranes eventually slough off and occlude the airway lumen or can be débrided mechanically with forceps through a bronchoscope. The tissue beneath it is frequently friable and erythematous. What Speiser and Spratling failed to include is that on occasion the necrosis extends through the full thickness of the bronchial or tracheal wall. In this catastrophic situation, not only the mucosal lining sloughs off but also portions of cartilaginous rings. Eventually the entire tracheal or bronchial wall dissolves, and a fistula develops into the mediastinum. In this setting, a frequent cause of death is massive hemoptysis due to continued erosion into major vascular structures. In some brachytherapy studies, the mortality rates from massive hemoptysis are as high as 29.4%, of which the vast majority are due to necrosis of the airway and adjacent structures.[3]

Speiser and colleagues report an incidence of 9% to 13% for the development of some degree of radiation necrosis after brachytherapy. Surprisingly, not all radiation necrosis develops acutely. There exist multiple examples of latent airway necrosis, which developed 6 to 9 months after the last radiation treatment. It has been shown that certain factors were associated with this complication. These factors include large cell carcinoma histology, curative intent, previous Nd:YAG laser photoresection, concurrent or previous external beam radiation, length of airway treated, location in the trachea or proximal bronchi, and contact by the brachytherapy catheter with the bronchial wall.[2-4] Certainly the total dose of radiation plays a big role in the development of this complication. The treatments are typically fractionated in an attempt to minimize the incidence and severity of complications. Routine brachytherapy dosimetry consists of a maximal dose of 2000 cGy divided into three treatment fractions.[5,6]

The histopathologic findings consist of severe inflammatory changes of the airway mucosa with an overlying amorphous fibrinous exudative layer. Present within the amorphous exudate is eosinophilic debris and varying amounts of entrapped white cells. Also present in some specimens are necrotic tumor cells admixed with granulation tissue.[2] In general, most cases of radiation necrosis fail to show viable neoplastic cells in the area of airway involvement.

The treatment options for this disease process are limited. Certainly further brachytherapy or external beam radiation to the area needs to be discontinued. In milder cases, the white fibrinous membrane can be débrided mechanically, and the process typically resolves. Anecdotal reports suggest some benefit from extended courses of corticosteroids, but no data support this. In the severe cases with full-thickness necrosis and fistulization through the bronchial wall, very little can be done. I have had some limited success using hyperbaric oxygen to stop the necrotizing process and promote healing of the tissues, but in general this is a devastating complication.[7]

REFERENCES

1. Hart GB, Mainous E: The treatment of radiation necrosis with hyperbaric oxygen. Cancer 37:2580-2585, 1976.
2. Speiser BL, Spratling L: Radiation bronchitis and stenosis secondary to high dose rate endobronchial irradiation. Int J Radiat Oncol Biol Phys 25:589-597, 1993.
3. Hara R, Itami J, Aruga T, et al: Risk factors for massive hemoptysis after endobronchial brachytherapy in patients with tracheobronchial malignancies. Cancer 92:2623-2627, 2001.
4. Perol M, Caliandro R, Pommier P, et al: Curative irradiation of limited endobronchial carcinomas with high dose rate brachytherapy. Chest 111:1417-1423, 1997.
5. Seagren SL, Harrell JH, Horn RA: High dose rate intraluminal irradiation in recurrent endobronchial carcinoma. Chest 88:810-814, 1985.
6. Schray MF, McDougall JC, Martinez A, et al: Management of malignant airway obstruction: Clinical and dosimetric considerations using an iridium-192 afterloading technique in conjunction with the neodymium-yag laser. Int J Radiat Oncol Biol Phys 11:403-409, 1985.
7. Kindwall EP: Hyperbaric oxygen's effect on radiation necrosis. Clin Plastic Surg 20:473-483, 1993.

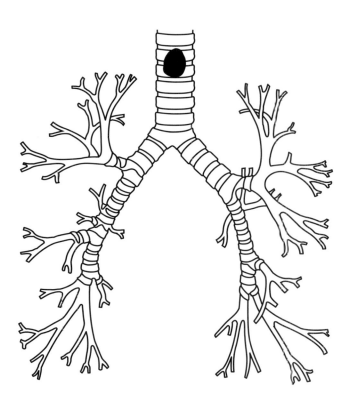

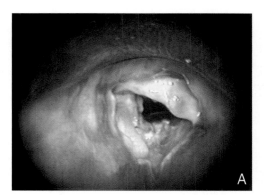

Figure 57-1. A, Necrosis and ulceration of the tracheal wall in a patient who received radiation therapy. A yellow-brown fibrinous exudate is seen covering a portion of the necrotic mucosa.　　　　*Continued*

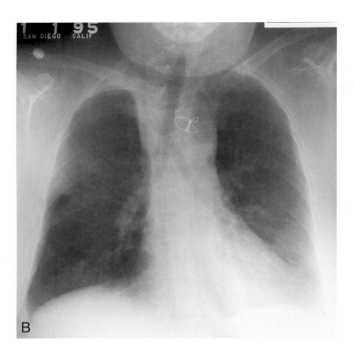

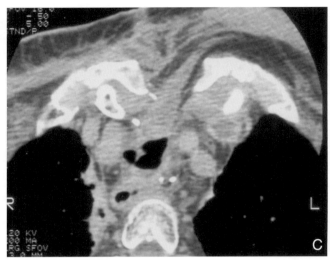

Figure 57-1, *cont'd.* **B,** The frontal radiograph demonstrates slight narrowing of the trachea at the level of the aortic arch. The apparent increase in the width of the mediasinum reflects postradiographic therapy changes with dense paramediastinal parenchymal consolidation. **C,** A single image from a CT study demonstrates marked soft tissue irregularity of the trachea with a soft tissue density present along the anterior surface. Increased density is present throughout the mediastinal fat that is consistent with postradiation therapy change.

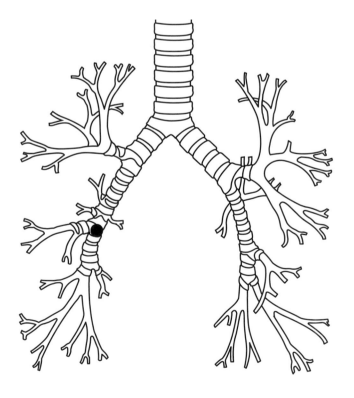

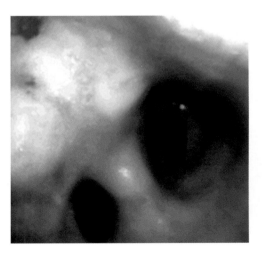

Figure 57-2. The typical whitish waxy debris that accumulates on the surface of the mucosa in the setting of radiation necrosis. This is a view of the superior segment and basilar segments of the right lower lobe.

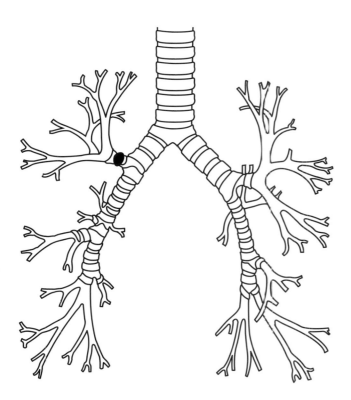

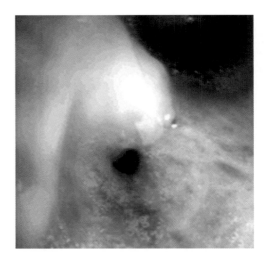

Figure 57-3. A large deposit of waxy, whitish, necrotic debris, which partially obstructs the orifice to the right upper lobe.

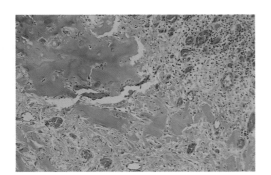

Figure 57-4. A portion of bronchial wall that sloughed off in a patient who received endobronchial brachytherapy for non–small cell lung cancer. Note the necrotic cartilaginous structures surrounded by an inflammatory exudate and vascular congestion with infarction.

CHAPTER 58

Saber Sheath Trachea

Jeffrey S. Prince

The saber sheath trachea is a deformity in the intrathoracic trachea that has a strong association with chronic obstructive pulmonary disease (COPD). The radiologic entity was described originally by Greene and Lechner as a fixed deformity of the trachea with coronal diameter one half or less the sagittal diameter. The unusual-shaped trachea abruptly changes to a rounded configuration at the thoracic outlet. Other characteristics are soft tissue thickening of the lateral walls and ossification of the cartilaginous rings.[1] In a later study, Greene found a 95% association between the presence of saber sheath trachea on chest radiograph and clinical COPD. The association with other radiographic signs of airway obstruction with COPD was much lower at 42%.[2]

The radiographic finding is defined by the tracheal index. The tracheal index is calculated as the ratio of the coronal diameter of the trachea on the posteroanterior radiograph of the chest to the sagittal diameter of the trachea on the left lateral chest radiograph. Measurements should be performed 1 cm above the aortic arch. Saber sheath trachea is defined as a tracheal index of less than 0.66.[1] The findings of a thickened lateral tracheal wall and ossification of the cartilaginous rings are frequently apparent on chest radiograph.

The finding of saber sheath trachea on CT has also been studied. Saber sheath trachea is defined in a similar manner on CT. Trigaux and colleagues showed there was a strong correlation with an elevated functional reserve capacity (FRC) on pulmonary function testing.[3] Arakawa and associates showed that the finding of saber sheath trachea on CT had a sensitivity of 40% and specificity of 90.9% for COPD.[4] Although thickening of the lateral walls of the trachea is described on chest radiograph, this finding was not confirmed on CT.[5]

Bronchoscopic findings in saber sheath trachea reflect those seen on chest radiograph. The tracheal lumen is significantly narrowed in a side-to-side direction when compared with the normal anterior-to-posterior diameter. There is no dynamic nature to these airway findings, unlike tracheomalacia, which varies with inspiration and expiration. The tracheal mucosa is completely normal in appearance. The distal trachea and mainstem bronchi typically retain the normal shape and caliber.

The etiology of saber sheath trachea remains unclear. Many theories have been expressed regarding the cause of the deformity. Some physicians feel that this may be due to cartilaginous remodeling of the trachea resulting from injuries caused by chronic coughing. The finding of heavy tracheal calcification is evidence of the chronic damage and repair suffered by the trachea.[2] Others believe that the saber sheath appearance is the result of constant extrinsic compression of the trachea by severely hyperinflated lungs in the setting of COPD.[3,6]

REFERENCES

1. Greene R, Lechner GL: "Saber-sheath" trachea: A clinical and functional study of marked coronal narrowing of the intrathoracic trachea. Radiology 115:265-268, 1975.
2. Greene R: "Saber-sheath" trachea: Relation to chronic obstructive pulmonary disease. Am J Roentgenol 130:441-445, 1978.
3. Trigaux JP, Hermes G, Dubois P, et al: CT of saber-sheath trachea: Correlation with clinical, chest radiographic and functional findings. Acta Radiologica, 35:247-250, 1994.
4. Arakawa H, Kurihara Y, Nakajima Y, et al: Computed tomography measurements of overinflation in chronic obstructive pulmonary disease: Evaluation of various radiographic signs. J Thorac Imaging 13:188-192, 1998.
5. Gamsu G, Webb WR: Computed tomography of the trachea: Normal and abnormal. Am J Roentgenol 139:321-326, 1982.
6. Callan E, Karandy EJ, Hilsinger RL: "Saber-sheath" trachea. Ann Otol Rhinol Laryngol 97:512-515, 1988.

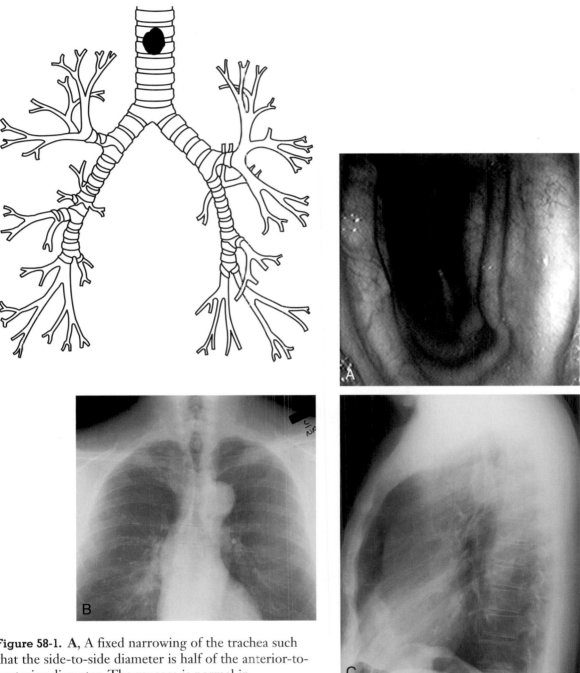

Figure 58-1. A, A fixed narrowing of the trachea such that the side-to-side diameter is half of the anterior-to-posterior diameter. The mucosa is normal in appearance, and the distal airways resume their normal circular shape. The tracheal abnormality is named for its similarity in shape to the sheath of a saber sword. Frontal (**B**) and lateral (**C**) radiographs demonstrate narrowing of the lateral dimension of the trachea with a slightly increased anteroposterior dimension.

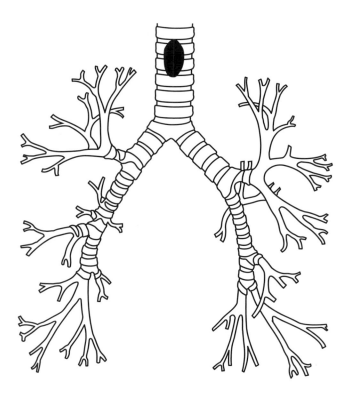

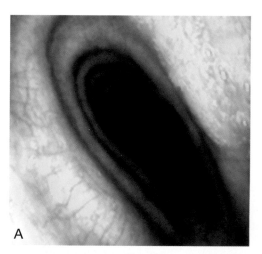

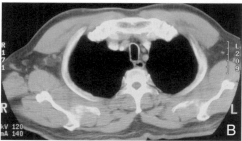

Figure 58-2. A, Extreme narrowing of the intrathoracic trachea consistent with a saber sheath abnormality in a patient with severe chronic obstructive pulmonary disease. **B,** A single image from a CT study demonstrates an increase in the anteroposterior dimension of the trachea relative to its lateral dimension.

CHAPTER 59

Manifestations of Fibrosing Mediastinitis on the Airway

Gehan Devendra

Fibrosing mediastinitis is a rare disorder caused by the proliferation of fibrous tissue in the mediastinum. Other names for this include sclerosing mediastinum or mediastinal fibrosis. The causative agent is unclear, but in the United States it is clearly associated with *Histoplasma capsulatum* infection.

The pathogenesis is speculated to be an abnormal host reaction to histoplasma antigens, resulting in a massive fibrotic response. Other associations to the development of fibrosing mediastinitis include treatment with methysergide,

rheumatic fever, trauma, radiation therapy, and autoimmune disease.[1]

The fibrosis can be intense and can cause stenosis of any of the mediastinal structures, including pulmonary arteries, superior vena cava, coronary arteries, esophagus and trachea, and bronchi. Also local matting of mediastinal nodes can result in the so-called mediastinal granuloma, which may be a precursor to mediastinal fibrosis; however, this is controversial.[2] The bronchoscopic manifestations are nonspecific. A splayed or distorted carina may be seen commonly. Extrinsic narrowing of the trachea or, more commonly, the bronchi is another finding. The airway mucosa at the site of narrowing is often bland to normal appearing. However, on occasion white, rock-hard granulomatous lymph nodes appear to erode through the bronchial wall.

Pathologic specimens of the mediastinal fibrosis will show paucicellular eosinophilic material. Occasionally, *H. capsulatum* organisms can be found. The most common clinical symptoms are cough or dyspnea. Chest pain, hemoptysis, superior vena cava syndrome, weight loss, and fever have also been reported. There is no gender predominance.

Chest radiography typically reveals widening of the mediastinum with calcification. In reference to airway complications, tracheal stenosis can be seen. On CT evaluation of the chest, stenosis of the trachea or bronchi can be seen. Other findings include mediastinal granuloma, which causes airway compression.[3] Treatment of tracheobronchial stenosis from fibrosing mediastinitis varies. Steroids have been tried to reduce the fibrosis but have not been shown to be beneficial.[4] Mediastinal granuloma can cause tracheal compression, which can be treated surgically with resolution of symptoms.[5] Other surgical approaches include decortication of the trachea, and radical procedures with allotransplanting of the trachea have been performed.[6,7] Nonsurgical approaches include bronchoscopic balloon dilation and or stent placement.[8]

REFERENCES

1. Rossi SE, McAdams HP, Rosado-de-Christenson ML, et al: Fibrosing mediastinitis. Radiographics 21:737-757, 2001.

2. Dines DE, Payne WS, Bernatz PE, Pairolero PC: Mediastinal granuloma and fibrosing mediastinitis. Chest 75:320-324, 1979.

3. Strimlan CV, Dines DE, Payne WS: Mediastinal granuloma. Mayo Clin Proc 50:702-705, 1975.

4. Dunn EJ, Ulicny KS Jr, Wright CB, Gottesman L: Surgical implications of sclerosing mediastinitis: A report of six cases and review of the literature. Chest 97:338-346, 1990.

5. Kalweit G, Huwer H, Straub U, Gams E: Mediastinal compression syndromes due to idiopathic fibrosing mediastinitis—Report of three cases and a review of the literature. Thorac Cardiovasc Surg 44: 105-109, 1996.

6. James EC, Harris SS, Dillenburg CJ: Tracheal stenosis: An unusual presenting complication of idiopathic fibrosing mediastinitis. J Thorac Cardiovasc Surg 80:410-413, 1980.

7. Levashov YN, Yablonsky PK, Cherny SM, et al: One-stage allotransplantation of the thoracic segment of the trachea in a patient with idiopathic fibrosing mediastinitis and marked tracheal stenosis. Eur J Cadiothorac Surg 7:383-386, 1993.

8. Sheski FD, Mathur PN: Long-term results of fiberoptic bronchoscopic balloon dilatation in the management of benign tracheobronchial stenosis. Chest 114:796-800, 1998.

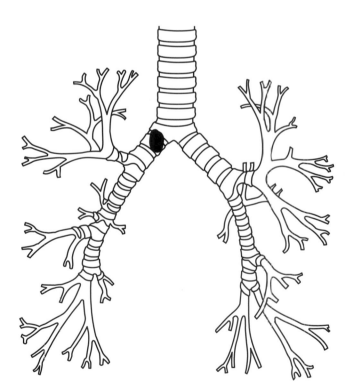

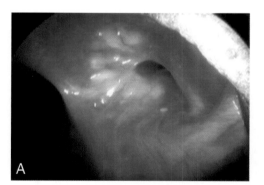

Figure 59-1. A, The proximal right mainstem bronchus at the level of the carina is narrowed from both endoluminal fibrotic scarring and extrinsic compression by calcified sclerotic mediastinal lymphadenopathy.

Continued

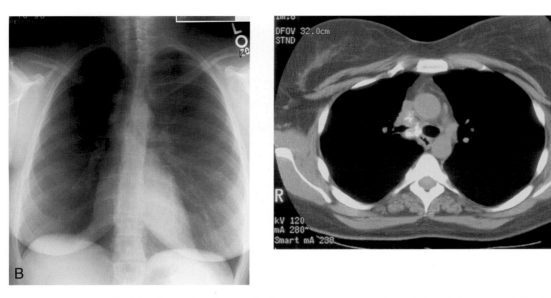

Figure 59-1, *cont'd.* **B,** The frontal radiograph demonstrates narrowing of the right upper lobe bronchus with slight rightward shift of the mediastinum. **C,** The CT image demonstrates narrowing of the right upper lobe bronchus. Increased soft tissue density is seen within the mediastinum. Calcified lymph nodes are present.

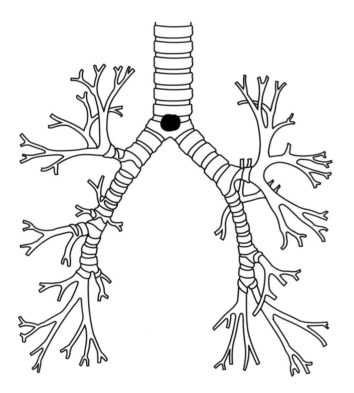

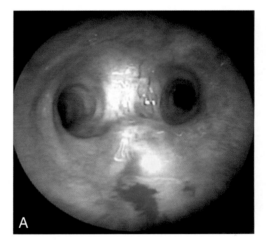

Figure 59-2. A, Splaying of the carina from massive subcarinal sclerotic lymphadenopathy in a woman with fibrosing mediastinitis due to histoplasmosis. **B,** The frontal radiograph demonstrates narrowing increased opacity within the right lower lobe with evidence of volume loss. The airway itself is not well visualized. **C,** The CT image demonstrates densely calcified subcarinal lymph nodes with slight narrowing of the bronchus intermedius. There is a slight shift of the mediastinum to the right.   *Continued*

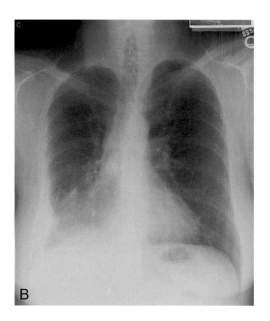

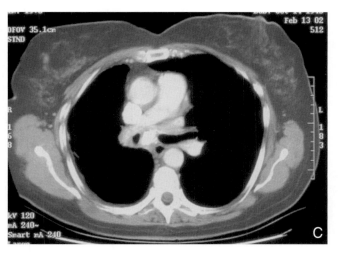

Figure 59-2, *cont'd.*

Figure 59-3. The lesion is composed of ropy collagen and nonspecific inflammatory infiltrates (H&E, ×100).

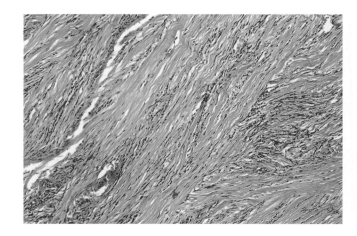

CHAPTER 60

Tracheobronchomalacia

David R. Duhamel

Tracheobronchomalacia is the result of congenital and acquired weakness in the tracheal and bronchial cartilage that supports the airway. This allows the anterior and posterior walls of the trachea and bronchi to collapse against one other with exhalation and coughing, resulting in symptoms of airway obstruction.[1] Tracheobronchomalacia is frequently misdiagnosed as chronic bronchitis, chronic obstructive pulmonary disease (COPD), or asthma and is erroneously treated with bronchodilators without benefit. This mistake is understandable though because the presenting symptoms are often the same: cough, sputum production, and dyspnea. Some patients may even present with frank stridor. Although the anatomic defect may appear trivial and typically escapes detection by conventional examination methods, the functional impediment to ventilation may be clinically significant with obstruction of expiratory airflow and interference with secretion clearance. The inefficient cough mechanism leads to retention of secretions, frequent pneumonias, and subsequent bronchiectasis. The true incidence of this disorder is unclear. Jokinen and associates reported a 23% incidence in 214 patients examined for chronic bronchitis.[2] Other studies reported an incidence of 1% to 4.5% in patients who underwent bronchoscopy for various pulmonary disorders.[3]

The etiologies of tracheobronchomalacia are variable. It is most often due to localized pressure necrosis of the trachea from the cuff of an endotracheal tube, thyromegaly, or vascular anomaly. It is also frequently seen at the site of an old tracheostomy stoma or after blunt trauma to the chest causing tracheal or bronchial disruption. Tracheomalacia may or may not be accompanied by tracheomegaly. Chronic and recurrent infections, radiation therapy, and relapsing polychondritis are all risk factors for the development of diffuse malacia.[2] It is believed that in a patient with chronic cough, the repetition of compressive forces generated by the cough eventually lead to flexibility and collapse of the supportive structures of the tracheal wall. There are also congenital forms of tracheobronchomalacia.[4] Williams-Campbell syndrome is due to the congenital deficiency of cartilage in the tissues of the tracheobronchial tree.[5] These congenital forms of malacia are frequently accompanied by other structural anomalies, including vascular rings, esophageal atresia, laryngomalacia, and cleft palate.

The bronchoscopic appearance can be variable. A diffuse process, of course, appears different from a localized process. It is very important to have an awake interactive patient during bronchoscopy to visualize these abnormalities. It is frequently necessary to have the patient forcibly exhale or cough to fully appreciate the extent of airway collapse. Collapse of up to 50% of the anterior-to-posterior diameter with coughing is considered to be normal. First-degree tracheobronchomalacia is defined as airway collapse from 50% to 75%, second degree from 75% to 100%, and third

degree is 100%.[6] The degree of impairment is proportional to the length of airway involved and the degree of airway collapse.[7] The most commonly encountered cause of localized tracheomalacia is probably at old tracheostomy sites. The surgical tracheostomies are particularly prone to this complication because a tracheal ring is often removed at the time of insertion. After decannulation of the tracheostomy, the unsupported tracheal wall will dynamically collapse into the airway lumen with respiration. The appearance of the lesion has been described as a second set of vocal cords in the proximal trachea. The incidence of this complication is lessening with the increased use of percutaneous dilational tracheostomy over traditional open surgical tracheostomy. One of the many advantages of this newer technique is that it leaves the cartilaginous structures intact.

Tracheomalacia is very difficult to diagnose with traditional radiography. The standard chest radiograph and routine inspiratory CT scan are limited by their inability to demonstrate the dynamic collapse of the airways. Fluoroscopy has been used to diagnose tracheal collapse in patients while they are performing various breathing maneuvers, such as forced expiration and cough. The newer CT technologies such as electron beam and spiral CT offer advantages over fluoroscopy. CT has the ability to image in the axial plane with the option to reconstruct the images in sagittal and coronal planes as well. The CT images are easily reproduced and can give information about parenchymal and mediastinal pathology. It is important that the patient be coached properly to perform the necessary breathing maneuvers when trying to elicit tracheobronchomalacia during a CT scan. One of the simplest and most accurate techniques for demonstrating collapsibility of the airways by CT scan is to measure the change between the inspiratory and end-expiratory cross-sectional areas of the trachea. Aquino and co-workers found that a change of 18% or greater in the upper trachea and 28% or greater in the midtrachea were highly predictive of tracheomalacia.[3]

The treatment options for tracheobronchomalacia are fairly simply. The weak and collapsible walls must be reinforced or removed. If the segment of malacic airway is short, it easily can be repaired with a sleeve resection.[2] The longer segments of diseased airway can be more difficult to manage. In these situations, the airway is reinforced either internally or externally. The external approach requires a major thoracic surgery with muscle and bone grafts to buttress the outer surface of the trachea and bronchi. This procedure called tracheopexy is performed infrequently and is typically reserved for the congenital forms of tracheobronchomalacia. A much simpler technique and one that is used much more frequently is that of internal stenting of the airway. The first stent was designed by Dr. Charles Stent in England around 1850. Nowadays, a stent refers to a hollow cylindrical prosthesis that maintains luminal patency of a tubular structure by opposing extrinsic compressive forces and providing internal support. The stents used in the airways fall into two separate categories: metal or Silastic. Each type of stent has its own advantages and disadvantages, but in general I prefer the Silastic stent for its ease of insertion and removal and its low incidence of granulation tissue.

REFERENCES

1. Nuutinen J: Acquired tracheobronchomalacia: A bronchological follow-up study. Ann Clin Respir 9:359-364, 1977.
2. Jokinen K, Palva T, Nuutinen J: Chronic bronchitis. A bronchologic evaluation. J Otorhinolaryngol 38:178-186, 1976.
3. Aquino SL, Shepard JO, Ginss LC, et al: Acquired tracheomalacia: Detection by expiratory CT scan. J Comput Assist Tomogr 25:394-399, 2001.
4. Cogbill TH, Moore FA, Accurso FJ, et al: Primary tracheomalacia. Am Thorac Surg 35:538-543, 1983.
5. Williams H, Campbell P: Generalized bronchiectasis associated with a deficiency of cartilage in the bronchial tree. Arch Dis Child 35:182-186, 1960.
6. Jokinen K, Palva T, Sutinen S, Nuutinen J: Acquired tracheobronchomalacia. Ann Clin Res 9:52-57, 1977.
7. Feist JH, Johnson TH, Wilson RJ: Acquired tracheobronchomalacia: Etiology and differential diagnosis. Chest 68:340-345, 1975.

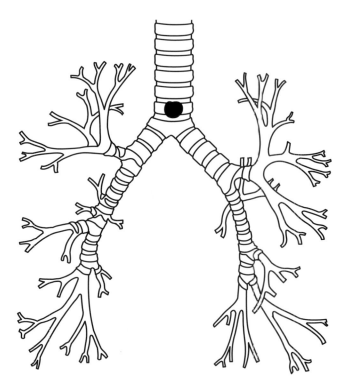

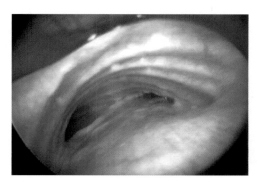

Figure 60-1. Near complete collapse of the tracheal and bronchial lumens during expiration in a patient with severe tracheobronchomalacia.

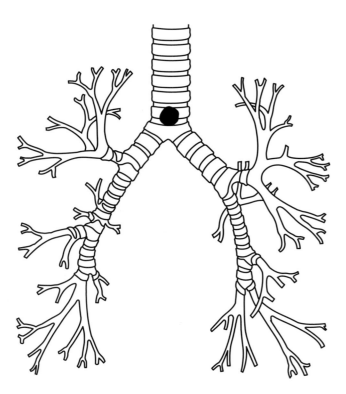

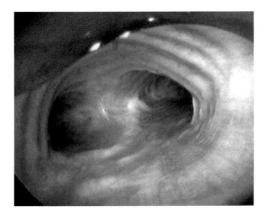

Figure 60-2. The same view of the distal trachea and bronchi now on inspiration. The tracheal and bronchial lumens appear normal in caliber.

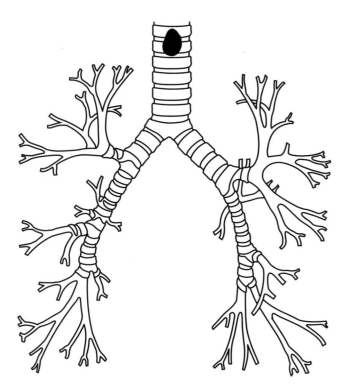

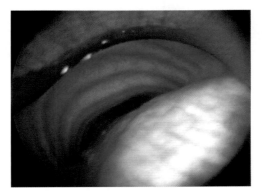

Figure 60-3. A view of the proximal trachea in the same patient demonstrating near complete collapse of the lumen during exhalation.

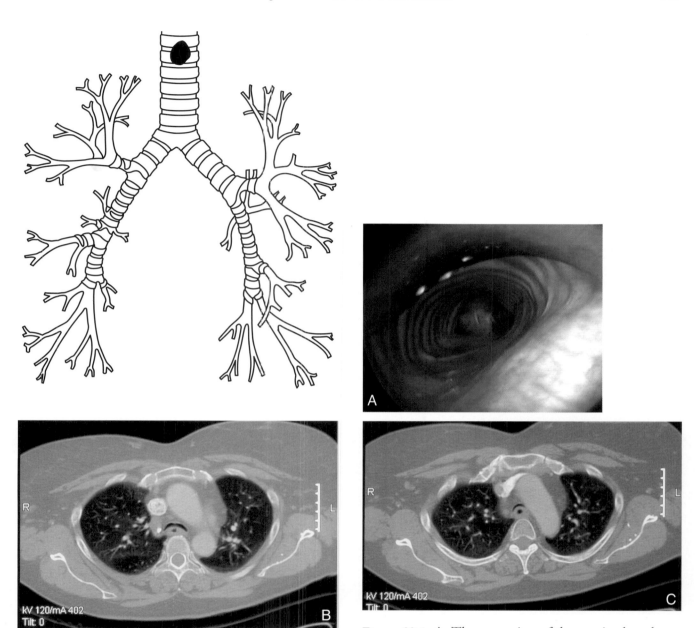

Figure 60-4. A, The same view of the proximal trachea now on inspiration. The tracheal lumen appears normal in diameter. Two images from a dynamic CT study demonstrate collapse during expiration at the level of the aortic arch (**B**) and the anteroposterior window (**C**).

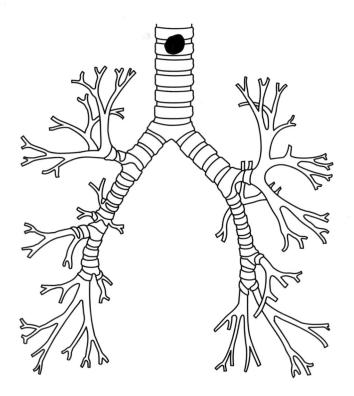

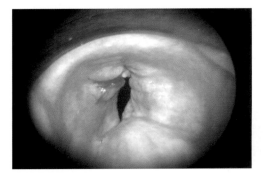

Figure 60-5. Localized tracheomalacia on inspiration at the site of an old tracheostomy stoma.

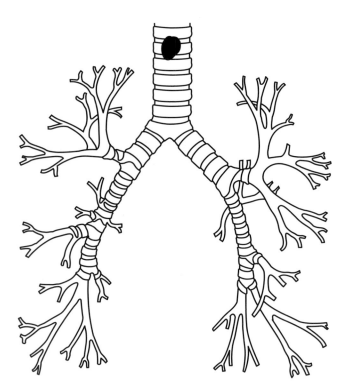

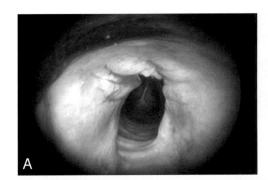

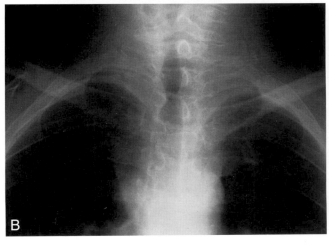

Figure 60-6. A, The same area of localized tracheomalacia seen on expiration, now with a much larger diameter lumen. **B**, Detail of trachea from a frontal radiograph demonstrates irregular, focal narrowing at the thoracic inlet.

CHAPTER 61

Endobronchial Aspergillosis

Gehan Devendra

Aspergillosis is a disease caused by a number of species of the genus *Aspergillus*, 95% of which are caused by *Aspergillus fumigatus*. The spectrum of illness and therefore the clinical manifestations are vast, from allergic reactions to colonization in immunocompromised hosts to invasive disease, sepsis, and rapid death.

Allergic Bronchopulmonary Aspergillosis

This form is an immunologic reaction to the fungus. Allergic bronchopulmonary aspergillosis (ABPA) is thought to have a frequency of 5% to 10% in steroid-dependent asthmatics.[1] It also has a high rate in patients with cystic fibrosis, by some accounts about 10%, whereas others describe colonization rates of 57%.[2,3] Pathogenesis is via *Aspergillus*-specific IgE, which causes mast cell degranulation and results in the clinical manifestations of wheezing, pulmonary infiltrates, and eosinophilia. Degenerating cells and inflammation result in the formation of mucous plugs.

Radiographic findings are consolidation, atelectasis, bronchectasis, and finger-like projections resultant from mucus impaction.[4] Most of these are more upper than lower lobe. Bronchoscopic findings include proximal bronchiectasis and mucoid impaction. Treatment is a combination of steroids and itraconazole.[5]

Aspergilloma

Aspergillomas are masses of fungus that grow in pre-established lung cavities caused by diseases such as old tuberculosis or chronic obstructive pulmonary disease (COPD). The clinical manifestations are variable and can range from incidental findings to scant hemoptysis to massive hemoptysis. The classic radiographic finding is a cavity with a mobile mass. Therapy is dependent on the clinical manifestation. Surgery in patients who can undergo lung resection is curative; however, many patients have underlying lung disease that prevents this treatment. Other modalities include bronchial embolization for hemoptysis or intracavitary instillation of antifungal medicine either percutaneously or bronchoscopically.[6,7]

Chronic Necrotizing Aspergillosis (Semi-invasive Aspergillosis)

This is a variant of aspergilloma, which results in the slow local destruction of lung parenchyma in patients with underlying lung disease.[8] Clinical manifestations include shortness of breath, cough, and sputum production. Radio-logic findings include upper lobe infiltrate with or without a fungus ball and pleural thickening that may go on to cavitation.[4] Treatment is with amphotericin B, which slows tissue destruction. Itraconazole can be used for mild cases after amphotericin B therapy.

Invasive Aspergillosis

Immunocompromised status is the greatest risk factor for developing invasive aspergillosis. The two main subtypes of invasive aspergillosis are parenchymal and tracheobronchial. Clinical manifestations are similar to those of an acute bacterial pneumonia in an immunocompromised patient. Viewed radiographically, the parenchymal disease demonstrates patchy infiltrates, with or without small nodules, lobar, segmental, or bilateral diffuse infiltrates.[4] These may go on to cavitate. Tracheobronchial disease usually occurs in the context of patients with parenchymal disease; however, 7% of invasive aspergillosis has isolated tracheobronchial disease.[9] Bronchoscopic descriptions of tracheobronchial disease include diffuse erythema, whitish plaques with a cobblestone appearance, ulcers, mediastinal lymph nodes eroding through the tracheal wall, necrotizing pseudomembranes, granulation tissue, or stricture formation.[10-12] Septated hyphae are found on histology with cultures positive for *Aspergillus* species. Treatment is with amphotericin B. Although the overall success rate is poor, newer therapies such as voriconazole have shown promise.[13] Stricture formation and granulation tissue can be treated with endobronchial stenting, laser ablation, rigid bronchoscopic dilation, and balloon dilation.[12]

REFERENCES

1. Henderson AH, English, MP, Vecht RJ: Pulmonary aspergillosis: A survey of its occurrence in patients with chronic lung disease and a discussion of the significance of diagnostic tests. Thorax 23:513-523, 1968.
2. Laufer P, Fink JN, Bruns WT, et al: Allergic bronchopulmonary aspergillosis in cystic fibrosis. J Allergy Clin Immunol 73:44-48, 1984.
3. Sammut PH, Howard ST, Linder J, Colombo JL: Unusual form of endobronchial aspergillosis in a patient with cystic fibrosis. Pediatr Pulmonol 16:69-73, 1993.
4. Gotway MB, Dawn SK, Caoili EM, et al: The radiologic spectrum of pulmonary *Aspergillus* infections. J Comp Assist Tomogr 26:159-173, 2002.
5. Stevens DA, Schwartz HJ, Lee JY, et al: A randomized trial of itraconazole in allergic bronchopulmonary aspergillosis. N Engl J Med 342:756-762, 2000.
6. Hargis JL, Bone RC, Stewart J, et al: Intracavitary amphotericin B in the treatment of symptomatic pulmonary aspergillomas. Am J Med 68:389-394, 1980.
7. Hamamoto T, Watanabe K, Ikemoto H: Endobronchial miconazole for pulmonary aspergilloma. Ann Int Med 98:1030, 1983.
8. Binder RE, Faling LJ, Pugatch RD, et al: Chronic necrotizing pulmonary aspergillosis: A discrete clinical entity. Medicine 61:109-124, 1982.

9. Clarke A, Skelton J, Fraser RS: Fungal tracheo-bronchitis: Report of 9 cases and review of the literature. Medicine 70:1-14, 1991.

10. Angelotti T, Krishna G, Scott J, et al: Nodular invasive tracheobronchitis due to *Aspergillus* in a patient with systemic lupus erythematosus. Lupus 11:325-328, 2002.

11. Verea-Hernando H, Martin-Egaña T, Montero-Martinez C, Fontan-Bueso J: Bronchoscopic findings in invasive pulmonary aspergillosis. Thorax 44:822-823, 1989.

12. Pervez NK, Kleinerman J, Kattan M, et al: Pseudo-membranous necrotizing bronchial aspergillosis. A variant of invasive aspergillosis in a patient with hemophilia and acquired immune deficiency syndrome. Am Rev Respir Dis 131:961-963, 1985.

13. Herbrecht R, Denning DW, Patterson TF, et al: Voriconazole versus amphotericin B for primary therapy of invasive aspergillosis. N Engl J Med 347:408-415, 2002.

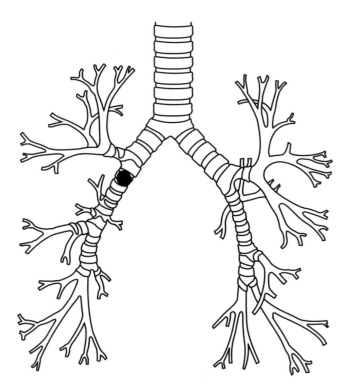

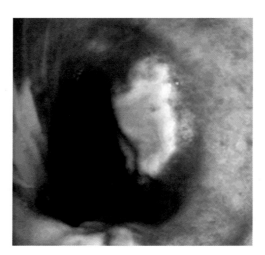

Figure 61-1. A view of the proximal right mainstem bronchus, which is completely coated with yellowish-green exudates. The underlying mucosa is inflamed and friable. A brushing of the area demonstrated septated hyphae consistent with *Aspergillus* infection.

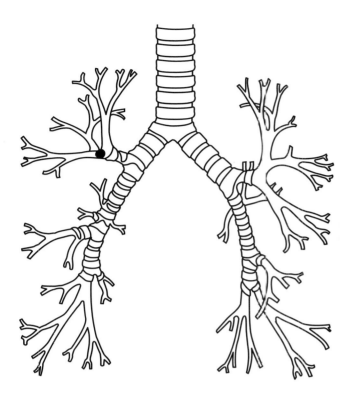

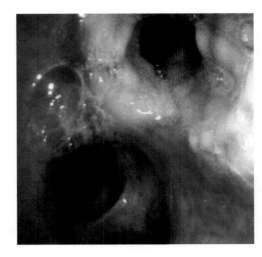

Figure 61-2. Yellow-green plaques on a red friable mucosa in the anterior segmental bronchus of the right upper lobe that is consistent with endobronchial aspergillosis.

Figure 61-3. Thin, uniform septated hyphae with acute-angle dichotomous branching in aspergillosis (Gomori methenamine, ×100).

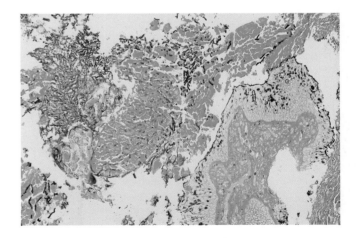

CHAPTER 62

Bronchial Webs and Adhesions

David R. Duhamel

Bronchial webs are thin membrane-like diaphragms that partially or completely occlude the airway. These lesions are typically congenital and extremely rare with only 10 cases reported in the world literature. The true incidence may be higher though because most go unrecognized.[1] The first case report of a congenital bronchial web was published in 1945.[2] Complete bronchial obstruction by a membranous web was diagnosed at autopsy in two neonates. Both children presented with respiratory compromise and lobar collapse by radiograph. The web was located in the proximal left mainstem bronchus in one child and the mid-right mainstem bronchus in the other. Interestingly, the airway distal to the obstruction was found to be completely normal in both cases. Kovitz and associates reported the finding of a bronchial web in a 71-year-old woman who had suffered significant blunt chest trauma 30 years previously.[1] Based on this case report, it seems possible that bronchial webs can develop in areas of bronchial disruption or mucosal trauma. Further support comes from my unpublished experience of a membrane-like web of tissue overgrowing the proximal end of a metallic stent and completely occluding the airway lumen.

The radiographic findings in the setting of an endobronchial web are not well described. A few references are made of lobar collapse and volume loss distal to the web. A partial or complete web may be associated with localized bronchiectasis or pneumonitis distal to the obstruction. There has been little mention of CT scan findings in the radiology literature, but a case report does describe a bronchial web diagnosed by contrast bronchograpy.[3] The bronchoscopic appearance of a endobronchial web can be fairly impressive. A thin, pinkish, elastic membrane circumferentially arising from the bronchial wall is described in most cases. The lesions can be managed endoscopically without much difficulty. An initial perforation is made in the center of the web using an aspiration needle. The aspiration of air suggests a patent lumen distal to the membrane. Next, a valvuloplasty balloon can be used to serially dilate and increase the diameter of the opening. An Nd:YAG laser can then be used to resect the remaining tissue, or a Silastic stent can be placed to maintain the patency of the lumen.

Another structural anomaly of the airway, which appears closely related to the bronchial web, is the bronchial adhesion or "string."[4] In a case report, Takayama and colleagues[4] described a thin, fibrous, bandlike structure spanning the lumen of an intermediate bronchus, which they termed a *bronchial string*. This lesion was thought to be congenital based on the lack of inflammation and scarring in the surrounding mucosa. The fibrous band was easily transected with biopsy forceps. Histopathologic analysis revealed a fibrous strip of tissue covered by ciliated epithelium without bronchial glands or cartilage and containing a lymphocytic infiltrate. I have identified identical bandlike adhesions in both the trachea and bronchi of patients with various traumatic, neoplastic, and inflammatory disease processes. These diseases and processes include Wegener's granulomatosis, thyroid cancer, postradiation therapy, endotracheal intubation, *Klebsiella rhinoscleromatis* infection, and airway stent placement. The adhesions are typically found incidentally and are not often associated with any clinical symptoms other than those of the associated illness.

Fibrous bands or adhesions have also been described in the larynx and upper airway. The vast majority of these lesions are congenital, and Cohen reports on 51 children with congenital glottic webs presenting to an inner city children's hospital over 32 years.[5] A glottic bar or adhesion is also known to develop following intubation.[6] These are usually described as pearly white fibrous connections between the vocal cords. The patients are typically asymptomatic with normal phonation and minimal shortness of breath. A fair number of cases have been identified of an anesthesiologist being unable to intubate the patient. The vocal cords are very susceptible to ischemia and pressure necrosis caused by the endotracheal tube. This often leads to ulceration and granuloma formation. One theory to account for the development of a glottic web is the formation of large vocal cord granulomas with subsequent fusion to the opposing areas of ulceration.[6] The lesions easily can be treated by dividing the band of tissue with a CO_2 laser.

REFERENCES

1. Kovitz KL, Foroozesh MB, Goyos JM, Rubio ER: Endoscopic management of obstruction due to an acquired bronchial web. Can Respir J 9:189-192, 2002.
2. Wallace JE: Two cases of congenital web of a bronchus. Arch Pathol 39:47-48, 1945.
3. Patronas NJ, MacMahon H, Variakojis D: Bronchial web diagnosed by bronchography. Radiology 121:526, 1976.
4. Takayama S, Miura H, Kimula Y: A case of "bronchial string"—A rare anomaly of the bronchus. Respiration 58:115-116, 1991.
5. Cohen SR: Congenital glottic web in children. Ann Otol Rhinol Laryngol 94:121-124, 1985.
6. McCombe AW, Philips DE, Rogers JH: Inter-arytenoid glottic bar following intubation. J Laryngol Otol 104:727-729, 1990.

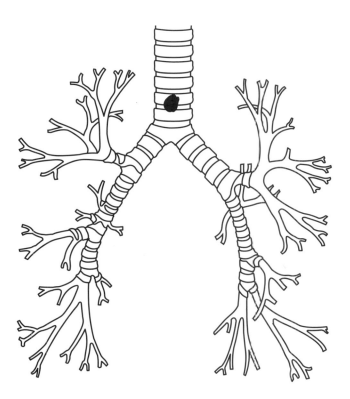

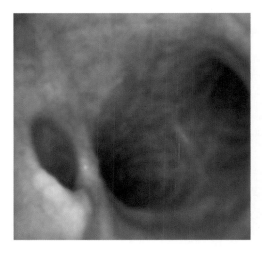

Figure 62-1. A thin, bandlike adhesion on the right lateral wall of the distal trachea.

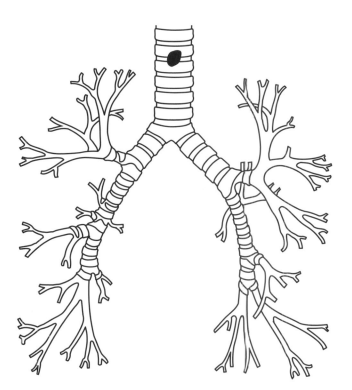

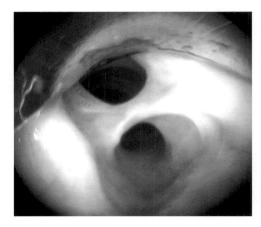

Figure 62-2. A thick adhesion connecting the anterior and posterior tracheal walls.

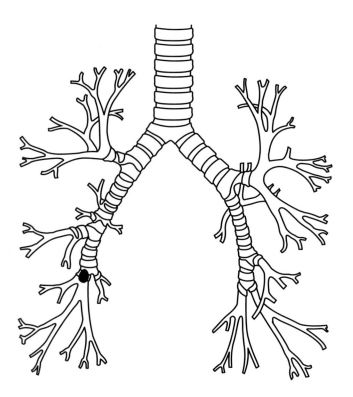

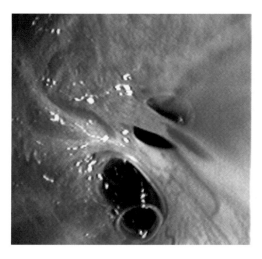

Figure 62-3. Several bandlike adhesions obscuring the basilar segments of the right lower lobe.

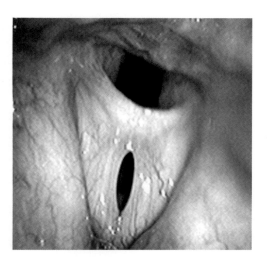

Figure 62-4. Fusion of the vocal cords due to a large central adhesion in a woman who was intubated for a prolonged period.

INDEX

Note: Page numbers followed by the letter f refer to figures and those followed by t refer to tables.